International Medical Graduates
in the United States

Hassaan Tohid • Howard Maibach
Editors

International Medical Graduates in the United States

A Complete Guide to Challenges
and Solutions

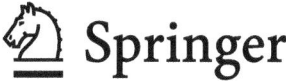 Springer

Editors
Hassaan Tohid
California Institute
of Behavioral Neurosciences
and Psychology
Fairfield, CA
USA

Howard Maibach
University of California
San Francisco, CA
USA

ISBN 978-3-030-62248-0   ISBN 978-3-030-62249-7   (eBook)
https://doi.org/10.1007/978-3-030-62249-7

This Springer imprint is published by the registered company Springer Nature Switzerland AG
The registered company address is: Gewerbestrasse 11, 6330 Cham, Switzerland

I dedicate this book to my lovely wife Sidra and my beloved daughter Ayla.

My wife Sidra helped me all the way in completing and editing this book with her valuable suggestions, ideas, and support. One of my favorite chapters on medical ethics was, in fact, her idea to be incorporated into this book. Her sacrifices for creating a helpful environment for me when working on this project is one of the most valuable memories of this book. It is rightly said, "Behind every successful man is a woman." This holds true for every step of completing the project of this book.

My daughter Ayla was just born when this project began. Because of my involvement in this project, I could not give her the attention she deserved. Now finally the book is completed, I will now be able to compensate for the loss of time spent with her.

Dr. Hassaan Tohid

Preface

"Success is a progressive realization of a worthy goal" – Earl Nightingale

According to this definition, success is a journey. It is not the achievement of your goal. The journey of international medical graduates (IMGs) applying for the US residency match begins the day they commence their medical school. Thousands of these IMGs apply for residency match each year, and many go unmatched. However, according to Earl Nightingale, anyone striving to achieve a goal is a success, regardless of the outcome. In my eyes, all the IMGs who try for residency match are success stories themselves. There are many challenges these IMGs face during this process and after the match cycle ends. There is not much information available on what should IMGs do, how do they go about this process, and what do they do in case they don't match. Amidst the uncertainty of what the future holds, lack of proper guidance, the difficulties faced by IMGs, and our consideration of these challenges, made this book a reality. We decided to write this book with a goal to help IMGs learn about various aspects of US residency, including the pre- and post-match process awareness on what they can do in order to have a fruitful career.

This book addresses all aspects of the life and journey of IMGs is discussed, from socio-cultural issues to medical ethics and problems like residency application or notable issues such as visa problems, and the solutions of these issues have been discussed in great details. This book is useful for anyone interested in the subject of IMGs and US clinical residency in the United States. The book will be helpful for all the IMGs applying for US residency match, and the scientists and researchers studying the influx of IMGs in the US. I highly recommend this book for all the IMGs applying for the match. The students should read this book and then start their journey for residency.

Just like any project, writing this book was a tough process. The initial challenge was how to finish the book before the deadline. Dr. Maibach and I had multiple meetings on how to make this book a reality. It was decided to start looking for authors who would assist in this project. Thus, a robust search was conducted to find appropriate authors. This process also led to some challenges of finding a right person for the right chapter. We wanted to include authors with high integrity and dedication; therefore, the authors were scrutinized with a careful consideration. After trial and error, we learned from our mistakes and eventually found all the right people for the book. The research process for the substance of the book was mainly relied upon literature review, interviews of relevant people and IMGs and physicians working in the US, and personal experiences of the authors. The entire process of writing and completing the book took a little over 2 years. Because of the wonderful team, we were able to complete the whole book from the first chapter to the last before the deadline, which we believe was a great achievement. I thank all the authors and congratulate them on finishing the task on time.

This first edition of *International Medical Graduates in the United States: A Complete Guide to Challenges and Solution* will be a great addition to Springer's publications and has a potential to serve millions of physicians and IMGs over the next few years and will be an important contribution to the United States Public Health. I wish good luck to all the IMGs and want to emphasize it again that their journey has just begun, and they are already successful regardless of the outcome of the match; they are an asset and we expect a great future ahead.

Sincerely,

Dr. Hassaan Tohid, MBBS, SUDCC, CCATP
TEDx Speaker, Neuroscientist, Substance Abuse Counselor
Chief Executive Office, California Institute
of Behavioral Neurosciences and Psychology
4751 Mangels Blvd
Fairfield, CA, 94533, USA
Contact: 707-999-1268
Website: www.cibnp.com; www.hassaantohid.com

Contents

About the Editors

Hassaan Tohid, MBBS, SUDCC, CCATP is a neuroscientist, a clinician, and an author. He is the founder of California Institute of Behavioral Neurosciences and Psychology, where he leads the organization as the CEO. He trains international medical graduates (IMGs) for research writing, publishing, and statistical data analysis through his courses and helps them achieve their goal of attaining US Clinical Residency. He has created many courses for medical students and IMGs related to research and career success. As an academic, he is a neuroscientist and delivered a TED talk on mirror neurons at TEDx UCDavissf and later dissociative identity disorder at TEDx UAlberta. He has published around 50 scientific articles and various blogs. Besides academia, Dr. Tohid is a substance use disorder treatment counselor and is California Board Certified in addiction counseling. After graduating as a medical doctor, he chose substance use disorder counseling as a domain for his clinical and counseling career. He was also awarded the honorary professorship and visiting professorship by various institutes internationally.

Howard Maibach, MD is a dermatologist and a professor of dermatology at the University of California, San Francisco (UCSF), with expertise in treating contact dermatitis (a rash caused by touching an irritating substance) and occupational dermatitis (a rash resulting from workplace exposure to an irritating substance). His specialties include allergic skin disorders and skin conditions caused by exposure to toxic substances. He also has an interest in dermatopharmacology, the study of medications for skin disorders. Dr. Maibach earned his medical degree from Tulane University School of Medicine. He completed a residency as well as a fellowship in dermatology at the Hospital of the University of Pennsylvania. Dr. Maibach has served on the editorial boards of more than 30 scientific journals. He is a member of 19 professional societies, including the American Academy of Dermatology, San Francisco Dermatological Society, and International Commission on Occupational Health. Dr. Maibach has published around 3000 research articles and has written over 80 books on dermatology.

Contributors

Noorulain Aqeel Napa State Hospital, Napa, CA, USA

Saïd C. Azoury, MD Division of Plastic Surgery, Department of Surgery, University of Pennsylvania, Philadelphia, PA, USA

Nitya Beriwal Lady Hardinge Medical College, New Delhi, India

Jonathan Bernad American Clinical Experience, Los Angeles, CA, USA

Ai-Tram N. Bui Harvard Medical School, Boston, MA, USA

Ivan Cancarevic California Institute of Behavioral Neurosciences and Psychology, Fairfield, CA, USA

Raguraj Chandradevan Graduate Medical Education-Internal Medicine, Northside Hospital Gwinnett, Lawrenceville, GA, USA

Nashit Chowdhury Department of Family Medicine, Cumming School of Medicine, University of Calgary, Calgary, AB, Canada

Turin Tanvir Chowdhury Department of Family Medicine, Cumming School of Medicine, University of Calgary, Calgary, AB, Canada

Department of Community Health Sciences, Cumming School of Medicine, University of Calgary, Calgary, AB, Canada

Steven R. Daugherty Medical School Companion, Chicago, IL, USA

Bruna Maria Castro de Oliveira Harvard Medical School, Boston, MA, USA

Department of Anesthesia, Critical Care, and Pain Medicine, Massachusetts General Hospital, Boston, MA, USA

David Dragas International American University College of Medicine, Vieux Fort, Saint Lucia

Mark Ekpekurede Alberta International Medical Graduates Association (AIMGA), Calgary, AB, Canada

Michael G. Fitzsimons Harvard Medical School, Boston, MA, USA

Division of Cardiac Anesthesia, Department of Anesthesia, Critical Care, and Pain Medicine, Massachusetts General Hospital, Boston, MA, USA

Shawn Forrester California Institute of Behavioral Neurosciences and Psychology, Fairfield, CA, USA

Lisa N. Guo Harvard Medical School, Boston, MA, USA

Sarah Hayek General Surgery, Geisinger Medical Center, Danville, PA, USA

Roohi Afshan Kaleelullah California Institute of Behavioral Neurosciences and Psychology, Fairfield, CA, USA

The University of North Carolina, Adam's School of Dentistry, Chapel Hill, NC, USA

Dong Hyang Kwon Georgetown University, Washington, DC, USA

Department of Pathology, MedStar Georgetown University Hospital, Washington, DC, USA

Deidre Lake Alberta International Medical Graduates Association (AIMGA), Calgary, AB, Canada

Michelle S. Lee Harvard Medical School, Boston, MA, USA

Department of Dermatology, Brigham and Women's Hospital and Harvard Medical School, Boston, MA, USA

Bilal Haider Malik CiBNP, Fairfield, CA, USA

Institute of Behavioral Neurosciences and Psychology, Fairfield, CA, USA

Internal Medicine, Research, California Institute of Behavioral Neurosciences & Psychology, Sacramento, CA, USA

Vinod E. Nambudiri Department of Dermatology, Brigham and Women's Hospital and Harvard Medical School, Boston, MA, USA

Chau Nguyen International American University College of Medicine, Vieux Fort, Saint Lucia

Bindu Pillai Laguardia Community College, Long Island City, NY, USA

Lucia Plichtová Hospital Department of Medicine, Bridgeport, CT, USA

Gokul Ramani Jacobi Medical Center/Albert Einstein College of Medicine, Department of Internal Medicine, Bronx, NY, USA

Arturo J. Rios-Diaz, MD Department of Surgery, Thomas Jefferson University, Philadelphia, PA, USA

Division of Plastic Surgery, Department of Surgery, University of Pennsylvania, Philadelphia, PA, USA

Ian H. Rutkofsky Department of Psychiatry, HCA – Aventura Hospital and Medical Center, Aventura, FL, USA

Department of Research, CiBNP, Fairfield, CA, USA

Kevin E. Salinas Harvard Medical School, Boston, MA, USA

Mohsen Shabahang General Surgery, Geisinger Medical Center, Danville, PA, USA

Haziq F. Siddiqi Harvard Medical School, Boston, MA, USA

Kumudhati Tiwari California Institute of Behavioral Neurosciences and Psychology, Fairfield, CA, USA

The University of North Carolina, Adam's School of Dentistry, Chapel Hill, NC, USA

Hassaan Tohid California Institute of Behavioral Neurosciences and Psychology, Fairfield, CA, USA

Syeda Sidra Tohid California Institute of Behavioral Neurosciences and Psychology, Fairfield, CA, USA

Chapter 1
International Medical Graduates (IMGs) and the Types of IMGs

Lisa N. Guo and Vinod E. Nambudiri

Who Are International Medical Graduates (IMGs)?

International medical graduates (IMGs) are graduates of non-US or non-Canadian medical schools, regardless of US citizenship status [1]. It is the location of the medical school – **not** the personal citizenship of the individual graduate – that determines whether an individual is considered an IMG. Thus, non-US citizens who graduated from medical schools in the USA and Canada are not considered IMGs, but US citizens graduating from medical schools outside of the USA and Canada are considered IMGs. IMGs are an integral part of the US physician workforce, representing roughly a quarter of active physicians [2]. IMGs hail from a wide array of countries all across the globe and bring with them diverse perspectives and unique experiences that greatly enrich the US healthcare provider population.

Level of training, experience, as well as ultimate career aspirations vary greatly among IMGs first coming to the USA. Many IMGs seeking to train in the USA are fresh medical school graduates without residency equivalent training in the country where they attended medical school, while others may have already had established medical careers. Some may have the ultimate goal of settling down and practicing in the USA long-term. Others may intend to return to their home countries to practice after training and gaining experience in the US medical system.

Reasons for pursuing additional training and/or medical careers in the USA vary greatly, encompassing both personal and professional motivations. "Pull" factors

L. N. Guo
Harvard Medical School, Boston, MA, USA
e-mail: lisa_guo@hms.harvard.edu

V. E. Nambudiri (✉)
Department of Dermatology, Brigham and Women's Hospital and Harvard Medical School, Boston, MA, USA
e-mail: vnambudiri@bwh.harvard.edu

© Springer Nature Switzerland AG 2021
H. Tohid, H. Maibach (eds.), *International Medical Graduates in the United States*, https://doi.org/10.1007/978-3-030-62249-7_1

attracting international graduates to the USA may include higher compensation for work, high-quality training, training that is not otherwise available in their home countries, better job opportunities for themselves and their families, improved quality of life and career structure, family ties to the USA, and peer pressure, among others. "Push" factors driving physicians to leave their home countries may include religious and political persecution, poor work conditions and quality of life, limited opportunities to pursue a desired specialty, and many more [3]. Whatever an individual's specific reasons are, they must be compelling enough for the individual to leave the familiar and pursue without guaranteed success the long, expensive, and challenging road that is entering the US graduate medical education and healthcare system as an international medical graduate.

Types of IMGs

IMGs can be categorized based on US citizenship status. *US IMGs* are US citizens or permanent residents who attended international medical schools. Conversely, *non-US IMGs* are non-US citizens or permanent residents who attended international medical schools [4].

Non-US IMGs outnumber US IMGs throughout the various stages of becoming a licensed physician in the USA. The Educational Commission for Foreign Medical Graduates (ECFMG) is the regulatory body that certifies prospective IMGs to be eligible to enter the graduate medical education application process, providing a level of standardization for candidates applying from countries in which the medical education and healthcare system may be different from that of the USA. Approximately two thirds of ECFMG certificants were non-US citizens in 2018 [5]. Among IMGs entering the 2018 Main Residency Match (the primary way by which residency positions are filled), about 58% of IMG applicants were non-US IMGs [4]. According to the American Medical Association (AMA), non-US IMGs make up roughly the same proportion of the IMG physician workforce in the USA [6].

In addition to citizenship status, there may be other differences between these two groups. Many US IMGs have spent the majority of their lives in the USA. Because of this, they may be more likely to have native proficiency in English and greater familiarity with American culture than non-US IMGs. US IMGs also often attend Caribbean medical schools, many of which are for-profit, private institutions. In fact, the majority of actively licensed graduates from Caribbean schools in the USA are US IMGs [7]. Some of these medical schools offer students the opportunity to rotate at US hospitals. Thus, US IMGs may also have greater familiarity with the US medical system [8].

In contrast, non-US IMGs come from countries all around the world. In 2016, the ECFMG certified citizens from a staggering 154 counties [9]. Other than the USA, the largest number of certificates were given to IMGs from India, followed by Canada, Pakistan, and China [5]. The profile of actively licensed IMGs practicing in the USA is similar. The largest number of actively licensed IMG physicians graduated from medical schools in India (23%), the Caribbean (18%, many of whom are US IMGs, but not all), the Philippines (6%), Pakistan (6%), and Mexico (5%) [6]. Because they are not US citizens, non-US IMGs in particular have to contend with the complexities of US immigration and visa requirements. Non-US IMGs may also have to learn and adjust to the American culture, medical education, and health system, all of which may be very different from what they are accustomed to in their home countries.

Role of IMGs in the US Healthcare System

IMGs are an important part of the US healthcare system. The proportion of the US physician workforce made up by IMGs has increased steadily from 10% in 1963 [10] to 24.5% of active physicians in 2017, with a total of 218,540 active IMGs as reported by the Association of American Medical Colleges (AAMC) [2]. Not only are IMGs a large portion of the workforce, but they also address critical physician shortages in fields such as primary care. IMGs are more likely to be primary care physicians than US graduates, with 62% of practicing IMGs in primary care fields, compared to 31% of US graduates [6]. Given AAMC projections of a shortage of 46,900 to 121,900 total physicians in both primary care and non-primary care specialties in the USA by 2032, their role will likely only grow in importance [11].

IMGs also help address gaps in underserved areas and settings that are relatively less attractive to US medical graduates. They are more likely to be located in urban areas of high poverty [12] and are disproportionally represented in US counties with high infant mortality rates and lower socioeconomic status [13]. Among critical access hospitals, which are small rural hospitals that often serve as safety net providers and the only hospitals in their communities, those in persistent poverty counties and with provider recruitment issues report more reliance on IMG physicians [14]. Regardless of urban or rural location, data from National Ambulatory Medical Care Surveys demonstrate that a higher percentage of office visits to IMGs are made up by Medicaid patients, and patients of IMG physicians are more likely to live in neighborhoods with lower median household incomes [15].

Overall, these statistics highlight the fact that the US healthcare system and the many patients it serves depend on IMGs to ameliorate provider shortages as well as deliver care to areas of need. The reasons for these observed patterns are complex and multifactorial, including visa requirements that encourage IMGs to practice in underserved areas. The role of IMGs in the US healthcare system is further discussed in Chap. 17 and may be mentioned throughout this text given its magnitude and importance.

Characteristics of IMGs in the USA

Diversity

Given the wide range of countries that IMGs come from, it is not surprising that IMGs are diverse racially, ethnically, culturally, and linguistically. A report on the race and ethnicity of ECFMG certificants from 2000 to 2005 demonstrated that IMGs were more likely than US medical graduates to self-report as Asian (39.2% versus 20%) or Hispanic (7.9% versus 6.4%). IMGs were also much less likely to be white than US medical graduates (27.8% versus 64%) and slightly less likely to be black (4.7% versus 6.5%). The same patterns were also noted among residents and fellows [16]. This racial and ethnic breakdown is mirrored in the patients that IMGs take care of, as Hispanic and Asian or Pacific Islander patients are more likely to see IMG physicians than US medical graduates [15]. This may be a reflection of the fact that concordant ethnicity improves patient-physician relationships [17]. In addition, 98% of IMGs speak at least two languages fluently [6]. Again, the impact of this may be seen in the IMG patient population, as patients of IMG physicians are more likely to live in neighborhoods with a greater proportion of non-English-speaking and foreign-born individuals [15].

Historically, the majority of IMGs have been male, but the share of female IMGs is growing. According to the AMA, the proportion of first-time medical licenses issued to female IMGs rose from 25% to 45% from 1990 to 2014, which is only slightly lower than the proportion of females among US medical graduates in 2014 (47%) [6].

Thus, IMGs greatly enrich the diversity of the US physician workforce. In an increasingly diverse and multicultural US patient population, this can translate into benefits for patients. Not only do concordant ethnicities appear to improve patient-physician relationships, but they are also associated with improved health outcomes [17]. Furthermore, the ability to speak in the preferred language of a patient may facilitate patient-provider communication and bolster therapeutic alliances and overall patient satisfaction with medical care. IMGs can also share their experiences and perspectives with fellow trainees and colleagues to improve and contribute to the overall cultural competency of the US physician population.

Practice Specialties

Certain specialties have greater representation of IMG physicians than others. As mentioned previously, a higher proportion of IMGs than US medical graduates practice in primary care fields. The top 5 specialties and/or subspecialties with the greatest IMG representation reflect this, with the greatest absolute number of active IMGs in 2017 practicing in internal medicine (45,274), family medicine/general practice (25,860), pediatrics (14,577), psychiatry (11,615), and anesthesiology

Table 1.1 Number and percentage of total active physicians and residents and fellows who are international medical graduates (IMGs) in 2017

Specialty	Total active physicians	Active IMGs	Percent IMG among active physicians	Total residents and fellows	IMG residents and fellows	Percent IMG among residents and fellows
All specialties	892,752	218,540	24.5	129,400	30,763	23.8
Allergy and immunology	4774	1093	22.9	285	48	16.8
Anatomic/clinical pathology	12,836	3932	30.6	2264	990	43.7
Anesthesiology	41,758	9017	21.6	5884	762	13
Cardiovascular disease	22,210	6738	30.3	2739	1113	40.6
Child and adolescent psychiatry	9204	2794	30.4	919	301	32.8
Critical care medicine	11,556	4741	41	2138	860	40.2
Dermatology	12,051	591	4.9	1383	49	3.5
Emergency medicine	42,347	2765	6.5	7077	357	5
Endocrinology, diabetes, and metabolism	7495	2969	39.6	671	344	51.3
Family medicine/ general practice	113,508	25,860	22.8	11,351	3280	28.9
Gastroenterology	14,743	4270	29	1536	487	31.7
General surgery	25,041	4904	19.6	8703	1324	15.2
Geriatric medicine	5598	2844	50.8	273	145	53.1
Hematology and oncology	15,407	5614	36.4	1728	706	40.9
Infectious disease	9134	3136	34.3	742	299	40.3
Internal medicine	115,539	45,274	39.2	25,773	9957	38.6
Internal medicine/ pediatrics	5122	551	10.8	1481	127	8.6
Interventional cardiology	3847	1724	44.8	303	161	53.1
Neonatal-perinatal medicine	5529	2131	38.5	739	211	28.6
Nephrology	10,796	5293	49	847	574	67.8
Neurological surgery	5530	681	12.3	1418	111	7.8
Neurology	13,716	4289	31.3	2595	867	33.4
Neuroradiology	3681	532	14.5	263	44	16.7

(continued)

Table 1.1 (continued)

Specialty	Total active physicians	Active IMGs	Percent IMG among active physicians	Total residents and fellows	IMG residents and fellows	Percent IMG among residents and fellows
Obstetrics and gynecology	41,654	5943	14.3	5227	492	9.4
Ophthalmology	18,817	1327	7.1	1314	53	4
Orthopedic surgery	19,001	988	5.2	3829	72	1.9
Otolaryngology	9526	603	6.3	1542	29	1.9
Pain medicine and pain management	5342	1482	27.7	311	47	15.1
Pediatric cardiology	2733	715	26.2	447	95	21.3
Pediatric hematology/ oncology	2794	711	25.4	506	96	19
Pediatrics	58,430	14,577	24.9	8748	1597	18.3
Physical medicine and rehabilitation	9340	2239	24	1288	156	12.1
Plastic surgery	7142	724	10.1	1072	87	8.1
Preventive medicine	6613	824	12.5	300	55	18.3
Psychiatry	38,201	11,615	30.4	5743	1522	26.5
Pulmonary disease	5265	1576	29.9	70	61	87.1
Radiation oncology	5027	597	11.9	742	16	2.2
Radiology and diagnostic radiology	27,719	3127	11.3	4464	681	15.3
Rheumatology	5880	1973	33.6	479	209	43.6
Sports medicine (orthopedic surgery)	2611	108	4.1	157	10	6.4
Thoracic surgery	4411	875	19.8	441	56	12.7
Urology	9921	1087	11	1301	49	3.8
Vascular and interventional radiology	3416	457	13.4	269	31	11.5
Vascular surgery	3688	642	17.4	536	88	16.4

Source: AAMC, 2017 [2]

(9017) (Table 1.1). Fields with the greatest percentage of IMGs among active physicians were geriatric medicine (50.8%), nephrology (49.0%), interventional cardiology (44.8%), critical care medicine (41.0%), and endocrinology, diabetes, and metabolism (39.6%). Conversely, fields with the lowest percentage of IMGs were sports medicine (4.1%), dermatology (4.9%), orthopedic surgery (5.2%), otolaryngology (6.3%), and emergency medicine (6.5%). These patterns may in part be due to the dynamics of the graduate medical education application process and the specialties in which IMGs are able to obtain residency or fellowship positions.

Geographic Distribution

IMGs practice all around the USA. Thirty-two percent work in the South, 28% in the Northeast, 20% in the Midwest, 17% in the West, and 3% in territories and the military [6]. IMGs from various countries are more likely to practice in certain parts of the USA. For example, Florida was home to relatively higher proportions of IMGs who had trained in Cuba (67%), Nicaragua (48%), Panama (33%), Venezuela (33%), and the Dominican Republic (32%) in 2001, which may reflect shared cultural and linguistic connections to communities in the state. Similarly, California had relatively higher percentages of IMGs from China (24%) and Hong Kong (32%). Graduates from Indian medical schools tended to be distributed evenly across the country [18].

Overview of Certification and Licensure Requirements

IMGs must complete a series of requirements to practice in the USA. All states require at least some graduate medical education (GME) training in the USA to be licensed (some states also accept Canadian GME training), and there are many states that require international medical graduates to complete a full residency training program before granting licenses, even if US medical graduates may be licensed sooner (see Chap. 23). Thus, IMGs must apply for residency (and/or fellowship, although this generally requires prior residency training in the USA to qualify), even if they have already completed similar training in their home countries. As mentioned previously, the regulatory body that certifies IMGs is the Educational Commission for Foreign Medical Graduates (ECFMG). IMG applicants must be certified by the ECFMG to be eligible to apply for an Accreditation Council for Graduate Medical Education (ACGME)-accredited US graduate medical education program. To be certified, the ECFMG requires applicants to satisfy a medical science examination requirement by passing US Medical Licensing Examination (USMLE) Step 1 and Step 2 Clinical Knowledge (CK) as well as a clinical skills requirement by passing USMLE Step 2 Clinical Skills (CS). This exam also has an English language proficiency evaluation component. IMGs must also complete at least 4 years of medical training from a medical school listed in the *World Directory of Medical Schools* [1]. In 2018, the ECFMG issued 9431 certificates [19].

Once ECFMG certification is acquired, participants can then apply for a residency position. During residency, many trainees will also complete USMLE Step 3, the last of the series of USMLE tests, for which ECFMG certification is also required as a prerequisite. Finally, after passing all licensing exams and completion of at least some GME training (requirements vary by state), individuals can apply for a state license to practice. Licensing considerations state by state are further discussed in Chap. 23.

IMGs and the Residency Application Process

Matching into a residency program is a major hurdle that all medical graduates face on the road to becoming licensed physicians. The main process by which most applicants, including IMGs and US medical graduates, obtain residency positions is through the Main Residency Match (with the exception of urology and ophthalmology, which have their own match process) organized by the National Resident Matching Program (NRMP). In 2018, out of the 37,103 total applicants who entered the Main Residency Match, 12,142 were IMGs (32.7%). Of these, 5075 (41.8%) were US IMGs, and 7067 (58.2%) were non-US IMGs [4].

Unfortunately for IMGs, match rates are lower for IMGs than US medical graduates. To illustrate, the PGY-1 (year 1 of GME training) match rate was 94.3% for US allopathic seniors in 2018, versus 57.1% for US IMGs and 56.1% for non-US IMGs [20]. However, certain clinical fields are known to be more "IMG friendly" in the match process than others. Figure 1.1 compares match rates between US allopathic

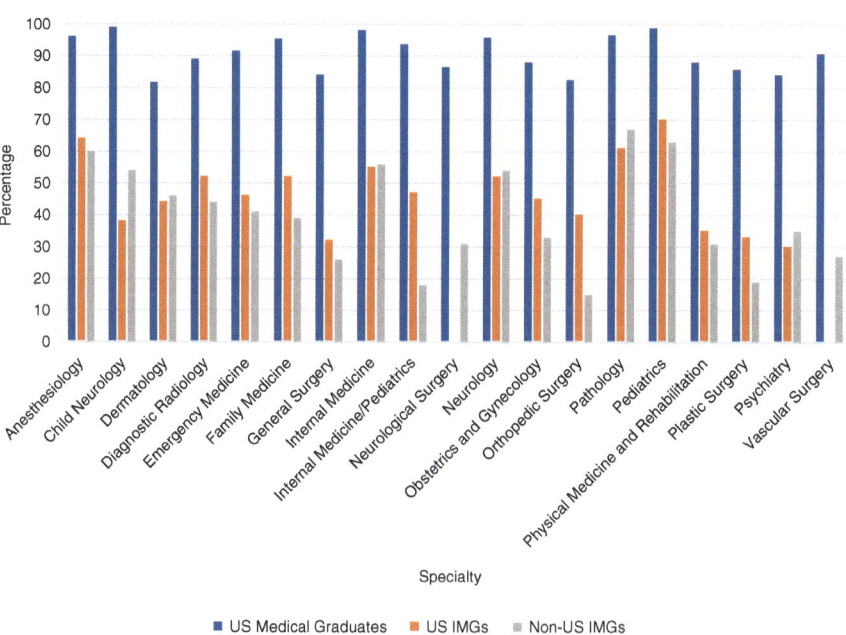

Fig. 1.1 Match rates by specialty for US medical graduates, US IMGs, and non-US IMGs in 2018. Only specialties with 50 or more positions and at least 7 matched or unmatched IMG applicants are included. Source: National Resident Matching Program (NRMP), 2018 [4, 25]

seniors, US IMGs, and non-US IMGs by specialty. Fields with the highest match rate for US IMGs were pediatrics (70%), anesthesiology (64%), and pathology (61%). Similarly, the highest match rates for non-US IMGs were in pathology (67%), pediatrics (63%), and anesthesiology (60%).

Comparing the types of IMGs, US IMGs have higher overall PGY-1 match rates than non-US IMGs, with dramatically higher match rates in certain individual fields, as shown in Fig. 1.1. However, US IMGs on average have lower mean USMLE Step 1 scores than non-US IMGs (222 versus 234 for matched applicants in 2018, respectively). US IMGs who matched in 2018 also had lower USMLE Step 2 scores (232 versus 240), fewer research experiences (1.7 versus 2.3), and fewer abstracts, presentations, and publications (2.5 versus 5.9) [4].

Examining the percentage of residents and fellows who are IMGs is another way to gauge "friendliness" of a particular field toward IMGs. Table 1.1 displays the number and percentage of residents and fellows who are IMGs for various specialties and subspecialties in 2017 as reported by the AAMC [2]. Excluding fellowship level subspecialties, pathology (43.7%), internal medicine (38.6%), neurology (33.4%), and family medicine/general practice (28.9%) had the highest proportions of IMGs among residents.

There are many complex drivers for the lower match rate of IMGs and the clustering of IMGs in certain specialties. For example, more competitive fields may be less reliant on IMGs to fill residency slots. Attitudes toward accepting IMGs into residency programs are also ambivalent. There may be a culture of stigma against IMGs as less desirable candidates. To illustrate, a survey of surgery residency program directors revealed that some program directors felt pressured to rank less-qualified US medical graduates above more qualified IMGs due to fear that the program would be perceived as weaker if they could not recruit US graduates [21]. There may also be bias against IMGs as less well trained. However, this has not necessarily borne out in terms of patient outcomes. A study of Medicare patients hospitalized from 2011 to 2014 and treated by international or US medical graduate general internists found that patients treated by IMGs actually had slightly lower 30-day mortality rates as compared to US graduates, with no difference in readmission rates, suggesting that quality of care is at least comparable between these two groups [22]. Despite this, biases likely still exist. Why US IMGs appear to do better in the match despite lower scores and other metrics of competitiveness is also difficult to explain. Issues pertaining to IMGs and securing residency positions are further discussed in later chapters.

Special Considerations for Non-US IMGs: Immigration and Visas

Non-US IMGs in particular face unique immigration-related challenges. In fact, this may be one of the most limiting barriers to entry. IMGs who are not citizens or lawful permanent US residents must obtain an appropriate visa to train in the USA. Several types of visas are possible, with the most common being J-1 (Exchange

Visitor) and H-1B (Temporary Worker) visas. The ECFMG can sponsor J-1 visas for those who are ECFMG-certified, but this type of visa requires visa holders to return to their home countries after residency for at least 2 years before applying for reentry to the USA. This requirement was instated in part to promote the transfer of skills acquired in the USA to home countries of IMGs and reestablish IMGs in their home countries to combat the phenomenon of "brain drain," in which skilled individuals leave lower-income countries for more developed nations, such as the USA [23]. However, for those wishing to stay and permanently immigrate to the USA, this can be a disruptive imposition.

This requirement can be waived in several circumstances. The residency requirement can be waived if a waiver applicant can demonstrate that he or she would experience persecution in his or her home country or if returning would bring exceptional hardship to the applicant's spouse and/or children who are US citizens or permanent residents. More commonly, IMGs can obtain J-1 waivers through sponsorship by an Interested Governmental Agency [24]. This sponsorship is generally obtained from federal governmental agencies such as the Departments of Health and Human Services, Veterans Affairs, and Housing and Urban Development if the IMG works for 3 years in areas with particular need for medical professionals, such as federally designated Health Professional Shortage Areas (HPSA) or Medically Underserved Areas (MUA). State health departments can also sponsor a maximum of 30 J-1 physicians each year, usually for practicing in underserved areas as well, known as the Conrad 30 program.

H-1B visas do not have this home residency requirement, but they are much rarer and harder to obtain. The applicant must have ECFMG certification, pass USMLE Step 1, Step 2 CK, Step 2 CS (these must be completed regardless to obtain ECFMG certification), and Step 3, obtain a state medical license, and match into the few programs that are willing and able to sponsor this visa.

Conclusion

The USA is a country of immigrants, and the physician workforce is no different. International medical graduates are an integral part of the US trainee and physician population, but the process of applying, entering, and staying in the USA can be difficult and uncertain. Even when an IMG physician successfully matches into a residency program, receives the necessary visa if applicable, and arrives in the USA, they may still face difficulties. These challenges and more, as well as possible solutions, will be further explored in subsequent chapters.

References

1. Educational Commission for Foreign Medical Graduates. 2020 information booklet [Internet]. Philadelphia: Educational Commission for Foreign Medical Graduates; 2019. [cited 2020 Feb 1]. 58p. Available from: https://www.ecfmg.org/2020ib/2020ib.pdf

2. Association of American Medical Colleges. Active physicians who are international medical graduates (IMGs) by specialty, 2017 [Internet]. Association of American Medical Colleges; 2017 [cited 2020 Feb 2]. Available from: https://www.aamc.org/data-reports/workforce/inter-active-data/active-physicians-who-are-international-medical-graduates-imgs-specialty-2017

3. Sheikh A, Naqvi SH, Sheikh K, Naqvi SH, Bandukda MY. Physician migration at its roots: a study on the factors contributing towards a career choice abroad among students at a medical school in Pakistan. Glob Health. 2012;8(1):43.

4. National Residency Matching Program. Charting outcomes in the Match: international medical graduates [Internet]. Washington, DC: National Residency Matching Program; 2018. [cited 2020 Jan 25]. 263p. Available from: https://www.nrmp.org/wp-content/uploads/2018/06/Charting-Outcomes-in-the-Match-2018-IMGs.pdf

5. Educational Commission for Foreign Medical Graduates. Top five countries of citizenship, certificates 1994–2018 [Internet]. Educational Commission for Foreign Medical Graduates; 2019 [cited 14 Feb 2020]. Available from: https://www.ecfmg.org/resources/Top5CitizenshipCountries1994-2018.pdf

6. O'Reilly KB. How IMGs have changed the face of American medicine [Internet]. Association of American Medical Colleges; 2019 [cited 2020 Feb 1]. Available from: https://www.ama-assn.org/education/international-medical-education/how-imgs-have-changed-face-american-medicine

7. Young A, Chaudhry HJ, Pei X, Arnhart K, Dugan M, Snyder GB. A census of actively licensed physicians in the United States, 2016. J Med Regul. 2017;103(2):7–21.

8. Halperin EC, Goldberg RB. Offshore medical schools are buying clinical clerkships in US hospitals: the problem and potential solutions. Acad Med. 2016;91(5):639–44.

9. Pinsky WW. The importance of international medical graduates in the United States. Ann Intern Med. 2017;166(11):840–1.

10. Salsberg ES, Forte GJ. Trends in the physician workforce, 1980–2000. Health Affairs. 2002;2(5):165–73.

11. Association of American Medical Colleges. 2019 Update: the complexities of physician supply and demand: projects from 2017 to 2032 [Internet]. Washington, DC: Association of American Medical Colleges; 2019. [cited 2019 Dec 5]. 72p. Available from: https://www.aamc.org/system/files/c/2/31-2019_update_-_the_complexities_of_physician_supply_and_demand_-_projections_from_2017-2032.pdf

12. Mick SS, Lee SY. International and US medical graduates in US cities. J Urban Health. 1999;76(4):481–96.

13. Mick SS, Lee SYD, Wodchis WP. Variations in geographical distribution of foreign and domestically trained physicians in the United States: 'safety nets' or 'surplus exacerbation'? Soc Sci Med. 2000;50(2):185–202.

14. Hagopian A, Thompson MJ, Kaltenbach E, Hart LG. The role of international medical graduates in America's small rural critical access hospitals. J Rural Health. 2004;20(1):52–8.

15. Hing E, Lin S. Role of international medical school graduates in providing office-based medical care: United States, 2005–2006 [Internet]. Hyattsville: National Center for Health Statistics; 2009. [cited 2020 Jan 10]. 7p. NCHS data brief no 13. Available from: https://www.cdc.gov/nchs/data/databriefs/db13.pdf

16. Norcini JJ, van Zanten M, Boulet JR. The contribution of international medical graduates to diversity in the US physician workforce: graduate medical education. J Health Care Poor Underserved. 2008;19(2):493–9.

17. Cooper-Patrick L, Gallo JJ, Gonzales JJ, Vu HT, Powe NR, Nelson C, et al. Race, gender, and partnership in the patient-physician relationship. JAMA. 1999;282(6):583–9.

18. Hart LG, Skillman SM, Fordyce M, Thompson M, Hagopian A, Konrad TR. International medical graduate physicians in the United States: changes since 1981. Health Affairs. 2007;26(4):1159–69.

19. Educational Commission for Foreign Medical Graduates. ECFMG fact card [Internet]. Educational Commission for Foreign Medical Graduates; 2019 [cited 14 Feb 2020]. Available from: https://www.ecfmg.org/forms/factcard.pdf.

20. National Residency Matching Program. Results and data: 2018 main residency Match [Internet]. Washington, DC: National Residency Matching Program; 2018. [cited 2020

Jan 30]. 116p. Available from: https://mk0nrmp3oyqui6wqfm.kinstacdn.com/wp-content/uploads/2018/04/Main-Match-Result-and-Data-2018.pdf

21. Moore RA, Rhodenbaugh EJ. The unkindest cut of all: are international medical school graduates subjected to discrimination by general surgery residency programs? Curr Surg. 2002;59(2):228–36.

22. Tsugawa Y, Jena AB, Orav EE, Jha AK. Quality of care delivered by general internists in US hospitals who graduated from foreign versus US medical schools: observational study. BMJ. 2017;356:j273.

23. Mullan F. The metrics of the physician brain drain. N Engl J Med. 2005;353(17):1810–8.

24. American Medical Association. Immigration information for international medical graduates. [cited 2020 Feb 10]. Available from: https://www.ama-assn.org/education/international-medical-education/immigration-information-international-medical-graduates

25. National Residency Matching Program. Charting outcomes in the Match: U.S. allopathic seniors [Internet]. Washington, DC: National Residency Matching Program; 2018. [revised 2019 Oct, cited 2020 Jan 30]. 215p. Available from: https://mk0nrmp3oyqui6wqfm.kinstacdn.com/wp-content/uploads/2019/10/Charting-Outcomes-in-the-Match-2018_Seniors-1.pdf

Chapter 2
Similarities and the Differences in the Education Systems Around the World

Ivan Cancarevic, Lucia Plichtová, and Hassaan Tohid

Education System of the United States

The US Education in General

The United States is home to some of the most elite universities in the world, which are also known for some of the most flexible curricula and widest range of available extracurricular activities. The United States is also the country that has given the world the greatest number of Nobel prize-winning scientists and the largest number of peer-reviewed scientific publications. While the United States does attract some of the most talented students from around the world, this is mostly based on the quality of higher education and, in particular, a smaller subset of universities in the United States. The United Kingdom is the most common international location where American students seek further education [1]. This should not come as a surprise as the two countries share the language and the United Kingdom is also home to some of the world's top universities. On the other hand, the stereotype of low-quality primary and secondary education is widespread, as is the perception of Americans lacking in basic general knowledge. The results of American students on international standardized examinations, while decent on a global scale, do lag behind students from many of the countries in the European Union or East Asia.

The federal government is not directly responsible for education at any level in the United States [1]. The roles of the Department of Education are as follows: establishing policies on federal financial aid and distribution of those funds, collecting data on schools, focusing on key educational issues, and prohibiting discrimination and ensuring equal access to education [2]. It is also responsible for executing

I. Cancarevic (✉) · H. Tohid
California Institute of Behavioral Neurosciences and Psychology, Fairfield, CA, USA

L. Plichtová
Hospital Department of Medicine, Bridgeport, CT, USA

© Springer Nature Switzerland AG 2021
H. Tohid, H. Maibach (eds.), *International Medical Graduates in the United States*, https://doi.org/10.1007/978-3-030-62249-7_2

the education policies of the president [1]. The education policy is shaped by the president and the cabinet, mainly the Secretary of Education [1]. The laws in the United States are passed by the congress, consisting of the House of Representatives and the Senate. Public policy debates are settled by the courts, the highest of which is the Supreme Court.

Homeschooling is legally recognized and regulated by the states. Usually, parents play the role of the teachers. The exact policies on homeschooling a child vary significantly between the individual states [1]. Homeschooling alone can rarely satisfy high school graduation requirements, although parent's certification that the student has completed the program is often recognized as equivalent [1].

Early Education

The lack of tradition of government involvement in everyday matters in the United States is often blamed for the perceived weakness of primary education [1]. All students are entitled to free public education for 12 years, and private school enrollment at this age is only around 10% [1]. The minimum school age is between 5 and 7, and 15 states require students to attend kindergarten [1]. English is the language of instruction with the exception of Puerto Rico, where Spanish predominates [1]. The kindergartens today focus mostly on reading and numeric skills with some implementation of music, art, and basic science [1]. In elementary schools, students generally receive education by the same teacher for the duration of the academic year, although some subjects may have special teachers [1]. The curricula are determined on a state level, and the implementation is generally decided by the individual schools and teachers [1].

The Middle School and High School

The middle school generally refers to grades 6–8 with some variations, starting around the age of 11. High schools refer to grades 9–12. Students mostly attend five or six class periods per day, and each teacher teaches one subject [1]. The curricula vary significantly between individual schools. The subjects students learn are typically English, mathematics, science, social science, fine arts, and physical education [1]. Most students also study foreign languages (the most common of which is Spanish) for at least 2 years, computer science for at least a year, and 2 or 3 years of other subjects [1]. The progress toward graduation is usually "measured" using a credits system with the states setting the minimum graduation requirements [1]. Most schools offer a range of extracurricular activities that many students participate in, both out of their own personal interest and in order to improve their university applications. They generally do not provide credit toward graduation and take place after the classes have finished [1]. High school students are often placed into different "tracks" depending on their future ambitions. These usually include general track, vocational track, and college-preparatory track aimed at satisfying most university admission requirements [1]. Some high schools offer an honors program for high-achieving students, where the curriculum is more demanding and the relative weight of the grades in those classes is often higher, enabling students to earn a grade point average above 4.0, which is typically seen as the highest [1]. Some schools also offer "advanced placement" courses where students take college-level courses that often count toward college graduation requirements as well as high school, and they are usually scored on a 5-point scale [1]. Individual colleges vary in their policies on accepting advanced placement courses [1].

Higher Education

There is a vast number of higher education institutions in the United States, and the courses they offer are as varied as the institutions themselves. Overall, American universities dominate most of the university rankings. In order to be recognized as universities, institutions have to offer, at minimum, bachelor's programs and some master's programs [1]. Colleges can offer associate degrees and bachelor's degrees [1]. The funding of higher education in the United States is extremely complex, and the funds typically come from a number of different sources, including private grants, tuition fees, state governments, and so on [1]. The private institutions are more reliant on private grants and tuition fees compared to public universities [1]. Ivy League is the term used to describe one of the most famous university alliances on the East Coast of the United States and comprises some of the most elite educational institutions in the world, including Harvard, Yale, Princeton, Columbia, Cornell, Brown, Dartmouth, and University of Pennsylvania [1]. It was originally formed as an athletic association but has grown to become one of the most recognized brands in the world of academia globally [1]. Admissions to Ivy League universities are highly competitive and prestigious, which has led to significant criticisms about the stress it puts on high school students. On the other hand, there are a number of for-profit higher education institutions in the United States, the quality of which may be questionable. There are a number of regulatory agencies overseeing and accrediting the universities. The enrollment at universities in the United States is increasing, and it is now frequently said that a degree is becoming almost essential to secure good jobs. Unlike universities in most other countries, the American university admission committees place a lot of value on extracurricular activities and letters of recommendation when it comes to offering admissions to students [1]. Admission to graduate programs, leading to master's and PhD degrees, is also competitive, and it is based on undergraduate performance, standardized test scores, letters of recommendation, essays, and samples of work, such as writing samples or research articles [1]. Interviews are also common [1]. The highest degree one can achieve in a field is a PhD degree. There are also a number of professional doctorates awarded to graduates of certain professional schools, such as "Juris Doctor" (JD), "Doctor of Medicine" (MD), or "Doctor of Public Health" (DPH), among others.

Medical Education in the United States

The Basic Structure

While some 6- and 7-year combined undergraduate and graduate medical programs exist in the United States, for the most part students apply to medical schools after graduating from college. Usually, students spend 4 years in medical school followed by several years in residency training, depending on their specialty of interest. License to practice is awarded by individual states.

Pre-medical Education

Pre-medical education refers to college education before applying for medical school. For most students that means obtaining a bachelor's degree in their field of interest while simultaneously satisfying the pre-medical requirements of medical schools that they plan on applying for. Those requirements are generally similar across schools although there may be small differences which prospective applicants need to be mindful of. Those who do not satisfy all the pre-medical requirements during their college years often go on to pursue post-baccalaureate programs in order to become eligible to apply to medical schools. Most medical schools require students to complete college courses in biology, chemistry, biochemistry, and physics [3, 4]. Advanced placement courses and courses from community colleges are not always considered sufficient to satisfy pre-medical requirements [3]. The pre-medical courses should also generally be completed at American or Canadian universities. Post-baccalaureate pre-medical programs are also becoming increasingly popular among students who have decided to pursue medicine later on. They can be expensive, often do not lead to a degree, and rarely guarantee admission to medical school, so enrolling in them is not a decision that should be taken lightly by prospective students [5]. Toward the end of their pre-medical education, most students sit the Medical College Admission Test (MCAT), a standardized exam required for admission to medical school in the United States [6]. The exam tests candidates on their knowledge of biology, chemistry, physics, behavioral science, and critical thinking and gives them numeric scores which help admission committees make decisions [6]. Those whose applications are considered strong enough are generally invited for in-person interviews at individual medical schools where final admission decisions are made.

Medical Education

Becoming a doctor in the United States takes a lot of time and money. As most medical schools last 4 years in addition to 4 years of college, the average students spends 8 years at university before earning their first salary. It is also expensive as the average first year medical student pays more than 36,000 USD per year in tuition, fees, and health insurance to attend a public medical school and almost 60,000 USD to attend a private medical school, meaning that the majority of students have to take significant loans to be able to pay for their education [7]. Many choose to attend more expensive medical schools due to their prestige and belief that that will increase their job prospects after graduation. There are many lists of "best" medical schools available online, the most famous of which is the "US News" [8]. American medical schools are moving toward more problem-based learning, in contrast to medical schools in some European countries that follow much more traditional curricula. The first 2 years are generally dedicated to basic sciences, such as anatomy, physiology, and pathology, although it varies by school. The third and fourth years are mostly spent at hospitals attending clinical clerkships [9–11]. Third year students usually complete a list of "core" or required clerkships in major medical disciplines, such as internal medicine, surgery, psychiatry, obstetrics and gynecology, pediatrics, and family medicine [7–9]. Fourth year clerkships are usually a series of electives, including rotations at hospitals affiliated with other schools where students hope to be offered residency positions. Obtaining strong letters of recommendation is crucial. American medical students also sit a number of medical licensing exams, known as the United States Medical Licensing Examination, or USMLE. The USMLE program consists of four exams, namely Step 1, Step 2 Clinical Knowledge (CK), Step 2 Clinical Skills (CS), and Step 3. The USMLE Step 1 is usually taken at the end of the pre-clinical portion of medical curricula and tests students on basic science knowledge [12]. It is a computer-administered whole-day exam [12]. The USMLE Step 2 CK is also a whole-day computer-administered exam which tests students on their knowledge of clinical subjects [13]. The USMLE Step 2 CS is a whole-day practical examination, administered in a few dedicated test centers in the United States, aimed at testing communication and clinical skills [14]. Passing those three exams is generally required to graduate from medical school. International medical graduates (IMGs), in addition to finishing accredited medical schools from abroad, also need to pass those three exams to obtain the Education Commission for Foreign Medical Graduates (ECFMG) certificate, which is a requirement to apply for residency programs in the United States [15]. The USMLE Step 3 is taken by medical school graduates, and it is one of the requirements for medical licensure [16].

Graduate Medical Education and Licensure

Medical licenses are given by individual states to physicians who satisfy the requirements. The requirements themselves are not uniform and depend on whether the applicant is an American or an international medical school graduate [17]. Some states also place a limit on the number of examination attempts for each step of the USMLE [17]. Specialty training or residency programs last at least 3 years and lead to recognition as a specialist through board certification. Once a year, students and graduates are able to apply to a centralized system which matches applicants with residency programs. Applicants register on the Electronic Residency Application Service (ERAS) website and select the residency programs they wish to apply to. The program directors then assess the individual applications and invite some applicants for in-person interviews. At the end of the process, applicants create ranking lists of programs, and programs create ranking lists of applicants. The computerized system then matches the applicants to programs based on preferences. Those who fail to secure jobs through the Match may be able to find one outside of the Match, although the vast majority of the positions are filled through the Match [18]. The working hours during residency are often long and the pay is significantly lower than that for specialists. Thousands of international medical graduates Match to residency programs in the United States. Those who do not have work authorization need to obtain visas. Internal medicine is the specialty most popular among international medical graduates. Surgical specialties are generally difficult to Match into and favor American graduates more strongly than internal medicine. Most of the international medical graduates find positions in the Northeast and Midwest, significantly fewer in the South, and very few on the West Coast [19]. The state of California even has its own list of international medical schools it recognizes, and only graduates of those schools are eligible to apply to Californian programs [20].

Medical Education in Canada

The structure of the curriculums of Canadian and American medical education systems is highly similar. Canada shares close cultural and economic ties with the United States, and Canadian medical graduates (CMGs) are not technically considered to be international medical graduates (IMGs) in the US medical system. Despite these close ties, however, only an exceedingly small percentage of annual US residency applicants are Canadian graduates [21]. As is the case around the globe, medical education in Canada can only be obtained after completing the compulsory prerequisite educational levels.

The compulsory educational system in Canada consists of both public and private institutions. Though the majority of Canadians attend public institutions, private schools are available to students at all levels of education. Canada contains ten provinces and three territories, and with education being managed on a provincial level, the systems within different provinces and territories often vary significantly. A rather unique feature of public schools in Canada is that they are largely managed on a local level by publicly elected school boards, rather than by a centralized institution. Thus, the curriculum and teaching methods may differ greatly, even within the same province [22]. Generally, education is divided into three levels: primary, secondary, and post-secondary education.

Primary education in Canada, referred to as elementary school, traditionally runs from kindergarten or grade 1 (age 5–6) through to grade 8 (age 13–14). The starting age of compulsory education ranges from 5 to 7 years, depending on the province or territory [23]. The school year begins in September and ends the following June. Most provinces also offer students the opportunity to attend middle school, also known as junior high school, which may run anywhere from grade 6 to grade 9. As Canada is a bilingual country, during the primary years all students in English-speaking schools are required to study French as a second language. French-language schools are also available, primarily in the francophone province of Quebec, but also in other provinces and territories.

Secondary education, also known as high school, lasts for 4 years in Canada, running from grade 9 to grade 12. Grade 12 is the final grade in all secondary school systems except in that of Quebec, where high school ends at grade 11 [24]. During high school, particularly the senior years (grades 11 and 12), students may enroll in a number of elective subjects of their choice, according to their professional aspirations. School attendance is mandatory up to the age of 16 in all Canadian provinces, with the exception of Ontario, Manitoba, and New Brunswick, where students must attend school either until the age of 18 or until a high school diploma is obtained [24]. During the final year of high school, students wishing to pursue a higher education prepare and send applications to the universities or colleges of their choice, learning their status of admission by the summer months.

Post-secondary education in Canada consists of a variety of institutions including universities, university colleges, and colleges. Students have the opportunity to earn bachelor's, master's, and doctoral degrees from universities, or diplomas and certificates from colleges. These institutions are funded largely by the provincial and territorial governments, but also rely on tuition fees and research grants for financial support [24].

Those interested in pursuing medicine as a profession typically must receive a bachelor's degree in another field prior to applying to medical school. Though a degree in any field may be considered, most medical schools require a minimum number of credits to be completed in various science courses; thus, most students naturally select a program in the biological sciences [25]. Though admission requirements differ according to the medical school, the vast majority of schools require completion of a 4-year undergraduate degree at an accredited university in order to consider the applicant. Though some schools may consider applicants with 3-year degrees, or even 2-year degrees in the case of western Canadian medical schools, such admissions are infrequent and are typically only seen in students with exceptional credentials and experience [26]. Additionally, most medical schools in Canada require applicants to have completed the Medical School College Admission

Test (MCAT). The MCAT is a multiple-choice computer-based exam which tests students' knowledge of the sciences as well as verbal reasoning skills. Students may take the exam more than once if they wish, but no more than three times in 1 year or seven times in a lifetime [27]. Overall, the most important criteria considered by the medical school selection committees are grade point average, MCAT scores, extra-curricular experiences, and interview performance. Attaining admission to a Canadian medical school is a strenuous process, and the acceptance rates range between less than 5% in Ontario and around 12% in the western provinces – a considerably lower rate than in the United States [28–30]. As a result, many Canadians prefer to study medicine abroad, most commonly at Caribbean medical schools or in the United States.

Canada houses a total of 17 medical schools which produce an average of 2900 medical graduates each year [31]. These schools are distributed amongst eight provinces, with the greatest number of spots available within the two most populated Canadian provinces – Ontario and Quebec. Traditionally, the duration of the medical school curriculum in Canada is 4 years. However, some universities, such as McMaster University in Ontario, have an accelerated 3-year program in which studies run for 11 months each year [32]. The first 2 years of the curriculum focus on teaching the core concepts of pre-clinical subjects such as anatomy, histology, physiology, and pharmacology, amongst others. The second half of the program consists of clinical rotations, where students learn and gain hands-on experience under the direct supervision of medical residents and physicians. Upon completion of their medical studies, graduates are awarded a Doctor of Medicine (M.D.) degree, or in the case of McGill University, a Doctor of Medicine and Master of Surgery (MDCM) degree. Every medical school in Canada is jointly accredited by two institutions – the Committee on Accreditation of Canadian Medical Schools (CACMS) and the US Liaison Committee on Medical Education [33].

Medical graduates in Canada must complete a residency program in order to become licensed physicians. Completion of an internship after medical school is not necessary – instead, students enter into a residency program immediately after graduation. Residencies are salaried postgraduate training programs which vary in duration. Most programs, such as general internal medicine, are 5 years long. On the other hand, family medicine residencies are 2-year programs, and some surgical residencies may last for 6 years [34]. Before applying for a residency, students must have passed two examinations: the National Assessment Collaboration (NAC) Examination, which consists of a series of stations in which various clinical scenarios are presented, and the MCCQE Part 1, a computer-based multiple-choice exam [35].

During autumn of the final year of medical school, CMGs apply for residency positions via the Canadian Resident Match Service (CaRMS), a system which works very much like its US counterpart – the National Resident Matching Program (NRMP). CaRMS is a computerized matching platform in which applicants, after attending interviews, rank programs in order of their preference in the form of a rank order list (ROL). Programs also create their own ROLs, ranking the applicants they have interviewed according to their preference. In the end, applicants are matched to programs via a computerized algorithm.

Most students apply through the R-1 Main Residency Match, which occurs in two iterations. During the first iteration, all Canadian or international medical graduates who have not completed any prior postgraduate training may apply. In contrast to the US system, CaRMS allots a certain number of separate positions only available to IMGs, for which CMGs may not apply. It is important to note that visa holders are not eligible for entry into the Match – only IMGs who are citizens or permanent residents of Canada are able to apply [36]. During the second iteration, applicants who failed to Match or those with prior postgraduate training may apply for those positions not filled during the first iteration. Applicants discover their residency placements on Match Day, which typically takes place during March. The Match rates for Canadian medical graduates are very high – upward of 95% [37]. For IMGs the Match rates are significantly lower, with around 61% of current year and 24% of previous year graduates matching [37]. In contrast, between 2016 and 2020, the number of active CMG applicants in the US NRMP Match ranged only from 11 to 22 students each year [21]. The Match is a binding contractual agreement, and as a result, after matching at a program, the doctor must commence his/her residency training with that program on July 1st of that year. After the completion of residency, the doctor is eligible for full licensure and independent practice.

Despite its vast size and great geographical variance in educational curricula, Canada, at all levels of government, continues to prioritize the delivery of a high quality of education to all of its citizens. With its well-funded public education system, Canadians wishing to pursue medicine are equipped with a strong base of knowledge and core competencies starting from childhood, which allows them to successfully navigate medical school and residency. Though the path to becoming a doctor is not an easy one, Canada remains committed to training highly skilled and independent physicians ready to serve the ever-changing needs of its diverse population.

European Education Systems

British Education System

Unsurprisingly, British education system produces some of the world's most renowned experts in most fields, including medicine. Britain is also home to one of the largest international student populations. There are minor differences between educational systems of Scotland and the rest of the United Kingdom. Compulsory elementary education lasts for 6 years, from the age of 5 to the age of 11, and compulsory secondary education lasts for 5 years thereafter. At the end of the secondary education, students sit General Certificate of Secondary Education (GCSE) exams. Those who wish to pursue higher education generally go on to spend another 2 years in pre-university programs. At the end of those programs, students generally take Advanced Level examinations (often referred to as A-levels). University admissions, managed by Universities and Colleges Admissions Service (UCAS), are partly dependent on the A-level examination scores and partly on the rest of the applicant's CV. Universities offer undergraduate and postgraduate programs. Some of them, notably medicine, require applicants to sit additional admission exams and attend interviews prior to being offered a place. The universities of Oxford and Cambridge have slightly different admission processes and students are generally limited to one application to one program at either Oxford or Cambridge. Higher education degrees are awarded as either "Pass" or "Honors" degrees. In Scotland, compulsory education generally consists of 7 years of elementary education and 4 years of secondary education [38].

Medical Education in Britain

Britain is home to some of the world's most famous medical schools. Medicine courses in the United Kingdom last between 4 and 6 years, with 4 years representing graduate-entry medicine programs, aimed at those with B.A. degrees in other fields, while 5- and 6-year programs refer to standard undergraduate entry medicine. Admissions are competitive and applicants can apply to a limited number of programs. Over the first 2 years, students usually study pre-clinical subjects, followed by 3 years of clinical rotations. Six-year courses usually offer an additional year of science, leading to a separate bachelor's degree in a related subject. Many medical schools in the United Kingdom have recently adopted problem-based learning approach to medical education. At the end of the final year, students generally sit their final exams [39]. Newly graduated physicians enter the workforce as "foundation doctors." They stay in that role for 2 years, during which they rotate through a number of specialties, both medical and surgical. At the end of the "foundation program," physicians apply to what would more closely resemble a residency program in other countries. Those choosing medical or surgical specialties usually spend 2 years as "core trainees," rotating through specialties within their field of interest before enrolling in a higher specialist training, eventually leading to becoming a specialist. Many choose to obtain additional postgraduate degrees. Foreign physicians may enter the training at different points. Physicians from outside the European Union generally have to sit the PLAB (Professional and Linguistic Assessments Board) examinations. Whether a test is introduced for European physicians following Britain's departure from the EU remains to be seen [40]. British training is among the best regarded around the world, and British specialists are usually eligible to work in any country in Europe, alongside Canada, Australia, and New Zealand.

German Education System

As one of the global leaders in technology, research, and development, there is little doubt that the German education system is capable of producing some of the most elite experts in the world. In general, the educational system is divided into five levels, from early childhood education all the way to university-level education and continuing education [41, 42]. Importantly, as is the case in most European countries, the education is mostly funded through taxes and the costs of pursuing higher education are minimal. Until the age of 6, most children in Germany attend kindergarten. Pre-school education is optional [42]. Most of the day-care centers in Germany are privately owned [42]. Many non-profit organizations, such as churches and Parent's Associations, provide some forms of early education in Germany as well [42]. The focus is mostly on improving the children's communication and language skills and motor development. An interesting aspect of early education in Germany is the focus on improving body awareness and self-acceptance. As toddlers approach school age, the focus shifts to teaching the basics of mathematics, science, and culture. Assessments in this age group are infrequent. The compulsory education starts at the age of 6 and lasts for 9 or 10 years [41, 42]. For the first 4 or 6 years, children attend mixed-ability classes for 5 or 6 days a week. Music, sports, foreign languages, and handicrafts are among the subjects taught, alongside languages and mathematics [41, 42]. The grading is mostly numerical [42]. Following primary education, at the age of 10, children move on to secondary education. There are three types of secondary schools that students are allocated to based on academic abilities [41, 42]. The most elite type, the "gymnasiums" provide deep general knowledge and prepare students to enter tertiary education at university level [41, 42]. Germany is home to some of the most prestigious universities in the world. Most students attend 3–5-year programs that lead to either bachelor or master's degrees in their fields of interest. Some students go on to pursue postgraduate education.

Medical Education in Germany

The medical education system in Germany differs significantly from that of the United States. Students enter medical schools after high school and spend 6 years there, compared to 4 years of post-college education in the United States. The admissions are based on the academic performance during secondary education. Most medical schools follow a pre-set curriculum, defined by the German government, where the first 2 years are dedicated to basic, pre-clinical sciences, and years 4–6 are dedicated to clinical rotations [43]. Medical schools in Germany are tax-funded, and besides minimal administrative costs, the students are not required to pay tuition fees. Up to a third of medical students in Germany do not graduate and do not enter the workforce [43]. A number of graduates decide to pursue careers in research and industry, leaving a massive shortage of physicians in Germany [43]. Students who want to pursue specialty training apply to individual hospitals for positions. Most specialty training programs last anywhere between 4 and 6 years, depending on the specialty [43]. Physicians often have to spend certain amounts of time in different hospitals to fulfill all the requirements of the training program [43]. Individual German states provide licensure to those who successfully complete their residency programs.

French Education System

Just like in Germany, education is for the most part free in France. Education is compulsory from the age of 6 until the age of 16 [44]. Many children enter pre-school at the age of 3, and the majority of high school graduates enter tertiary education [44]. The schools are secular and most are state-run. There are also some private schools. Students spend between 24 and 26 weeks per year in school with 4 or 5 school days per week, depending on the region [44, 45]. The system is based on strict discipline and traditional learning methods. The authority of teachers is generally significantly higher than in the United States, and the academic expectations in France are high [45]. Pre-schools provide care for children until they are old enough to enter school at the age of 6 [44, 45]. The main aim of the curricula of the pre-schools is to prepare children for primary schools. Primary school children go through five educational levels from the age of 6 to the age of 11 [44, 45]. Primary schools often do not work on Wednesdays. Children are taught literacy, basic mathematics, and a foreign language, most commonly English. Up to a third of students have to repeat a year at some point [45]. Between the ages of 11 and 15, students attend middle schools, which consist of four educational levels. Middle schools provide students with general education in a number of fields [44, 45]. At the end of middle school, students sit an exam in which they are tested on French, mathematics, history or geography, foreign language, and computer science. From the age of 15 to the age of 18, students attend high school, consisting of three levels, with the aim of preparing them for university entrance. At the end of high school, the students sit another round of exams, which determine their academic futures [44, 45]. Most high school graduates enter universities, which generally follow the typical structure of higher education programs in Europe.

Medical Education in France

The medical education in France is provided in three cycles and by a number of different universities. The first 2 years are spent teaching basic sciences outside of the hospital setting [46]. At the end of the first year, students are required to sit a difficult and competitive exam [46]. The results of this exam determine which career the students are able to pursue afterward (e.g., research, clinical care, biology, etc.) [46]. The second phase lasts 4 years, the first of which is spent teaching general medicine, followed by 3 years of "pathology and therapeutics" [46]. Most of the courses are provided in hospitals. Once the students finish the second phase of the education, they can enter one of two major career paths: general medicine third cycle or specialized medicine third cycle [46, 47]. The general medicine cycle lasts 2 years and prepares the students for a career as a general practitioner [46, 47]. The specialized medicine cycle lasts 4–5 years and prepares the students for a career in one of the medical specialties [46, 47]. Additional subspecialty programs are available to those who wish to pursue them. The traditional style of didactic teaching is still the most prevalent in France, and the newer methods of problem-based learning are not being readily accepted by universities [47]. Nevertheless, there is little doubt that the French system produces some of the best physicians in the world today.

Italian Education System

Similarly to France and Germany, education in Italy is compulsory from the age of 6 until 16. Those aged between 3 and 6 go to kindergartens with the aim of preparing them for primary schools. Between the age of 6 and 11, students attend compulsory primary schools followed by secondary schools between the ages of 11 and 14 [48, 49]. Those wishing to study music can forego secondary schools and go straight to conservatories [48]. This is followed by upper secondary or vocational training [48, 49]. Those 19 or older can enter universities if they successfully complete upper secondary education and pass the required examinations. The universities generally follow the standard European framework, which is even named after a famous Italian university in Bologna. The schools and universities are monitored and financed by the government.

Medical Education in Italy

Like in the rest of Europe, students enter medical school at the age of 19 in Italy. Unlike France and Germany, Italy is one of the smaller number of European countries which offer medical education programs in English, mostly aimed at foreign students. The tuition fees are minimal. Medical schools also generally last 6 years, the first 2 of which are mostly based around basic sciences followed by an increasingly clinical curriculum toward the end of the program [50]. Newly graduated physicians enter specialty training programs with the aim of becoming either a general practitioner or a specialist in any field. The ranking on the national exam determines the specialty physicians can pursue and the location they can pursue it at [50]. Further specialization is also possible for those who desire it.

Education Systems in Latin America

Education System in Mexico

As the geographically closest Latin American country to the United States, we will begin our analysis of Latin American education systems by taking a look at Mexico. It consists of three distinct levels: primary education, secondary education, and higher education. Formal basic education includes pre-school, elementary, and lower secondary school [51]. It is compulsory for children to attend primary school from the age of 6. Pre-school before that is private and optional. The education is secular and religious instruction is banned in public schools [51]. Children remain in primary schools until the age of 12, meaning they spend the total of 6 years as primary school students. Primary schools are free. An interesting fact is that in many schools half the classes are taught in Spanish and the other half is taught in a foreign language, often English. Following primary school, children attend 3 years of secondary school where they learn most of the basic subjects such as sciences and history [51]. It is followed by 3 years of high school or "preparatory school," which has recently also become compulsory [51]. These schools either prepare students for university admissions or provide vocational training for those wishing to seek employment. Based on the academic abilities some go on to pursue higher education at one of the Mexican universities. Overall, the quality of education may not be up to western standards, especially in more rural areas, and many students do not complete their schooling. The things are changing for the better, though, and it is expected that by 2035 Mexico is going to become one of the top 20 countries globally by the number of students attending higher education [51].

Medical Education in Mexico

Mexico also has a large number of medical schools that train the country's physicians. These programs generally last between 4 and 5 years [52]. After graduating, most physicians spend a year working as interns and another year as rural general practitioners before sitting the national examination in order to pursue postgraduate training. The passing rate on those exams is very low, and the majority of physicians do not pursue residency training [52, 53]. Those who pass the exam are able to choose further specialty training, with at least one quarter of those physicians choosing to train in internal medicine. For example, surgeons spend another 4 years doing specialty training and on top of that an additional 2 years pursuing sub-specialty training [52, 53]. Just like in many other Latin American countries, a number of young physicians are interested in seeking further training in the United States due to perceived high quality of training, good working environment, and future earnings potential [54].

Education System in Brazil

The public education system in Brazil is facing political challenges depending on the government in charge. Recently, the newly elected Brazilian president Bolsonaro has demanded the "banishment of the ideologies of the left" from Brazilian schools which has led to decreased funding [55]. The system is divided into stages, starting with early childhood education at the age of 4 and 5, followed by elementary education for 9 years and secondary education in grades 10–12 [55]. After finishing those 12 years, students can pursue higher education in form of vocational or university-level programs. Compulsory education includes early childhood and secondary education and is provided free of charge. The national curriculum determines the standards that children are required to meet prior to finishing school [55]. Participation in elementary education is almost universal. Most of the education is in Portuguese, although some of the indigenous populations have secured the rights to use their own languages [55]. The compulsory subjects include Portuguese, mathematics, history, geography, science, and physical education. Recently, English has become mandatory. Secondary education is provided at general academic schools, technical schools, and military schools [55]. There are also a number of international schools. Students who wish to pursue higher education sit the National Examination of Secondary Education (ENEM) [55]. The universities consist of smaller autonomous units, faculties. Many are private and the majority are for-profit. There is fierce competition for the limited number of seats at public universities. There are great geographical differences when it comes to access to education, and most universities are located in more affluent parts of the country.

Medical Education in Brazil

Like in most other countries, medical schools in Brazil are undergraduate-level university courses that last 6 years [56]. The curricula and the approaches to education of individual medical schools vary widely. It is believed that the quality control is lacking. Nevertheless, Brazil manages to educate some excellent physicians as there are a number of highly respectable institutions in the country. Over 50% of medical students attend private medical schools, which stands in contrast to countries like Mexico and Argentina where most of the university-level education is provided by public institutions [57]. After graduating from medical school, physicians in Brazil also pursue residency training programs to gain further experience and expertise in one of the medical specialties.

Education System in Argentina

Lack of technological advancements and inefficiency of the educational system are often cited as the reasons for slower economic growth in Argentina during the twentieth century when compared to some other, mostly Asian countries. Despite that fact, the Argentinian education system overall outperforms most of the other Latin American systems, and the literacy and school enrollment rates are overall high. The number of university graduates is lower than in other major Latin American countries, and the performances of Argentinian students on standardized tests are less than ideal [58]. Students in urban centers generally receive higher quality of education than those in more rural parts of the country. All children in Argentina are required to attend 2 years of early childhood education before starting elementary school. Most of the country follows a 7 + 5 model where students spend 7 years in elementary school followed by 5 years in secondary school [58]. This varies by the province, though. The elementary education starts at the age of 6 [58]. The compulsory subjects include Spanish, English, science, mathematics, social sciences, arts, technical education, and physical education [58]. Many reforms are underway aimed at standardizing the school curricula across the country. When it comes to secondary education, besides more general academic programs, aimed at preparing students for university admissions, vocational or technical programs exist as well. All secondary school graduates are technically allowed to enroll in higher education in Argentina [58]. There are no entrance exams for universities, so the admission criteria vary significantly between institutions [58]. Besides universities, there are also post-secondary programs aimed at vocational education. Private universities also exist, although they are in the minority. The number of students attending higher education is increasing every year. Almost 80% of the university students attend public universities [58].

Medical Education in Argentina

Argentinian medical schools generally offer 6-year undergraduate-level programs that consist of 3 years of basic sciences followed by 2 years of clinical sciences and 1 year of internships [59, 60]. The admission requirements are university-dependent. Annually, approximately 5000 physicians graduate from Argentinian medical schools out of 12,000 who matriculate into medical schools [60]. The class sizes in some universities are unmanageably large. Problem-based learning is minimally implemented. The admission requirements for residency programs are even more strict, and fewer than 50% of the medical school graduates are able to obtain residency positions [60]. Those who fail to obtain residency positions generally undergo further education in science or undertake unaccredited healthcare works in hopes of improving their CVs for future residency applications [60]. The selection process for residency programs involves an exam and, at some institutions, an interview [60]. Most residency programs are 4 years long. Roughly two-thirds of residents are thought to be in basic specialties, while a third is in subspecialties [60]. Although there still appears to be plenty of room for improvement, overall it cannot be denied that Argentina has a better healthcare system than most of the neighboring countries.

Education Systems of Australia, Japan, and China

Education System of Australia

As one of the wealthiest countries in the world, it comes as no surprise that Australia is able to provide world-class education to its citizens, and a number of foreigners choose to study in Australia every year. Although immigration has become a heated political topic in Australia in recent years, the country continues to show its support for high-skilled individuals by promoting the easy immigration of professionals into the country. The education system is decentralized, and individual states and territories have their own departments of education [61]. Most of the funding comes from states, while roughly a quarter comes from the federal government, and it is mostly given to private schools [61]. School is compulsory from the age of 5 until the age of 16, and tuition fees are charged even in public schools. The details of the curricula vary by state, but children mostly receive the basic education in English, mathematics, science, humanities, computer science, and physical education [61]. Some of the more prestigious lower secondary schools require students to sit entrance examinations in order to achieve admission [61]. The upper secondary education is not compulsory, but a large majority of students choose to attend, and most can do it at the same schools where they did their lower secondary education [61]. Many vocational programs are available both at the secondary and post-secondary levels [61]. Universities are usually autonomous and able to select their students according to their own eligibility criteria. Admissions are commonly based on the Australian Tertiary Admissions Rank (ATAR), which ranks students in comparison to their peers according to final year grades and examination results [61]. Individual states are responsible for approving and licensing universities within its borders. Most of the funding for higher education institutions comes from tuition fees and external, usually private sources [61].

Medical Education in Australia

The medical education system in Australia is constantly changing. Traditionally, it followed the British model of undergraduate medicine courses of 5–6 years in duration. Nowadays, more and more medical schools are offering graduate-level courses in a manner similar to the medical schools in the United States. More and more rural clinical schools are opening nowadays [62]. After graduating from medical schools, young doctors undergo a year of professional training called an internship. Interns follow a pre-set curriculum where they are required to spend a certain number of weeks in internal medicine, surgery, emergency medicine, and a range of other specialties [62]. After internship, most physicians spend a few years working as "Resident Medical Officers" or "House Medical Officers" doing a variety of placements in order to improve their CVs. They then apply for "Registrar" posts, which are specialty training posts that lead to being licensed as specialists in their field of interest [62]. Some physicians then go on to pursue PhDs, especially if they are interested in more competitive jobs [62]. The professional registrations are awarded by the Medical Board of Australia. Several international medical graduates are interested in moving to Australia, but their career paths are extremely difficult due to oversupply and a limited number of training jobs. Those who have trained in New Zealand, the United Kingdom, Ireland, the United States, or Canada are typically seen more favorably compared to others [63].

Education System of Japan

As one of the global leaders in education and technology, there is no question about the ability of the Japanese education system to produce some of the world leaders in science and technology. Compulsory education begins at the age of 6, although most of the children attend kindergarten. Most kindergartens are private, and many are highly selective [64]. Unlike kindergartens, almost all primary schools are public, charge no tuition fees, and last 6 years [64]. The curriculum includes Japanese, mathematics, natural sciences, social sciences, art, music, moral education, home-making, life environment studies, special activities, and periods of combining skills learned in different classes [64]. Lower secondary education is also compulsory and lasts for 3 years. The achievements during lower secondary education determine the child's prospects of enrolling in upper secondary education and, in extension, good university and career [64]. Upper secondary education has academic and vocational streams, with the academic streams generally being more competitive. Approximately 30% of upper secondary schools are private [64]. Higher education in Japan is provided by a few different institutions, the most prestigious ones of which are universities. Almost 80% of all higher education enrollment is at private institutions [64]. The admissions are based on the upper secondary education results and on competitive examinations. Students often must sit two different sets of examinations: national university admission examination plus the admission tests administered by individual universities [64]. Those who wish to specialize further attend master's and PhD courses after graduating from universities.

Medical Education in Japan

Japanese healthcare system is one of the most advanced in the world, and Japanese doctors are well trained. Unlike higher education in general, many places at medical schools are offered by public institutions [65]. Graduate-entry medicine represents only about 10% of all medical school admissions in Japan [65]. In recent years, many Japanese medical schools have started offering more integrated curricula and problem-based learning principles, and clinical education is increasingly offered in forms of clinical clerkships [65]. Similarly, to American medical students, Japanese students also sit a number of standardized examinations throughout their medical training and the pass rates are high [65]. The residency training for graduates is obligatory and lasts at least 2 years. The first 2 years are spent rotating through various specialties [65]. Legally, residents must be paid reasonably well and extra hours are outlawed [65]. Despite that, there are reports of physicians being overworked and underpaid [66]. Advanced training programs are available to those who want to pursue it [65]. A lot of focus is placed on graduate, non-clinical education as well [65].

Education System in China

Those who follow the international competitions in mathematics or sciences will know that Chinese students tend to represent the majority of medal-winners in most disciplines. Also, the number of Chinese students attending elite universities in the west is vast, and the results of Chinese students on Programme for International Student Assessment (PISA) testing have been exceptional. Part of the reason for that is surely the large population of China, but the ability of its education system to produce excellent results should not be underestimated. The system is administered at three levels: by the country's Ministry of Education, the departments of education of individual provinces, and the counties and municipalities on the local level [67]. All children must complete 9 years of schooling, starting no later than the age of 7, three of which are spent in lower secondary education [67]. While most of the schools are public, a third of them are private which may charge tuition fees, although all schools are required to follow the standardized curriculum [67]. Around 60% of those who choose to attend upper secondary education go to general high schools following successful completion of an admissions test [67]. Historically, students have had to choose between science and arts streams, although in recent years there has been a drive to allow more flexibility [67]. Many reforms are currently underway. Vocational high schools train mid-level technicians while simultaneously providing an alternative pathway to higher education [67]. Many international schools are opening in China. University admissions are dependent on high school performance and admission test results [67]. The admission test is delivered nationally over 2 days every academic year although the details of it vary by province [67]. Most of the universities are public, but many of the vocational colleges are private [67]. Students with bachelor's degrees can pursue master's and PhD programs if they choose to do so.

Medical Education in China

The number of students choosing to study medicine in China is increasing every year. Traditionally, most universities were offering undergraduate medicine courses that last 5 or 6 years, although recently some graduate-entry, 4 + 4 programs have been introduced [68]. Many of the programs offer the degree in English. The early years mostly focus on basic sciences, while later years are mostly devoted to clinical training. After graduating from medical schools, students can pursue master's or doctorate-level training [69]. National standards are starting to be implemented with the general aim of matching the western standards when it comes to medical education [70]. Traditionally, this has been difficult due to large numbers of students and relative poverty in much of China [70].

Indian and Pakistani Education System

A huge percent of international medical graduates are from India and Pakistan. As of 2020, India alone had around 542 medical schools [71, 72]. These medical schools are usually called Medical Colleges in India, and collectively, these medical schools produce over 80,000 medical doctors each year [72]. With India being the second largest country in terms of population as of 2020 and very soon expected to be the most populated country in the world, it obviously needs more doctors, and this number is in no way able to fulfill the need of doctors across India. Many of these graduates leave India and move to the United States and try to get the US clinical residency. This does affect India; however, it could have been a blessing for the United States because the United States itself is in dire need of qualified hardworking doctors [73, 74]. These students want to move to the United States for various reasons, such as higher income, high quality of life, higher quality medical healthcare system, and many more reasons [75]. However, not all the graduates successfully practice medicine in the United States, some do go back to India, but many remain in the United States and either switch their careers or still keep applying for the Match each year and remain unsuccessful. Eventually, they too give in and choose some other professions. In the end, a huge chunk of doctors does not practice medicine in India nor in the United States. This causes a huge loss of doctors from the society.

A similar situation is in Pakistan, as of 2020 there are 114 medical colleges in Pakistan, out of which 44 are government owned, while 70 are private [76]. Therefore, around 13,700 doctors graduate each year. Pakistan is also a highly populated country with over 200 million people. This number 13,000 plus is in no way enough to counter the increased patient load. Yet, thousands of these graduates try to move to the United States. This does create a dearth of doctors practicing in Pakistan which leads to a serious brain drain [77]. However, most of these doctors from both countries cannot successfully practice medicine in the United States, a big reason being the difference in education system in India and Pakistan versus the educational system in the United States and especially the United States Medical and Licensing Exam (USMLE). The end result is that many doctors do not practice medicine at all because either they have left their countries for good because of the permanent residency in the United States or maybe they switch profession because of the time-consuming process of USMLEs and the residency.

The question is that why so many graduates from India or Pakistan do not successfully pass USMLE? If it is not the personal choice, then what is in the Indian and Pakistani education system that hinders the success of these graduates in attaining the residency slot? In order to understand this, we need to look at the educational system of both countries in depth.

The Indian Education System

India is a huge country with a population of over 1.2 billion people as of 2020. It is expected that in some years India will supersede China and will become the most populated country in the world. The Indian education system is well designed and planned; yet, because of the increased population, the country has people with all socioeconomic statuses; therefore, naturally the country has an education system that supports lower-middle-class families and middle-class families, and there is parallel system for financially stable families.

The education system in India has pre-primary education (pre-elementary school), primary education (elementary school), upper elementary or middle school, secondary, higher secondary, and university education like most countries of the world. Moreover, like any other developing country, the schools are also divided into privately owned and government-operated (public schools). Only the privileged minority of students join private school because of higher tuition fee. Therefore, it is quite natural to expect that the students graduated from the private schools tend to speak and write better English than the students from the government schools. Another challenge many students could face is the medium of education, because not all the schools are English medium, and it is obvious that a student studying in an English medium school will have better English skills in comparison to the one graduating from a Hindi medium or local language medium schools [78].

The students when admitted to the medical college must study medicine in English, which gives the students of English medium and private schools system an edge over others. Many students who speak and understand English language can take USMLE or PLAB exams and start their clinical career in the United States or the United Kingdom, respectively. Unfortunately, the students graduating from non-English medium schools do have difficulty in understanding medical books in English language in their medical colleges, if they do get admission to the medical college. The difficulty for these students who have difficulty in speaking and writing English is not over here; another challenge for them is to pass USMLEs or PLAB exams. Therefore, a huge percentage of highly qualified physicians graduating in India do not pass the exams like USMLE and another huge percentage of the students cannot apply for these exams due to the financial constraint. This does benefit India in a sense that these students can work and practice in their home country because India also needs a huge population of doctors to serve the Indian patients. However, it hurts the US healthcare system because the United States also needs foreign doctors.

Now let us analyze the system and see how it shapes the medical education and the production of medical doctors each year.

Pre-primary Education (Pre-elementary)

As the name suggests, the pre-primary education is the stage of education before the primary education. It is not a mandatory part of the education and is not available in all the locations. It could be considered as the pre-school counterpart of the US education system, which is an optional part of the education for children, and it is solely up to the parents whether the children should enroll into the pre-school or they do not. The pre-primary school grades are usually named as prenursery, nursery, and junior and senior kindergarten [78].

Elementary or Upper Elementary/Middle School

The Indian education system also has a primary system (elementary) that is divided into lower and upper primary education. The grades from 1 to 5 are the usual lower primary, while the grades from 6 to 8 are the upper primary (elementary) or middle school.

Secondary and Higher Secondary Education

The primary education is followed by secondary education. The secondary education is also divided into two parts where grades 9 and 10 are the first half (secondary) followed by 11th and 12th grades (higher secondary). The students take the board exam at the end of the 10th grade and at the end of the 12th grade. After the 12th grade is passed with good scores, the students apply for university admissions. The students take a pre-admission exam to apply for the university despite passing 12th grade [78].

University or Medical College

After the 12th grade education and the medical admission exams, the students are admitted to the medical colleges or universities. The same goes for the engineering and other fields. As of 2020, there are over 800 universities in India, of which nearly 40% are privately owned. University Grants Commission established Medical Council of India (MCI) which oversees accreditation status of universities and registers the physicians across the country [72]. The medical degree that the recent graduate doctors receive is called as Bachelor of Medicine and Bachelor of Surgery

(MBBS). The students are supposed to complete 1-year clinical internship after the 5 years of MBBS.

As of 2020, there are around 353 medical colleges in India offering 91,490 seats. Therefore, the system produces less than 100,000 doctors each year in a country with a population of over one billion.

The curriculum offered by the Indian Medical Colleges is almost similar to most countries in South Asia. The students are enrolled for 5 years followed by 1 year of mandatory clinical internship. The subjects required to graduate as a doctor are as follows:

- The MBBS course in India comprises total 4.5 years of theoretical plus 1 year of mandatory clinical internship (usually 6 months are mandatory). The first year is called First Professional or MBBS 1. In which the students learn anatomy, histology, physiology, and biochemistry.
- The First Professional Year is followed by Second Professional Year or MBBS 2, which is also almost 18 months in length. The subjects covered during this phase are pathology, microbiology, pharmacology, and forensic medicine.
- The Second Professional is followed by Third Professional (MBBS 3) which is divided into two parts. In the first part the subjects taught are ophthalmology; ear nose, and throat (ENT); and community medicine, while the second part of MBBS 3 curriculum comprises medicine, surgery, pediatrics, and gynecology and obstetrics. After passing the exams, the students are just provisionally registered but cannot get the license until they complete the mandatory 1-year clinical internship known as Compulsory Rotatory Resident Internship (CRRI). Moreover, the degree is also not awarded until the student completes CRRI [72].

This system along with the mode of exams is different from the US system. But many other issues such as corruption and low-quality education in some medical schools make it difficult for the students to compete at the international level [71]. Moreover, not all students are fluent in conversational and written English due to different cultural background or the level of primary education or many other reasons. All these reasons combine, make it challenging for many doctors to pass USMLE and get the clinical residency position in the United States.

The USMLE Journey

The Indian system just like any system poses some challenges for the young doctors. The difference in the USMLE question style and the emphasis on critical thinking makes it difficult for many of the graduates to handle the exam. Moreover, not all medical graduates have a firm grip on the English language, which makes it difficult for them to pass such an exam. Many students who do not have such difficulty may face another challenge of the financial constraint because the USMLE is an expensive route for these students.

The Education System of Pakistan

In Pakistan, the education system is divided into various kinds – the private English medium education (mainly known as matric system), the public Urdu medium system (which also contains the matric system), and the private Cambridge system (where the board of education is totally foreign and it is linked to Cambridge, United Kingdom; this is highly expensive and not affordable for the majority of the population). In order to understand how it effects the IMGs, we will have to understand the system in detail.

The Pre-primary and Primary Education

The pre-primary education starts at the kindergarten or before kindergarten called the nursery. Both private and public schools have this primary system. The students study multiple subjects like any primary system of the world. The pre-primary is followed by primary just like the Indian system. The grades 6–8 are the middle school [79].

The system usually relies on students memorizing long notes and paragraphs word for word. They must write those long-memorized paragraphs as their answers in a 3-hour exam.

The students also must take Urdu, the national language of Pakistan, as a compulsory subject regardless of the type of school they belong to, whether private or public school. The national language of the country is Urdu; therefore, most of the time of the students' life inside the school and outside is spent speaking Urdu language, so it is logical to assume that the students have far stronger grip on Urdu language than English language. Majority of the students, even if they are from private English-speaking schools, are not fully fluent in English nor their English language skills are in any way equal to the language skills of a native English speaker. However, the topmost students usually do have strong writing and reading skills, yet very few topmost students are fully fluent in spoken English.

The Secondary Education

The secondary education in Pakistan starts after the eighth grade. The students usually remain in the same school and continue the studies. The ninth and tenth grade exams are not administered by the school, but the exams are organized and arranged by a local city board.

The ninth and tenth grades are usually controlled by the central educational board of each city that arranges the final exams which are called matriculation exams.

Each city has its own secondary board. Once the students pass this exam, they graduate from the school. Then they start their college life (the college in Pakistan is for 2 years and is equivalent to the high school 11th and 12th grade of the United States).

Higher Secondary Education or Intermediate College Education

The college or higher secondary education is a 2-year period, and the students' performance in these years mainly determines the decision of medical school admissions.

Just like the matriculation board (secondary school certificate), the college education is controlled by the Higher Secondary Board. The exam is called HSC exams, and the system of exams is quite like the matriculation exams.

The system has divided it into pre-medical and pre-engineering categories. The pre-medical students apply for the medical schools, while the pre-engineering students can only apply for engineering schools. There are other categories for non-science students like commerce and arts. However, we are focused on medical students mainly in this chapter.

Alternate Education System

Pakistan is unique in a sense that besides the regular metric and intermediate education system, there is alternate education system in Pakistan that runs parallel to the existing system. It is known as the Cambridge system. The high school ninth and tenth equivalent exams are called as O-Level examinations, while the higher secondary education examinations are called as A-Level examination. These exams and the system overall is fairly expensive; therefore, usually the student from the rich or upper-middle-class families get this education. This education system does improve the English language of the student because of being affiliated with Cambridge; however, these students after A-Levels cannot get into medical colleges without the scoring conversion. This conversion reduces their scores and makes them less competitive for the medical college admissions. Yet every year many A-Level students are successful in getting admission into the medical college. However, their percentage is less in comparison to the students coming from the HSC system (inter or matric system).

There are some recent advancements in the education system and some new boards were introduced such as Agha Khan Board; however, how much are these systems successful is yet to be determined.

The University or Medical School Life

Once the students graduate from the Intermediate Board (HSC), they take a pre-admission entry test, and the top candidates who collectively score the highest combining the HSC scores and the entry test scores are selected for the admissions. The medical school is either called medical college or a university. Usually a university has multiple medical colleges affiliated with it. The degree is not awarded by the medical college but the parent university.

Pakistan has four provinces and the medical education is regulated by the provincial department of health. In order to be recognized by the government, the medical college must meet the criteria set by a central regulatory authority called Pakistan Medical and Dental Council (PMDC) and by Higher Education Commission Pakistan.

The medical college or university education is monitored by the Pakistan Medical and Dental Council (PMDC), which is the central registration council for all the doctors in the country. The medical education comprises 5 years of total education, with the first 2 years of basic science subjects such as anatomy, physiology, and biochemistry. After the first 2 years, students usually start hospital rotations and study clinical subjects such as general pathology; systemic pathology; ear, Nose, and throat (ENT); ophthalmology; forensic sciences; and community medicine, while clinical medicine, pediatrics, surgery, and gynecology and obstetrics are taught in the final year of medical college [80].

There are total of 114 medical schools in Pakistan as of 2020, of which 44 are public (government), while 70 are private.

The examinations are usually multiple choice question (MCQ) style; however, some private universities still have a mixture of MCQs and writing long answers as the mode of exams.

After graduation the students are required to complete 1 year of clinical internship known as House Job, which is needed to practice medicine in the country [79]. This is required by the PMDC. However, the students who are planning for USMLE and want to move to the United States do not need to complete this internship year. However, for the British system it is needed.

This system and culture create some serious problems for the students:

1. The examination system where you just memorize and write it down deprives the students from critical thinking and analysis skills.
2. Despite being a school graduate, the students are merely fluent and struggle in speaking and listening skills. (If the student is from an Urdu medium school, they obviously are way behind in writing, speaking, listening, and reading English skills.)
3. Another problem is that the students are habitual of taking exams with the format of writing long answers on the answer sheets. MCQ-type exam is just a small part of the exam.

Now when such students take exams such as USMLEs where the students' critical thinking and analysis skills are tested, most such students cannot handle such a situation. Moreover, the developing infrastructure and widespread corruption in the country in different sectors is also visible in the education system, which makes it difficult for the students to compete at the international level.

Other South Asian Countries, Middle East, and Nearby Countries

Other South Asian countries such as Bangladesh, Nepal, Afghanistan, Sri Lanka, and Myanmar have very much the similar medical education system with almost the similar subjects and quite similar challenges after graduation like the financial constraint, English language fluency, the difference in the exam style, widespread corruption in all sectors including education system, and so on [81]. Quite similar is the situation with the Middle Eastern countries such as Saudi Arabia, Lebanon, the United Arab Emirates (UAE), Qatar, Bahrain, Saudi Arabia, Iraq, Egypt, excluding Israel (which is becoming very much Americanized gradually), and Turkey [82].

Iran medical education system is robust and produces high class doctors; however, the problem remains with the Irani graduates is the language issue mainly because of the mode of education mainly is in Persian and the traditional US–Iran political rivalry makes it difficult for the Irani students to get the visa; same is the situation with the countries with the US visa ban like Syria and Libya.

These issues will persist for a long time as we do not see any recent advancements on the visa restrictions by the United States nor do we see and expect to see drastic changes in the education system of these countries that will make the journey of residency for the IMGs easy. Looks like the IMGs of banned countries will have to wait for the ban to be over and the students of South Asian countries will have to keep trying and find ways to improve their language and exam skills, and arrange finances or find alternate countries to start their clinical careers or just stay in their countries as an option. One thing is for sure, if they stay in their countries, it is good for their countries, but it is not good for the US healthcare system because the United States needs more doctors. In the end, the one who suffers the most is the qualified physician who wanted to move to the United States for a better future.

Education in Africa

Africa is home to around 1 billion people, and the differences in development between individual African countries are vast. On the one hand, the Republic of South Africa is widely seen as a country with high standards of medical care and education. On the other hand, many countries in Sub-Saharan Africa are affected by extremely high poverty levels and as much as one-third of children grow up malnourished [83]. The access to education is also unequal, and many children struggle to obtain even elementary education. High crime and corruption rates in many parts of Africa make it difficult to judge the quality of some universities and medical schools. In addition, the prejudice against African physicians in the west makes it difficult for them to secure good jobs. Nevertheless, some countries such as Nigeria manage to educate large numbers of physicians who enter the workforce in the United States and the United Kingdom [84, 85]. The education systems of individual nations in Africa often depend on its history as some follow more typically British education models, while others are more strongly associated with systems in other countries, such as France.

Conclusion

The education system around the world varies: some countries do have similarities with the US education system and the language, while most countries around the world do not have English as the official language nor as the lingua franca. The education system also varies in terms of examination model, like some countries rely on writing long notes as the answers to the questions in the examination room, while some rely on multiple-choice questions on paper. The USMLE is a computer-based exam where the students must sit for long hours in front of computer screens and answer the multiple-choice questions; this kind of computer-based exam is new for most IMGs. Therefore, it is quite natural to expect that most IMGs around the world will face difficulty passing the USMLEs.

The proper solution is to get acclimatized with the US education system and prepare for the exams and practice the way the USMLEs are taken. The IMGs coming from non-English-speaking countries should also practice communication skills and improve their English language comprehension and speaking, in order to overcome the disadvantage. This in some way will help many IMGs; however, it is not a permanent solution for this issue because learning a new language takes considerable amount of time. Some experts believe that the US exam should be in the IMGs' own language, but this has its own drawbacks because once the IMGs are accepted by a US residency program, the majority of patient population will be English-speaking (some will be Spanish-speaking). It is rare that the patients will speak their own language (if they belong to a non-English-speaking or Latino country). Until then relying on the current system is the only solution, and we hope for the positive changes in the system for the IMGs in the near future.

References

1. Education in the United States of America [Internet]. WENR. 2018 [cited 2020 May 30]. Available from: https://wenr.wes.org/2018/06/education-in-the-united-states-of-america.
2. Overview and Mission Statement | U.S. Department of Education [Internet]. [cited 2020 May 30]. Available from: https://www2.ed.gov/about/landing.jhtml.
3. Pre-medical Requirements [Internet]. Medical Education at Yale. [cited 2020 May 30]. Available from: https://medicine.yale.edu/education/admissions/requirements/.
4. Majors: Pre-Medical Studies [Internet]. [cited 2020 May 30]. Available from: https://www.mycollegeoptions.org/content/research/major/Description/Pre-MedicalStudies.aspx.
5. Considering a Postbaccalaureate Premedical Program [Internet]. [cited 2020 May 30]. Available from: https://students-residents.aamc.org/content/article/considering-postbaccalaureate-premedical-program/.
6. What You Need to Know About the MCAT® Exam [Internet]. [cited 2020 May 30]. Available from: https://students-residents.aamc.org/choosing-medical-career/article/preparing-mcat-exam/.
7. Is Medical School Worth the Cost? [Internet]. The Balance. [cited 2020 May 30]. Available from: https://www.thebalance.com/average-cost-of-medical-school-4588236.

8. Best Medical Schools in 2021 – US News [Internet]. [cited 2020 May 30]. Available from: https://www.usnews.com/best-graduate-schools/top-medical-schools.
9. Years 1 and 2 [Internet]. Medical School – University of Minnesota. 2018 [cited 2020 May 30]. Available from: https://med.umn.edu/admissions/curriculum/years-1-and-2.
10. Years 3 and 4 [Internet]. Medical School – University of Minnesota. 2018 [cited 2020 May 30]. Available from: https://med.umn.edu/admissions/curriculum/years-3-and-4.
11. Curriculum I School of Medicine [Internet]. [cited 2020 May 30]. Available from: https://www.bumc.bu.edu/busm/admissions/curriculum/.
12. United States Medical Licensing Examination I Step 1 [Internet]. [cited 2020 May 30]. Available from: https://www.usmle.org/step-1/.
13. United States Medical Licensing Examination I Step 2 CK (Clinical Knowledge) [Internet]. [cited 2020 Oct 28]. Available from: https://usmle.org/step-2-ck/.
14. United States Medical Licensing Examination I Step 2 CS (Clinical Skills) [Internet]. [cited 2020 May 30]. Available from: https://www.usmle.org/step-2-cs/.
15. Certification – Requirements For Certification [Internet]. ECFMG. [cited 2020 May 30]. Available from: https://www.ecfmg.org/certification/requirements-for-certification.html.
16. United States Medical Licensing Examination I Step 3 [Internet]. [cited 2020 May 30]. Available from: https://www.usmle.org/step-3/.
17. FSMB I State Specific Requirements for Initial Medical Licensure [Internet]. [cited 2020 May 30]. Available from: https://www.fsmb.org/step-3/state-licensure/.
18. The Match: Getting into a Residency Program [Internet]. [cited 2020 May 30]. Available from: https://www.aafp.org/medical-school-residency/residency/match.html.
19. Resources: Residency Match [Internet]. ECFMG. [cited 2020 May 30]. Available from: https://www.ecfmg.org/resources/data-residency-match.html.
20. Medical Schools Recognized I Medical Board of California [Internet]. [cited 2020 May 30]. Available from: https://www.mbc.ca.gov/Applicants/Schools_Recognized/.
21. National Resident Matching Program. Results and Data: 2020 Main Residency Match. Washington, D.C.: National Resident Matching Program; 2020 p. 22.
22. Council of Ministers of Education, Canada [Internet]. CMEC. 2020 [cited 27 May 2020]. Available from: https://www.cmec.ca/299/Education-in-Canada-An-Overview/index.html.
23. The Canadian Education System [Internet]. Canadavisa.com. 2020 [cited 27 May 2020]. Available from: https://www.canadavisa.com/canadian-education.html#gs.6v00p3.
24. Robson K. Sociology of education in Canada [Internet]. 1st ed. Toronto, Ontario; 2013. [cited 27 May 2020]. Available from: https://ecampusontario.pressbooks.pub/robsonsoced/chapter/__unknown__-4/.
25. The Association of Faculties of Medicine of Canada. Admission Requirements of Canadian Faculties of Medicine: Admission in 2020 [Internet]. Ottawa, Ontario: The Association of Faculties of Medicine of Canada; 2019. Available from: https://afmc.ca/en/news-publications/admission-requirements.
26. Canadian Medical School Profiles [Internet]. Oxfordseminars.ca. 2020 [cited 27 May 2020]. Available from: https://www.oxfordseminars.ca/MCAT/mcat_profiles.php.
27. MCAT FAQs [Internet]. Students-residents.aamc.org. 2020 [cited 27 May 2020]. Available from: https://students-residents.aamc.org/applying-medical-school/faq/mcat-faqs/.
28. The University of British Columbia, Faculty of Medicine. Statistical Data on Application and Admissions – 2019 (MED 2023) [Internet]. The University of British Columbia; 2019. Available from: https://mdprogram.med.ubc.ca/admissions/admissions-statistics/.
29. McMaster University. McMaster University Undergraduate Medical Program Class of 2022 [Internet]. McMaster University; 2019. Available from: https://mdprogram.mcmaster.ca/md-program-admissions/how-we-select.
30. Schulich Medicine & Dentistry. Schulich Medicine MD Program Admission Statistics, Class of 2022. 2019.

31. Sanfilippo A. Is every Canadian medical school graduate entitled to become a practicing physician? [Internet]. Undergraduate School of Medicine Blog. 2017 [cited 27 May 2020]. Available from: https://meds.queensu.ca/ugme-blog/archives/3568.
32. MD Program [Internet]. Mdprogram.mcmaster.ca. 2020 [cited 27 May 2020]. Available from: https://mdprogram.mcmaster.ca/md-program.
33. MD Program Accreditation I NOSM [Internet]. Nosm.ca. 2020 [cited 27 May 2020]. Available from: https://www.nosm.ca/education/md-program/md-program-accreditation/.
34. Residency levels [Internet]. Postgraduate Medical Education. 2020 [cited 27 May 2020]. Available from: https://www.mcgill.ca/pgme/programs/residency-programs/residency-program-levels.
35. Eligibility criteria – CaRMS [Internet]. CaRMS. 2020 [cited 27 May 2020]. Available from: https://www.carms.ca/match/r-1-main-residency-match/eligibility-criteria/.
36. How do I apply to CaRMS if I am an IMG? [Internet]. Canadian Resident Matching Service. 2020 [cited 27 May 2020]. Available from: https://carms.zendesk.com/hc/en-us/articles/115004093363-How-do-I-apply-to-CaRMS-if-I-am-an-IMG-.
37. The Canadian Resident Matching Service. 2020 CaRMS Forum [Internet]. The Canadian Resident Matching Service; 2020 p. 9, 11. Available from: https://www.carms.ca/pdfs/2020-carms-forum.pdf.
38. Education in the U.K. [Internet]. WENR. 2016 [cited 2020 Jun 21]. Available from: https://wenr.wes.org/2016/02/education-in-the-u-k.
39. Studying medicine [Internet]. The British Medical Association is the trade union and professional body for doctors in the UK. [cited 2020 Jun 21]. Available from: https://www.bma.org.uk/advice-and-support/studying-medicine.
40. How specialty training (residency) works in the UK: A complete beginner's guide – The Savvy IMG [Internet]. [cited 2020 Jun 21]. Available from: https://thesavvyimg.co.uk/specialty-training-residency-in-the-uk/.
41. Education in Germany [Internet]. [cited 2020 May 26]. Available from: https://wenr.wes.org/2016/11/education-in-germany.
42. Education System in Germany – Overview of the German School System [Internet]. [cited 2020 May 26]. Available from: https://www.studying-in-germany.org/german-education-system/.
43. Zavlin D, Jubbal KT, Noé JG, Gansbacher B. A comparison of medical education in Germany and the United States: from applying to medical school to the beginnings of residency. Ger Med Sci. 2017;15:Doc15. Published 2017 Sep 25. https://doi.org/10.3205/000256.
44. Education in France – WENR [Internet]. [cited 2020 May 26]. Available from: https://wenr.wes.org/2015/09/education-france.
45. The French education system: a guide for expat parents I Expatica [Internet]. Expat Guide to France I Expatica. [cited 2020 May 26]. Available from: https://www.expatica.com/fr/education/children-education/french-education-system-101147/.
46. The French and U.S. approaches to training doctors – Scope [Internet]. [cited 2020 May 26]. Available from: https://scopeblog.stanford.edu/2009/11/10/the_french_and/.
47. Segouin C, Jouquan J, Hodges B, et al. Country report: medical education in France. Med Educ. 2007;41(3):295–301. https://doi.org/10.1111/j.1365-2929.2007.02690.x.
48. Italy – Education I Britannica [Internet]. [cited 2020 May 26]. Available from: https://www.britannica.com/place/Italy/Education.
49. Education in Italy [Internet]. WENR. 2004 [cited 2020 May 26]. Available from: https://wenr.wes.org/2004/05/wenr-mayjune-2004-italy.
50. Italy I Medical Mobility [Internet]. [cited 2020 May 26]. Available from: https://www.medicalmobility.eu/italy.
51. Education in Mexico [Internet]. WENR. 2019 [cited 2020 May 25]. Available from: https://wenr.wes.org/2019/05/education-in-mexico-2.
52. Centro Medico Internacional I World Class Healthcare in Matamoros Mexico [Internet]. [cited 2020 May 25]. Available from: http://www.cmi-matamoros.com/c_process.html.

53. Medical Education in Mexico | June 2018 | ACP [Internet]. [cited 2020 May 25]. Available from: https://www.acponline.org/membership/medical-students/acp-impact/archive/june-2018/medical-education-in-mexico.
54. Quality of medical education in Mexico – The Lancet [Internet]. [cited 2020 May 25]. Available from: https://www.thelancet.com/journals/lancet/article/PIIS0140-6736(04)16114-X/fulltext.
55. Education in Brazil [Internet]. WENR. 2019 [cited 2020 May 25]. Available from: https://wenr.wes.org/2019/11/education-in-brazil.
56. dos Santos RA, do PT Nunes M. Medical education in Brazil. Med Teach. 2019;41(10):1106–11.
57. Scheffer MC, Dal Poz MR. The privatization of medical education in Brazil: trends and challenges. Hum Resour Health. 2015;13(1):96.
58. Education in Argentina [Internet]. WENR. 2018 [cited 2020 May 25]. Available from: https://wenr.wes.org/2018/05/education-in-argentina.
59. IFMSA Exchange Portal [Internet]. [cited 2020 May 25]. Available from: https://exchange.ifmsa.org/exchange/explore/nmo/1047.
60. Centeno AM. The programs and context of medical education in Argentina. Acad Med. 2006;81(12):1081–4.
61. Education in Australia [Internet]. WENR. 2017 [cited 2020 May 29]. Available from: https://wenr.wes.org/2017/12/education-in-australia.
62. Prideaux D. Medical education in Australia: much has changed but what remains? Med Teach. 2009;31(2):96–100. https://doi.org/10.1080/01421590802509171.
63. Becoming a Doctor [Internet]. Australian Medical Association. 2018 [cited 2020 May 29]. Available from: https://ama.com.au/careers/becoming-a-doctor.
64. Education in Japan – WENR [Internet]. [cited 2020 May 29]. Available from: https://wenr.wes.org/2005/05/wenr-mayjune-2005-education-in-japan.
65. Kozu T. Medical education in Japan. Acad Med. 2006;81(12):1069–75. https://doi.org/10.1097/01.ACM.0000246682.45610.dd.
66. Nakamura A. Hospital doctors feeling the strain [Internet]. The Japan Times. 2008 [cited 2020 May 30]. Available from: https://www.japantimes.co.jp/news/2008/04/12/national/hospital-doctors-feeling-the-strain/.
67. Education in China [Internet]. [cited 2020 May 30]. Available from: https://wenr.wes.org/2019/12/education-in-china-3.
68. Wang C, Chen S, Zhu J, Li W. China's new 4 + 4 medical education programme. Lancet. 2019;394(10204):1121–3. https://doi.org/10.1016/S0140-6736(19)32178-6.
69. Medical Degree and Education in China | BestEduChina [Internet]. [cited 2020 May 30]. Available from: http://www.besteduchina.com/medical_degree_in_china.html.
70. Lam TP, Wan XH, Ip MS. Current perspectives on medical education in China. Med Educ. 2006;40(10):940–9. https://doi.org/10.1111/j.1365-2929.2006.02552.x.
71. Bearak M. How bad are most of India's medical schools? Very, according to new reports. The Washington Post. April 20, 2016. Available at https://www.washingtonpost.com/news/worldviews/wp/2016/04/21/how-bad-are-most-of-indias-medical-schools-very-according-to-new-reports/.
72. Medical Council of India. Available at https://www.mciindia.org/CMS/.
73. Pasko T, Smart DR. Physician characteristics and distribution in the US, 2004 edition. Chicago, IL: American Medical Association; 2004.
74. Cooper RA, Stoflet SJ, Wartman SA. Perceptions of medical school deans and state medical society executives about physician supply. JAMA. 2003;290:2992–5.
75. Fuller Torrey E, Torrey BB. The US Distribution of Physicians from Lower Income Countries. PLoS One. 2012;7(3):e33076. Published online 2012 Mar 21. https://doi.org/10.1371/journal.pone.0033076.
76. Pakistan Medical & Dental Council. Available at http://www.pmdc.org.pk/AboutUs/RecognizedMedicalDentalColleges/tabid/109/Default.aspx.
77. Mullan F. The metrics of the physician brain drain. N Engl J Med. 2005;353(17):1810–8. https://doi.org/10.1056/NEJMsa050004.

78. Trines S. Education in India. World Education News + Reviews. Available at https://wenr.wes.org/2018/09/education-in-india.
79. Hunter R. Education in Pakistan. World Education News + Reviews. Available at https://wenr.wes.org/2020/02/education-in-pakistan.
80. Pakistan Medical & Dental Council. Available at http://www.pmdc.org.pk/.
81. Asia Pacific. Available at https://wenr.wes.org/category/education-system-profiles/asia-pacific-education-system-profiles.
82. Middle East. Available at https://wenr.wes.org/category/education-system-profiles/middle-east-education-system-profiles.
83. On the poorest continent, the plight of children is dramatic [Internet]. SOS-US-EN. [cited 2020 Jun 22]. Available from: https://www.sos-usa.org/SpecialPages/Africa/Poverty-in-Africa.
84. Top 10 NHS Doctors Nationalities Across the UK | ProMedical [Internet]. [cited 2020 Jun 22]. Available from: https://promedical.co.uk/top-10-nhs-doctors-nationalities-across-the-uk/.
85. Resources: Data – ECFMG J-1 Visa Sponsorship [Internet]. ECFMG. [cited 2020 Jun 22]. Available from: https://www.ecfmg.org/resources/data-sponsorship.html.

Chapter 3
Healthcare Systems Around the World

Ivan Cancarevic, Lucia Plichtová, and Bilal Haider Malik

The General Outline of the US Healthcare System

The US Healthcare System

It is frequently said that the USA is the only developed country in the world without a universal healthcare system and that medical bills are among the leading causes of bankruptcy, poverty, and even homelessness in the USA. Currently, the World Bank defines 80 countries around the world as "high-income economies," and their healthcare systems vary widely [1]. Some systems are entirely or almost entirely governmental and funded through taxes, while the rest involve some mix of private and public healthcare. In that aspect, the USA is no exception to the rule. While most Americans receive healthcare through their employers, a number of Americans are insured through one of the taxpayer-funded programs, such as Medicare or Medicaid.

I. Cancarevic (✉)
California Institute of Behavioral Neurosciences and Psychology, Fairfield, CA, USA

L. Plichtová
Hospital Department of Medicine, Bridgeport, CT, USA

B. H. Malik
CiBNP, Fairfield, CA, USA

Institute of Behavioral Neurosciences and Psychology, Fairfield, CA, USA

Internal Medicine, Research, California Institute of Behavioral Neurosciences & Psychology, Sacramento, CA, USA

© Springer Nature Switzerland AG 2021
H. Tohid, H. Maibach (eds.), *International Medical Graduates in the United States*, https://doi.org/10.1007/978-3-030-62249-7_3

Private Healthcare

Most health insurance in the USA is offered by a number of private insurance companies. Most Americans receive healthcare through their employers, while a significantly smaller number pays for the insurance individually, out of pocket. Students often receive health insurance through colleges they attend. A number of different health insurance plans exist, and they differ based on the costs and the amount of coverage that is provided. It should be noted that health insurance companies in the USA are for-profit institutions [2, 3]. The existence of "networks" is one of the unique features of the US healthcare systems. Insurance companies have networks of providers that they are affiliated with and whose services they cover. Seeing an out-of-network physicians is often either not covered by the insurance company or covered to a much smaller extent than seeing a physician in-network [2, 3].

Different employers may offer widely different healthcare plans. Moreover, the physician networks that the insurance companies are affiliated with may be very different, impacting the continuity of care when changing employers. Those who lose their jobs may be at risk of losing health insurance unless they purchase individual plans. The coverage of preexisting conditions has been a topic of much debate as most insurance providers used to reject patients with preexisting conditions or at least rejected the coverage of any complications that may be deemed related to those conditions. In 2010, the Affordable Care Act (ACA) was signed into law during the presidency of Barack Obama (sometimes referred to as "Obama Care") which aimed to fix some of the aforementioned issues. It provided tax credits and certain cost reductions for low-income families. It also requires most individuals to purchase health insurance and penalizes many of those who do not. Large employers are now required to offer health insurance, and the insurance companies' ability to reject people based on preexisting conditions was limited. It also expanded some of the taxpayer-funded programs [3].

Even those who have health insurance are frequently required to pay significant fees when seeing their physicians, in form of deductibles and copayments [2, 3]. Deductibles refer to the amounts patients are required to pay before the insurance starts covering their bills, while copays refer to payments associated with individual visits. There are often additional costs associated with prescription drugs, emergency services, and vision and dental care. Many individuals purchase additional vision and dental insurance.

Most of the hospitals in the USA are nonprofit private institutions with a number of for-profit and government-run hospitals. The majority of physicians in the USA practice in small offices rather than large hospitals [3].

Medicare

Medicare is the most widely known governmental health insurance program in the USA. It covers individuals over the age of 65, those with certain disabilities and end-stage renal disease (ESRD). Approximately 16% of American citizens receive healthcare coverage through Medicare [3]. Medicare A, B, and D plans are defined. Plan A covers hospital stays, care in nursing facilities, hospice care, and some home healthcare. Plan B covers outpatient care, preventive care, and medical supplies. Part D adds coverage for prescription drugs. It should be noted that Part D is offered through private companies approved by Medicare. It should be noted that the individuals who receive healthcare through Medicare are not exempt from all further healthcare costs and some deductibles and copays still apply to them [4].

Medicare is overall very popular and most of the enrollees are satisfied with the coverage they receive. A high satisfaction rate among Medicare users has prompted a national debate on switching to "Medicare for All," a governmentally funded single-payer healthcare system. The idea was first brought to public attention by the 2016 (and 2020) presidential candidate Bernie Sanders and has become more mainstream ever since. A number of other high-profile politicians now support moving toward universal healthcare, including 2020 presidential candidates senator Elizabeth Warren and New York mayor Bill de Blasio. The polls on the issue are mixed but it is clear that the policy is gaining more and more public support.

Medicaid

Medicaid is the largest federal and state program that aims to provide health insurance to those with insufficient incomes to pay for regular private insurance. It is means tested and currently covers those with incomes up to 133–138% of the poverty line. It was significantly expanded during the implementation of the Affordable Care Act in terms of both funding and eligibility [3]. Unlike Medicare, Medicaid funding comes both from the federal government and from individual states. Therefore, the exact details of Medicaid benefits differ between individual states [3]. Many consider it to be inadequate in terms of providing healthcare to those most disadvantaged. Also, a number of people are likely to lack resources to pay for private health insurance despite earning more than what would make them eligible to enrol in Medicaid.

Veterans Health Administration

Veterans Health Administration is a nationalized health insurance program aimed at providing healthcare to veterans. It is entirely operated by the federal government, rather than private companies. All the hospitals in the system are owned by the government, and the physicians working in those facilities are paid by the government. There are no deductibles, although some copayments may exist [5]. Questions remain about the quality of care received by those in the system as well as about the timely access to healthcare. Despite those concerns, a large majority of veterans is not dissatisfied with the quality of healthcare received through the program.

Furthermore, the majority of patients reported improved quality of care received over the last decade, and most reported having no issues obtaining appointments in timely manner [6].

The Affordable Care Act Debate

Healthcare is among the most heated political topics in the USA at the time of this writing. The approach to healthcare in general differs significantly between the voters of the two main political parties. The majority of the Republican politicians and voters believe that the government should not be involved in providing healthcare to citizens and would prefer the system to be left to the private market. On the other hand, most Democratic politicians and voters believe in much stronger safety nets and fear that leaving the system to the market could lead to large numbers of avoidable deaths and disabilities. Most Democratic politicians support significant expansions to the current governmental system, with most supporting the introduction of the "public option" – a governmentally funded healthcare plan that individuals could enrol in [7]. A few prominent politicians, such as Bernie Sanders and Elizabeth Warren, believe that the ultimate goal needs to be the implementation of a universal healthcare system, such as "Medicare for All" [7].

Such large differences in opinion have led to years of debate following the passage of the Affordable Care Act. The administration of president Donald Trump has promised to turn back the clock on the ACA and came within one senate vote of successfully doing so. Despite being unable to completely transform the system, the administration did manage to eliminate the "individual mandate" as well as the cost-sharing reduction subsidies to insurers. The funds to ease new sign-ups to the plan have been significantly reduced, and individual states have been allowed to add "work requirements" to Medicaid eligibility [8].

Healthcare Outcomes in the USA

Healthcare outcomes are difficult to compare between countries, in part because it is difficult to establish the appropriate criteria and the number of possible confounding variables is significant. The life expectancy at birth in the USA is around 79 years compared to 80 in the European Union and 82 in Canada [9]. The infant mortality rate in the USA is higher than in most other high-income countries [10]. It is estimated that tens of thousands of Americans die every year due to inadequate health coverage. The chronic disease burden and obesity rates are higher in the USA than in comparably wealthy countries, and the rates of violent crime and suicide are higher. Cancer survival in the USA is often considered among the best, if not the best in the world. Interpreting such data is tricky, however, as cancer survival rates depend heavily on the age when the cancer was first diagnosed, whether all institutions in the country are equally likely to report the cases they encounter and what other risk factors might impact cancer survival. While the rates of obesity in the USA are among the highest in the world, many European countries have higher tobacco and alcohol consumption rates than the USA, and their populations may be older. However, as home to some of the most elite research institutions in the world, the USA is at the forefront of medical research, and it has more Nobel laureates in physiology and medicine than any other country. The availability of some of the novel treatments may be higher in the USA than in the other countries [11]. The exact impact of that on morbidity and mortality is difficult to quantify, but it may very well be the case that the USA offers the best healthcare for those who can afford it.

Costs of the US Healthcare System

The Total Spending

The US healthcare system is among the most expensive in the world. While the exact costs are difficult to determine, a mix of administrative, legal, and medical costs is what makes the system that expensive [3].

The US spending on healthcare grows every year, and it reached 3.6 trillion US dollars in 2018, which equates to over 11,000 USD per person per year [3, 12]. It accounts for anywhere between 15 and 20 percent of the nation's gross domestic product (GDP). The average annual growth rate is at over 5 percent, meaning that it is expected that by 2028 the total healthcare spending could rise to over 6 trillion US dollars [13]. Such growth is higher than the average GDP growth, meaning that the percentage of GDP that is spent on healthcare is likely to increase as well. Female healthcare spending is on average higher than male healthcare spending (56% to 44%), and it holds true in all age groups except for children [14]. The spending also varies significantly between individual states, with the states in New England and Mideast reporting on average the highest levels of total per capita personal healthcare spending. Utah reported the lowest levels [15].

It should also be noted that the total spending varies depending on the payer. It is expected that Medicare spending is going to increase significantly due to aging of the population. This is especially evident in the eastern USA, with New Jersey being the state with the highest Medicare spending per enrollee.

The total spending in other developed countries is generally lower than in the USA. The UK spends less than 10% of its GDP on healthcare, which in 2017 turned out to be under 4000 USD [16]. In Canada the number is under 5000 USD, and in Australia it is under 6000 USD [16]. Swiss healthcare spending at around 10,000 USD per capita per year was the second highest in the world [16]. The World Bank average for high-income economies was 5179.67 USD [16].

How Much Individuals Spend on Healthcare

Almost 10% of the US population is considered uninsured [3]. This population is at constant risk of bankruptcy or even homelessness as a result of illness. A significant portion of those who have insurance are considered "underinsured," meaning that their insurance is likely inadequate to cover their healthcare needs. While insurance companies, and especially Medicare, are able to negotiate the prices with healthcare providers, individuals who have to pay out of pocket generally are not able to do so. As a result, patients who pay out of pocket tend to pay more than what an insurance company would pay for the same procedure or treatment [3].

The costs of individual procedures or treatments in the USA are also generally higher than in other developed countries. For example, an MRI scan in the USA on average costs over 1100 USD, while in Australia it costs under 200 USD [17]. In some countries, such as Spain, the number is even lower [17]. Surgical procedures in the USA are also significantly more expensive than in the rest of the developed world. Hip replacement surgeries cost on average 10,000 dollars more than in Australia [17]. Prescription drug costs in the USA are also generally much higher than in the other countries. On average, prescription drug prices in the USA are 3–4 times higher than elsewhere [17].

Can Americans Afford These Costs?

Anywhere between 25% and 50% of personal bankruptcies in the USA include significant medical debts [18]. Just having health insurance is often not enough for individuals to be able to afford healthcare in the USA. The significant deductibles, copays, and rising premiums make it unaffordable for many. Only about four in ten Americans say they would be able to cover a 1000 dollar emergency, such as an unplanned medical bill, using their own savings [19]. The average deductible is over 4500 USD [20]. This suggests that the majority of Americans would have to take out loans to pay for any medical bills as insurance typically does not cover any expenses until the annual deductible is met. That is on top of the average insurance premium of $440 per individual per month [21]. Even once the deductible is met, the patients are still required to pay copays for every visit until they meet their out-of-pocket maximum, which can be significantly higher than the deductible.

Moreover, a unique characteristic of US health insurance system is that many insurance companies offer different levels of health coverage at different price points. They may offer "bronze," "silver," "gold," and "platinum" plans with varying degrees of benefits. Some expats have compared it to choosing a credit card [22]. A paradox is that those with limited financial abilities are most likely to choose the cheapest plans which offer the fewest protections and tend to have the highest deductibles, meaning any unplanned healthcare costs may lead to debt and even bankruptcy.

Medicare and Medicaid Spending

In 2018 the US federal government spent over 750 billion US dollars on Medicare and 597 billion US dollars on Medicaid. Medicaid saw a significant increase, likely due to increased enrolment due to the Affordable Care Act [3, 23]. New Jersey is the state with the highest Medicare spending per enrollee at over 12,600 USD, while Montana is the state with the lowest Medicare spending per enrollee at just over 8200 USD [23]. For Medicaid, the state with the highest spending per enrollee was North Dakota at over 12,400 USD, while the state with the lowest spending was Illinois at under 5000 USD [23].

What Makes the US Healthcare System So Expensive?

There are many possible explanations of the high costs of healthcare in the USA when compared to similarly developed countries. Compared to most other countries, the administrative costs in the USA are much higher. Part of the reason is the existence of many different networks and insurance companies. Insurance companies also make large profits. Another possible cause of high administrative costs is the number of staff required to deal with complicated billing systems. The costs of individual treatments and procedures can vary greatly between institutions. Moreover, the frequency of lawsuits against physicians in the USA is higher than in most other countries. As a result of that, physicians often have to purchase expensive malpractice insurance to protect themselves. The fear of lawsuits also leads to increased practice of defensive medicine, meaning that patients are often subjected to a larger number of unnecessary tests in order to exclude unlikely diagnoses and decrease the likelihood of a lawsuit against the physician. Americans on average consume more diagnostic tests than patients in other high-income countries. To make matters more complicated, the medical education system in the USA is extremely expensive. Many medical schools charge more than 50,000 USD per year in tuition alone. Physician salaries are also higher than in most other countries. Most agree that a lot of that money is "wasted" and that the inefficiency of the system contributes to the costs [24].

Would Universal Healthcare Be More Expensive?

A major political debate is ongoing on whether implementation of the universal healthcare system would be a cheaper alternative in the USA. Many studies suggest that implementation of a "Medicare for All" system would lead to significant savings and drastically reduce the healthcare costs in the USA [25]. Such system would eliminate the premiums, deductibles, and copays while introducing a new form of tax. The proponents of the change claim that such system could make US healthcare spending more in line with that of the other countries such as Canada or Australia. The opponents of the system claim that this is a false assumption as there is no clear evidence to suggest that just changing the way the system is financed would reduce the costs that significantly. Also, the current Medicare costs do not necessarily match the costs in those countries, and the proposed system goes beyond what current Medicare covers. The ultimate costs of such system would be difficult to determine as they would largely depend on the way drugs are obtained, the cuts to the administrative costs, and possible changes to the salaries of health-care workers. Many physicians fear that a cut to their salaries could make it difficult for them to pay off significant student loans that they graduated with. It should be noted, however, that politicians most supportive of a switch to "Medicare for All system" also support free public universities and some forms of student loan for-giveness [7, 25].

Medical Workforce in the USA

The Number of Healthcare Workers in the USA

The global shortage of healthcare workers is a frequently discussed topic in the news. Most developed countries around the world report healthcare worker short-ages especially in more remote and rural areas. The USA is no exception to that rule. At the end of 2015, there were just under 900,000 actively licensed physicians in the USA [26]. That includes both Doctors of Medicine and Doctors of Osteopathy. The vast majority of US physicians are allopathic [26]. It should be noted that in the USA, unlike most other countries, osteopathic physicians are allowed to practice medicine on the same terms as the allopathic physicians. They are not limited to practicing only osteopathic manipulation techniques. The number of physicians in the USA has increased by 12% between 2010 and 2016 [27]. There are currently around three million registered nurses (RNs) in the USA [28]. There are a number of reports warning of severe upcoming workforce shortages. In fact, over the next decade, the USA may need as many as 100,000 additional physicians [29]. Besides physicians and nurses, a number of other healthcare workers play an important role in the system. They include midwives, radiology technicians, laboratory personnel, speech therapists, physical therapists, occupational therapists, and many others. A recent report by CNN suggested that the USA is going to need to hire as many as 2.3 million additional healthcare workers by 2025 to keep up with the demand [30]. With the population that is rapidly increasing and getting older, there is no question that the USA is in dire need of recruiting new healthcare workers to fill the current skill gap and provide healthcare to the population.

Most of the physicians in the USA have specialized in family medicine or inter-nal medicine (either general internal medicine or one of the subspecialties) [26]. Hundreds of thousands of physicians work in those fields. Some other fields are, comparably, smaller. For example, there are just over 10,000 dermatologists and 7000 plastic surgeons currently in the USA [26]. Despite those numbers, it is projected that it is the primary care physicians who are going to be needed the most in the upcoming years. Part of the reason for that is the necessity for providing primary care to the population in all parts of the country, while specialist services can be based in fewer areas.

How the USA Compares with the Other Developed Countries

There are currently 2.6 physicians per 1000 residents in the USA [31]. That number is about the average for high-income economies. It is somewhat lower than the numbers reported by many countries in the European Union and slightly lower than in Australia, comparable to that in Canada and higher than in Japan [31]. An interesting fact to keep in mind is that the US population is on average younger than the population of many of the aforementioned countries. As such, it can be concluded that while the shortage of physicians in the USA is significant, the situation is not likely to be much worse than in most of the other comparably wealthy countries. Recently, the Guardian reported that anywhere between 25% and 50% of job openings for consultants (referred to as attendings in the USA) remained unfilled in the last year [32]. The shortage of nurses in Britain is also concerning, with some estimates projecting the need to hire up to 5000 additional nurses annually, which is three times the number that is hired today [33]. Following the British vote to leave the European Union, the risk of serious health staff shortages has increased dramatically as fewer European citizens feel welcome in Britain. The situation in continental Europe could worsen rapidly as well. In some countries as much as 55% of primary care physicians are older than 55. German health minister went as far as to suggest introducing regulations that would stop healthcare professionals from emigrating after a large number of German healthcare workers emigrated to Switzerland which offered significantly higher salaries. The shortage of physicians in Germany was then managed by recruiting physicians from less wealthy EU member states, which in turn ended up unable to fill the positions [34]. Romania, for example, lost almost half of its physicians in a 5-year time period [35].

The International Medical Graduates (IMGs) in the USA

For decades, similarly to most other high-income countries, the USA has relied on immigrant workers to fill the shortages in its healthcare system. However, in order for foreign physicians to be able to gain licensure to practice medicine independently in the USA, they are required to pass a series of exams taken by medical students at American medical schools followed by finishing the entire residency (specialty training) program, regardless of whether the physician in question was already a licensed specialist in another country. With very few exceptions, all physicians in the USA have to do the entirety of their training after medical school in the USA. Therefore, the data from each year's residency application process can provide valuable insight into the extent to which the USA relies on IMGs. In 2019, almost 3000 US citizen IMGs and over 4000 non-US citizen IMGs matched into residency programs [36]. Since the match rate for graduates of US medical schools is extremely high and very few applicants fail to match every year, it appears that the USA needs to hire about 7000 physicians who have graduated abroad in order to fill their residency programs [36]. And even with all the residency positions filled, it is likely that the USA will face a significant physician shortage over the next decade.

According to the data released by the Educational Commission for Foreign Medical Graduates (ECFMG), which processes visas for foreign physicians working in US residency programs, the largest number of visas was sponsored to candidates from Canada and India with over 2300 visas for both countries, followed by Pakistan at around 1000 visas. It should be noted that some residency programs choose to sponsor their residents' visas themselves, which is not included in the statistics released by the ECFMG so the real numbers are likely to be higher. Such high reliance on healthcare workers from such a small number of countries is potentially hugely troublesome in case the supply from any of those countries decreases for any reason [37]. Physicians from India and Pakistan in particular have traditionally also moved to the UK in large numbers. As the UK becomes less attractive to physicians from continental Europe, it is likely to hire more physicians from India and Pakistan who are going to move there. Since the process of getting their credentials verified in the UK is widely considered to be easier than in the USA, it remains to be seen if a larger proportion of physicians from those countries chooses to find work in the UK. Moreover, the recent political changes may play a significant role in what happens to the physician workforce. The anti-immigrant sentiment in the USA is often perceived to be targeting communities of non-European descent, while the sentiment in the UK mostly relates to its relationship with the European Union. Such perceptions could significantly affect the physician migration in years to come.

Increased Medical School Enrolment and International Medical Graduates

For many years there have been talks about the bleak future for international medical graduates in the USA due to increased enrolment at medical schools in the USA. Due to the expected physician shortage, a number of medical schools have opened, and many of the existing ones have increased their class sizes. As such, it is expected that within the next few years, a significantly greater number of physicians are going to graduate from medical schools within the USA [38]. The number of available residency programs has not increased by a comparable margin. Since the match rate for graduates of American medical schools is significantly higher than for graduates of foreign schools, many believe that it is going to become progressively more difficult for foreign graduates to get jobs unless the number of jobs increases proportionally. Moreover, many American physicians are opposed to increasing the number of residency programs as they fear that the relationship between supply and demand would change to their disadvantage and that their standard of living would, consequently, suffer. Some also claim that the real problem in the USA is not that the total number of physicians is too small but that the distribution of them is inappropriate. Looking at international statistics, it is easy to see where such beliefs come from. The USA has more physicians per capita than a number of other wealthy countries. It should, however, be noted that the population density in the USA is significantly lower than in most European countries so it is likely that more physicians would be needed per capita in the USA than in Europe. Australia, a country with a significantly lower population density than the USA, has more physicians per capita. Also, while increasing access to primary care in rural and remote communities is important, there are times when emergency treatment cannot be adequately provided by general internists and family physicians, and speedy access to specialist treatment may be essential.

Salaries of Physicians and Nurses in the USA

High Salary, Expensive Living

It is generally well known that physician salaries in the USA are among the highest in the world. That is especially true for specialists in some fields. Anesthesiologists, cardiologists, radiologists, and surgeons are especially highly paid, although emergency medicine physicians and dermatologists also earn more than most physicians. Many argue that such high salaries are necessary due to the debt burden most American medical school graduates enter the workforce with. Also, the costs of malpractice insurance and health insurance are high and there is a relative lack of safety nets. The costs associated with raising a family in America are also often significantly higher than in most other countries as good nurseries and schools in major metropolitan centers are expensive. Therefore, American physicians often face costs that may be either nonexistent or much lower in other developed countries.

Resident/Fellow Salaries

The first year of residency, generally referred to as "internship," is when most US medical school graduates enter the workforce. Salaries of interns are significantly lower than those of the attending physicians, and the discrepancy is higher than in many countries. There are no significant differences between what interns make depending on the specialty they are training in. The average salary in the first year of residency is around $55,000 [39]. It should be noted that this is the gross income and taxes are deducted from it. Also, oftentimes residents have to pay portions of their own healthcare and educational costs. Nevertheless, it is still significantly higher than the median salary in the USA. In fact, the median household income in the USA is barely higher than the salary of an intern, at $63,000 [40]. Generally, the salary of residents and fellows in the USA rises every year. The average for all years of training is around $61,000, and the average for residents or fellows toward the end of their training is around $68,000 [41]. However, only around 50% of medical residents feel they are fairly compensated for their work, mostly because of the number of hours they spend at work. Around 40% of residents report spending over 60 hours a week seeing patients, and 60% report spending at least 50 hours per week seeing patients. The benefits that medical residents receive are also significant when compared to what most American workers receive. Almost all of the residency programs provide health insurance (including vision and dental) and paid time off. The majority of the programs also offer travel allowances, meal allowances, liability coverage, retirement plans, and book allowances. It should be noted, however, that medical residents often have to pay off significant amounts of student loan debt. Around a quarter of residents report having over $300,000 of debt and only 22% reported having no debt at all. Around half of all residents have more than $200,000 of debt to pay off [39].

Compared to the residents in the majority of the other high-income countries, the residents in the USA earn a good salary. The basic salary of medical residents in Australia is between A$73,000 and A$86,000. The overtime usually adds 25–50% extra [41]. Considering that the US dollar is worth more than the Australian dollar, the salaries of residents in the two countries are comparable, with Australian residents possibly earning slightly more. The salaries of trainee doctors in Germany are around 52,000 euros, which is slightly less than what residents in the USA earn [42]. In the UK the base starting salary for a newly qualified physician is around 28,000 GBP with annual increases [43]. Overtime adds to the salary and the final numbers are also similar or slightly lower than in the USA. The one country where the numbers are significantly higher is Switzerland, where residents can make more than 100,000 Swiss francs annually [44].

Attending Salaries

Once residents finish their programs and pass their specialty exams, they become attending physicians, most of whom work in hospitals and clinics around the country. The salaries of attending physicians in the USA are generally significantly higher than in the other developed countries. The average salary of primary care physicians in the USA was reported to be $237,000 per year and for specialists $341,000. On average, orthopedic surgeons reported the highest earnings, at $482,000 per year, whereas public health/preventive medicine specialists and pediatricians reported the lowest incomes at just over $200,000. Despite the high debt burden of physicians in the USA, it is worth noting that even the lowest paid physicians earn, on average, more than three times the average household income in the USA. There is a significant gender gap. Male physicians earn on average 50,000 dollars more than female physicians. Caucasian physicians also earn on average more than others. Self-employed physicians earn on average $70,000 more than those who work for an employer. The top-earning states for physicians are Oklahoma, Alabama, Nevada, Arkansas, and Florida. Depending on the specialty, between 40% and 70% of physicians believe they are fairly compensated for their work. Emergency physicians and preventive medicine physicians are the most likely to report being satisfied with their compensation, while infectious disease specialists are the least likely. Interestingly, infectious disease specialists are also the most likely to say they would choose medicine again if they were to go back to school [45].

Those salaries are significantly higher than in the other countries. For example, in the UK, newly qualified consultants (attending physicians) earn just under 80,000 GBP per year, while those with 19 or more years of experience as consultants earn around 108,000 GBP. They can earn additional income through "clinical excellence awards" and work in private practice. It should be noted, however, that even experienced consultants in the UK earn on average less than lowest paid specialists in the USA [46]. The salaries in Australia are somewhat higher than in the UK but lower than in the USA. Senior specialists in Australia do sometimes earn close to what physicians in the USA make [47]. In Germany, salaries largely depend on the seniority and the practice setting. The average surgeon earns around 103,000 euros per year before tax, which is similar to the salaries in the UK [42]. The one exception is Switzerland where independent specialists earn on average 257,000 Swiss francs, while gastroenterologists and neurosurgeons earn more than 600,000 Swiss francs [44]. It should be noted, though, that costs of living in Switzerland are among the highest in the world, on average much higher than in the USA.

Salaries of Nurses in the USA

Nurses in the USA are also decently paid, earning significantly more than the national average. The median salary of registered nurses in the USA is around $72,000, which is higher than the median household income in the country. The state where nurses earn the most on average is California where the average annual salary is almost $107,000, almost twice as high as in the lowest-paying state, South Dakota. In general, nurses earn the most in the states on the east and west coast [48].

The starting salaries of nurses in the UK are around 25,000 GBP. The average salary is around 37,000 GBP and some senior nurses earn over 50,000 GBP [49]. With the exception of newly qualified nurses, most earn more than what is the median salary for all UK workers at around 30,000 GBP [50]. The average salary for a nurse in Australia is around A$65,000, which considering the currency difference between AUD and USD or GBP is comparable to the salaries in the UK and lower than the salaries in the USA [51]. It should also be noted that the median income in Australia is A$48,000 [52]. The average salary for a nurse in Germany is around 30,000 euros, which is below the average wage [53]. Overall, it is clear that in most developed countries, nurses earn more than the majority of the population. In the USA, their earnings are overall comparable to those in the other countries. Nurses in the more expensive regions of the Northeastern and Western USA earn more on average, but the cost of living reduces their purchasing power.

Healthcare System in Canada

A Brief History

In early Canadian history, healthcare was administered and funded largely on a private level. This proved to be highly problematic for a large portion of the population, as unpredictable illnesses and accidents often lead to dire medical and financial consequences for middle- and lower-class citizens. It was only during the 1940s that the first provinces began to implement universal health coverage [54]. The first provincial universal healthcare plan was introduced in the province of Saskatchewan in 1947, followed closely by the Western provinces of Alberta and British Columbia in 1950 [54]. These early publicly funded plans were rather limited, initially covering only inpatient hospital-based care. The introduction of the *Medical Care Act* by the federal government in 1966 set a precedent for the national universalization of healthcare and the provision of a more comprehensive coverage of health services [54]. This bill extended publicly funded health coverage to outpatient physician services on a cost-sharing basis. Over the coming years, this new comprehensive public medical insurance program, now known as Medicare, began to gain traction across the nation and by 1972 was implemented by all of Canada's ten provinces and three territories [55].

The Role of the Government

Healthcare in Canada is regulated by three levels of government: federal, provincial or territorial, and municipal. Duties are divided between the three levels by the Canadian Constitution [54]. The role the federal government plays in healthcare is twofold. First, it funds medical services across the country by making transfer payments to its provinces and territories [54]. Second, the federal sector plays the imperative role of setting national healthcare standards and guidelines and ensuring that the core principles of Canadian healthcare are observed by all provinces and territories. The *Canada Health Act*, a pivotal legislation passed by Parliament in 1984, defines these principles as five conditions – public administration, universality, comprehensiveness, portability, and accessibility – which a province or territory must meet in order to receive federal funding [54]. Although the federal government's involvement in the day-to-day functioning of healthcare is minimal, it does directly oversee the delivery of health services to select population groups such as First Nations and Inuit communities, as well as members of the military and inmates of federal prisons [56].

The direct delivery of most health services, on the other hand, is organized and managed by provincial and territorial governments. In accordance with the *Canada Health Act,* all services which are deemed to be medically required or necessary must be fully covered by provincial health insurance plans [56]. Each province or territory has the authority to decide which services are considered medically necessary, and as a result, coverage for various medical services has great geographical variance. The largest government health program is Medicare, which consists of ten provincial and three territorial insurance programs that must comply with the *Canada Health Act* standards [55]. While Medicare accounts for the vast majority of health spending, there are many other small public insurance programs in existence as well.

Funding and Expenditures

The Canadian healthcare system is known as a single-payer system – in which healthcare is funded publicly by the government, but most healthcare services are provided by the private sector. The amount of money Canada spends on healthcare has been steadily increasing since the 1970s. In 1975, Canada spent 39.7 billion CAD on healthcare – 7% of the total GDP, averaging 1715 CAD per person [57]. To compare, in 2019 Canada's total health expenditure was 264 billion CAD (growing by 4.2% from 2018), 11.6% of the GDP, and 7068 CAD per person [57, 58]. Total health spending is highest in older age groups, and the average spending on residents over age 80 is 7 times greater than for those below age 65 [59]. Nearly 60% of the total health expenditure is spent on three categories of services: 26% on hospitals, 15% on pharmaceuticals, and 15% on physicians [57]. Since the 1970s, the share of expenditures for hospitals and physicians has been steadily declining, while the share spent on prescription drugs continues to increase [57].

Publicly funded healthcare accounts for 70% of the total health expenditure – approximately 184 billion CAD [57]. Within the public health system, provincial governments are the primary financers, constituting around 93% of total spending [56]. Provincial government insurance programs, in turn, are funded by income tax revenues and transfer payments from the federal government [54].

Alternately, private healthcare accounts for 30% of total healthcare spending [57]. Within the private sector, just under one-half of the funding comes from out-of-pocket spending, followed by approximately 40% coming from private health insurance [57]. Two-thirds of all Canadians have supplementary private health insurance in addition to universal healthcare, in order to cover for services which are not reimbursed by the *Canada Health Act* [56]. Private insurance expenditures are increasing by the highest rate annually, though out-of-pocket spending continues to increase as well [57].

Coverage of Services

All medically necessary hospital, physician, and diagnostic services are covered under the *Canada Health Act* for every eligible resident. As previously mentioned, what constitutes medically necessary services differs according to province or territory. Public insurance plans must provide first dollar coverage for all such services – where the insurance pays for the full service up front without copays or deductibles, as long as the service is medically necessary in that province or territory [56]. For example, one of the largest public health insurance plans in Canada is the Ontario Health Insurance Plan (OHIP) – for which all Canadians who permanently reside in the province of Ontario are eligible. Some of the services fully covered by OHIP include all medically necessary doctor's visits, hospital admissions, prescription drugs given in hospitals, abortions, eligible dental surgery and optometry, as well as preventive care such as annual physical exams, screening tests, and vaccinations [60].

Most provincial plans do not cover or only partially cover services such as dental and vision care, prescription drugs prescribed outside of the hospital, nonhospital institutions, long-term care, and ambulance care. Such services may be fully covered by the government in certain population groups, and coverage may vary greatly between different provinces. For instance, OHIP fully covers prescription medications for residents below age 25 and over age 65, as well as annual eye examinations for those below age 19 and over age 65 [60]. However, a large portion of the population are not covered for these services and, as a result, either purchase additional private insurance to cover these costs or pay out of pocket. In Canada, there are no caps in place for cost-sharing and out-of-pocket spending for uninsured services [56].

Structure of Canadian Healthcare Services

The primary care setting is typically the first point of contact for most Canadians with healthcare services. In 2018 Canada had 89,911 physicians – coming out to 2.4 doctors per 1000 people [61]. Around half of these doctors are general practitioners who provide primary care, with the second half being specialists. Medical specialists are typically secondary care providers, with the greatest proportion of them (65% in 2014) working in hospitals and the remainder in private offices or clinics [56]. Hospitals in Canada can be either private or public, the predominance of which varies significantly according to the province. In provinces like Ontario, private nonprofit hospitals are most common, while other provinces more commonly house hospitals which are publicly owned and managed by regional health authorities [56].

The number of physicians in Canada continues to grow each year at a much faster rate – double – that of the general population [61]. In 2018, 42% of physicians were female, continuing the upward trend of an increasing female physician proportion, most noticeably in certain disciplines such as family medicine [61]. Around 25% of Canadian physicians received their medical degree outside of Canada, a figure which has remained relatively stable over the past decade [61].

Most physicians work in private practices and are compensated via the fee-for-service (FFS) payment model. This is a traditional form of payment in which services such as consultations and procedures are billed individually and comprised 73% of total payments in 2018 [61]. However, the use of alternative payment plans (APPs) has been steadily increasing over the past decade, particularly among certain physician subsets such as those working in clinics or group practices [54]. Various forms of APPs include capitation, where doctors receive annual fees for each patient registered to them, salaries, and numerous combined models. In 2018, 27% of physicians were compensated by APPs, and these alternative methods of payment continue to increase in popularity, particularly among younger physicians [61]. Physician incomes in Canada are among the highest in the world with the average gross clinical payment being 281,000 CAD per family physician and 360,000 CAD per medical specialist in 2018 [61].

Performance of Canadian Healthcare: Going Forward

Albeit inclusive and universally accessible, Canada's healthcare system is not without its faults. Some of the issues currently at the forefront of concern include long wait times and poor availability of resources. Despite spending more on healthcare than most OECD (Organization for Economic Co-operation and Development) countries, Canada has one of the longest wait times for diagnostic imaging, elective procedures, and specialist appointments – ranking last out of ten countries with similar healthcare systems in the latter two categories [62]. Additionally, Canada continues to exhibit substantial deficits in availability of human and financial resources relative to other developed countries. Per 1000 people of the population, among 28 OECD countries, Canada stands 26th for number of physicians, 25th for number of psychiatric care beds, and 25th (out of 26) for number of acute care beds [62]. It also performs far below the OECD average in number of MRI and CT machines available per one million people of the population [62]. Clinical performance and quality in Canada remain variable. Canada ranks above average in certain health indicators, for example, performing well in 5-year survival rates for certain common cancers such as breast cancer. On the other hand, in other areas such as perinatal and infant mortality rates, Canada performs very poorly relative to other OECD countries [62]. Other issues most commonly cited as key concerns by Canadians include a lack of dental and prescription drug insurance coverage, as well as inconsistent access to primary care in certain geographical areas, especially rural communities.

In spite of its downfalls, Canada's universal healthcare system continues to receive a relatively high level of public support among its citizens. The inclusivity of the system is a defining point of pride for most Canadians, and the move toward strict privatization is currently relatively opposed by the public. However, many Canadians believe that the current costly system will not survive in the future. With incoming data shedding light on its inadequacies, the Canadian government aims to shift its focus toward structuring a more cost-efficient system, one in which the amount of money Canada spends on the system is matched by the delivery of a higher quality of care to all of its citizens.

The NHS

The UK has got one of the most robust healthcare systems in the world. It consists of both public sector and private sector entities. The public sector-/government-funded health system is called the NHS – National Health Service. The private sector comprises of different clinics and hospitals which supplement the role of the NHS. On the 5th of July 1948, a historic moment occurred in British history, a culmination of a bold and pioneering plan to make healthcare no longer exclusive to those who could afford it but to make it accessible to everyone. The NHS was born. The National Health Service, abbreviated to NHS, was launched by the then Minister of Health in Attlee's postwar government, Aneurin Bevan, at the Park Hospital in Manchester. The motivation to provide a good, strong, and reliable healthcare to all was finally taking its first tentative steps.

Costs

NHS net expenditure has increased from £78.881 billion in 2006/2007 to £120.512 billion in 2016/2017. Planned expenditure for 2017/2018 is £123.817bn and for 2018/2019 is £126.269bn. In real terms the budget is expected to increase from £120.512bn in 2016/2017 to £123.202bn by 2019/2020. Health expenditure per capita in England has risen from £1879 in 2011/2012 to £2106 in 2015/2016. The NHS net deficit for the 2015/2016 financial year was £1.851 billion. The provider deficit for the 2016/2017 financial year has been confirmed at £791m. CCG investment in mental health was £9.148bn in 2015/2016 and a planned £9.500bn in 2016/2017 [63].

NHS Sites

In England alone there are 207 clinical commissioning groups, 135 acute nonspecialist trusts (including 84 foundation trusts), 17 acute specialist trusts (including 16 foundation trusts), 54 mental health trusts (including 42 foundation trusts), 35 community providers (11 NHS trusts, 6 foundation trusts, 17 social enterprises, and 1 limited company), 10 ambulance trusts (including 5 foundation trusts), 7454 GP practices, and 853 for-profit and not-for-profit independent sector organizations, providing care to NHS patients from 7331 locations [63].

Workforce

In March 2017, across Hospital and Community Healthcare Services (HCHS), the NHS employed (full-time equivalent) 106,430 doctors; 285,893 nurses and health visitors; 21,597 midwives; 132,673 scientific, therapeutic, and technical staff; 19,772 ambulance staff; 21,139 managers; and 9974 senior managers. There were 10,934 additional HCHS doctors (FTE) employed in the NHS in March 2017 compared to March 2010 (11.45 percent). In the past year, the number has increased by 2.29 percent. There were 2197 more ambulance staff in March 2017 compared to 7 years earlier (12.50 percent). In the past year, the number has increased by 7.48 percent. There were 145 fewer psychiatrists across all grades (FTE) in March 2017 than March 2010 (1.64 percent decrease). 54.06 percent of NHS employees across HCHS are professionally qualified clinical staff, as of March 2017. In March 2017, 61,934 EU staff were working across HCHS – equivalent to 5.22 percent of the headcount. This equates to 57,737 FTE, which is 5.51 percent. Between March 2010 and March 2017, the number of professionally qualified clinical staff across HCHS has risen by 5.89 percent. In March 2017 there were 33,423 full-time equivalent GPs (excluding locums), which is a reduction of 890 (2.59 percent) on March 2016. Medical school intake rose from 3749 in 1997/1998 to 6262 in 2012/2013 – a rise of 67.0 percent. 7112 graduates were accepted on to foundation programs across the UK in 2016. The pay in the NHS for doctors can range from £22,000/annum (for foundation year 1 doctors) to £75,000/annum (for newly appointed consultants) [63].

The Healthcare System of India

India with a population of 1.3 billion is the second most populous country in the world just behind China. India is a booming economy, but as per the international reports, there is still a considerable percentage of population that lives below poverty line, which causes its own problems for the healthcare system. In India there are two sectors that provide healthcare to the public: one is public sector which is government funded, and the other is private sector to which people prescribe to out of their own pockets. Despite the two sectors, most of the people use the public sector healthcare facilities as the private sector insurers fees can be out of the reach of majority of population.

As per the estimates, Indian government spends $53 billion to fund its public sector healthcare facilities which makes 1.28% of the country's GDP. Of a total of 628,708 government beds, 196,182 are in rural areas. Government hospitals operate within a yearly budget allocation.

It is estimated that there are around 850,000 doctors available for active service in India, with a doctor-population ratio of 1:1596, which is much below the WHO standards. India has recently looked into its medical workforce development and opened new medical colleges to fulfil this shortage of doctors in the country. India has as dependent on different states a structure of training for doctors in different specialities. The base of the doctors working in the public sector can vary, but there is a consensus that they are not as well-paid as the doctors working in the private sector. There is also a shortage of professional development activities. All these factors contribute to a lot of doctors leaving for Western healthcare systems like UK and the USA which contributes to a significant brain drain from India.

The Healthcare System of Pakistan

Pakistan has a population of 220 million. Majority of the population lives in the rural areas. Like India there is a considerable percentage of people that live below the poverty line and don't have easy access to healthcare facilities. Pakistan has a mixed health system that includes public, parastatal, private, civil society, philanthropic contributors, and donor agencies. In Pakistan, healthcare delivery to the consumers is systematized through four modes of preventive, promotive, curative, and rehabilitative services. The private sector attends 70% of the population through a diverse group of healthcare members (some might be medically trained but there is a proportion of providers who are not adequately trained in the field of medicine).

Pakistan spends more than 50 billion PKR each year on its healthcare system which is 0.4% of its GDP. There are 924 public hospitals, 4916 dispensaries, 5336 basic health units, and 595 rural health centers.

As per estimates there are 139,555 doctors, 9822 dentists, and 69,313 nurses in Pakistan. This shows that there is a considerable shortage of trained healthcare staff to provide safe care to the patients in this region of the world. Pays for government-appointed healthcare staff have risen recently but are still considered to be one of the lowest in the region. There is somewhat a structured training process in place in Pakistan through college of physicians and surgeons of Pakistan. Keeping in mind other factors, there has been a brain drain of doctors from Pakistan to Western healthcare systems in search of better careers and professional development.

Healthcare Systems in Continental Europe

The European Union

Twenty-seven countries are members of the European Union. Liechtenstein, Norway, and Iceland are outside of the European Union but members of the European Economic Area. The UK has withdrawn from the European Union in 2020 following a referendum in 2016. Every country in the European Union and

European Economic Area has a unique healthcare system. What they all have in common is that regardless of the way they are funded, the healthcare is provided to all individuals. The European Health Insurance Card (EHIC) ensures citizens of one EU member state are able to get necessary healthcare in any other member state.

The German Healthcare System

Germany has a multi-payer universal healthcare system. Health insurance is mandatory for all citizens and permanent residents of Germany [3]. There are two systems providing health insurance in Germany. One of them is the competing, not-for-profit, nongovernmental health insurance funds ("sickness funds") in the statutory health insurance, and the other is the private health insurance. Most of the major academic hospitals are owned by the government. The government, however, has very little role in financing of healthcare [3]. The contributions to the sickness funds are mandatory and deducted as a percentage of gross wages up to a certain amount [3]. All employed individuals earning less than a threshold are mandatorily covered through sickness funds. Those who earn above the threshold can choose to remain covered by sickness funds or purchase private health insurance. Overall, 86% of the population is covered through sickness funds [3]. Those who opt out of the sickness funds and civil servants are covered by private health insurance. The insurance companies are regulated by the government to ensure that large premium increases for those insured do not occur. Inpatient and outpatient visits, mental healthcare, dental care, optometry, physical therapy, prescription drugs, medical aids, rehabilitation, and hospice and palliative care are covered [3]. It also covers sick leave compensation [3]. The copayments for the most part do not exceed 10 euros [3]. The sickness funds also cover obstetric care, although some private insurers do not. Emergency contraception is easily obtainable [3].

While most of the hospitals are owned by the government, most of the ambulatory physicians work in private practices. They are generally members of regional associations that negotiate contracts with sickness funds. Patients are free to choose their own primary care physicians, specialists, and hospitals. Family doctors have no formal gatekeeping function. The regional physician associations also ensure access to after-hours care for those in need. About half of all the hospitals are public, a third is private not-for-profit, and the rest are for-profit private hospitals [3]. Despite such system, the average per capita out-of-pocket spending in Germany was only $664 [3]. Life expectancy in Germany is 81 and the infant mortality rate is 3.22/1000 live births [9, 10].

The French Healthcare System

The French healthcare system is widely considered to be among the best in the world, and many consider it to be the best model for countries to follow. It is universal and for the most part funded through taxes, although private health insurance exists. The statutory health insurance (SHI) provides universal and compulsory coverage [3]. Very few individuals can opt out of SHI, usually those employed by foreign companies [3]. The government covers more than three-quarters of healthcare costs in France [3]. Most of the private health insurance in France is complementary, covering copayments for usual care, vision and dental care. Most of the voluntary health insurance is provided by not-for-profit, employment-based associations, which are allowed to cover only copayments for the services provided by the statutory health insurance [3]. The services which are covered through the SHI are defined by the government and do not vary based on the region [3]. Outpatient and inpatient care, including any rehabilitation services, are covered by the SHI [3]. Most appliances and prescription drugs are covered as well [3]. The hospice and mental healthcare are partially covered [3]. Most out-of-pocket spending is for dental and vision care, although the fees are generally minimal [3]. In fact, the average out-of-pocket healthcare spending in France is 305 USD per person per year [3].

The gatekeeping system at the level of the primary care is voluntary, and financial incentives are provided to those who choose to register with a primary care physician [3]. Physicians are also given financial incentives to work in areas lacking medical workforce [3]. Many of the physicians are paid on a fee-for-service basis [3]. The rest are either fully or partially salaried. For the most part, patients are free to choose the specialist once they are referred [3]. The after-hours care is generally accessed through emergency departments of public hospitals or private hospitals that have signed agreements with their Regional Health Agencies [3]. About two-thirds of all the hospitals are public institutions with the rest being a mix of private for-profit and private not-for-profit institutions [3]. Gynecologists can be freely chosen and referrals are not necessary. Contraception is readily available and most of the cost is usually reimbursed. Life expectancy in France is 83 and the infant mortality rate is 3.12/1000 live births [9, 10].

The Italian Healthcare System

The Italian healthcare system is a regionally based National Health Service (NHS), which provides universal coverage to all legal residents, mostly free of charge [3]. It is largely funded through taxes, which get distributed to the regional governments [3]. In addition to that, the individual regions are allowed to generate additional revenue [3]. There are no provisions for people to opt out of the system [3]. Therefore, while supplemental and complementary insurance do exist, substitutive private insurance does not. Some minor copays do exist [3]. The role of private healthcare is limited and it accounts for approximately 1% of all healthcare costs [3]. Some of the things that may be covered by private insurance include higher standard of comfort and privacy during hospital stays, some copays may be covered, and patients may be compensated during their stay at the hospital. The total out-of-pocket expenditure per capita is around $700 per year [3]. Most primary care physicians, including pediatricians, are self-employed or independent and are paid a capitation fee based on the number of patients they care for [3]. Overall, the earnings of primary care physicians in Italy are reasonable at around 100,000 euros per year before tax. Patients are required to register with a primary care physician who also serves as a gatekeeper [3]. Physicians are incentivized to limit prescribing and referrals only to medically necessary cases [3]. Local health units also often provide outpatient specialist services [3]. Once referred, patients can usually choose the hospital but not necessarily the individual specialist they see [3]. After-hours care is generally provided by the emergency medical service [3]. There is a significant number of private accredited hospitals [3]. Mental healthcare is fully covered and so are many of the rehabilitation facilities [3]. Long-term care is generally considered to be worse than in most other wealthy European countries [3]. Obstetric and gynecological care is readily available and so is contraception, including emergency contraception. Life expectancy in Italy is 83 and infant mortality is 2.7/1000 live births [9, 10].

The Swedish Healthcare System

The Swedish healthcare system is highly regarded worldwide. Healthcare in Sweden is organized on three levels: national, regional, and local [3]. The system is universal and all residents have access to it. Employers and employees contribute into the public fund [3]. Small copays are associated with many of the services, usually the equivalent of 20–40 USD [3]. Nationally, the annual out-of-pocket costs are capped [3]. Private insurance, in form of supplementary coverage, accounts for less than 1% of healthcare spending in Sweden [3]. All the services are covered by the public system and there is no pre-set list of defined benefits [3]. Dental care, vision care, long-term care, patient transport services, and hospice care are all covered [3]. There is no formal gatekeeping function of the primary care physicians [3]. Traditionally, long waiting lists have been a cause of dissatisfaction among the Swedish population so a new set of rules was released guaranteeing that specialist care must be accessible within 90 days and any surgeries must be carried out within 90 days from when it is determined that they are medically indicated. Urgent care is easily accessible at the time of the need [3]. Multiple primary care providers generally work together in larger practices [3]. Most patients register with a practice, rather than with an individual physician. Primary care providers also provide after-hours care [3]. Most physicians in Sweden earn around 6000 euros a month. Outpatient specialist services are offered at hospitals and private clinics. The majority of hospitals are public, with only a few private hospitals in the country [3]. Gynecologists generally work as primary care physicians and women's health services are easily accessible. Birth control is readily available. The life expectancy in Sweden is 82 and the infant mortality rate is 2.2/1000 live births [9, 10].

Healthcare Systems in Latin America

The Latin American Healthcare Systems

Although many still consider Latin America, consisting of Central and Southern America, to be a part of the developing world, a number of countries in the region report life expectancies comparable to many countries in the west. Moreover, Latin American healthcare systems are frequently discussed in the US politics, both in terms of the positives and the negatives. The universal systems of socialist countries like Cuba and Venezuela have frequently been used as examples of the disaster that might happen to the American public if the USA were to ever adopt a universal healthcare system. The proponents of switching to a universal system in the USA, on the other hand, tend to argue that they want the USA to be more like western and northern Europe. Meanwhile, some prominent personalities in the USA, such as the filmmaker Michael Moore, have spoken very highly and even recorded documentaries praising the Cuban healthcare system. In this chapter we are going to take a closer look at a number of countries in the region and analyze their healthcare systems.

The Mexican Healthcare System

It makes sense that Mexico is the first country that we are going to look at as it is not only one of the largest Latin American countries but it also shares a land border with the USA meaning that a number of people frequently travel between the countries. Mexico has achieved universal healthcare coverage through the public healthcare system that all employees contribute to. The Mexican constitution guarantees healthcare to all citizens. Those who are unemployed, such as many of the expats, are able to pay for access to the system. While the quality of healthcare in the public system is generally adequate, there is also a private healthcare system. The service is also inconsistent between different parts of Mexico. There is a separate system in Mexico for those with chronic conditions or those unable to pay, called "Seguro Popular." Only around 6% of GDP is spent on healthcare. The costs for any medical services are overall usually less than half of those in the USA. The same applies to most drugs. Overall, the system is far cheaper than that of the USA. Despite that, out-of-pocket expenditures are still significant compared to the total costs of healthcare. Both government-run and private hospitals operate in Mexico [64, 65]. Life expectancy in Mexico is 76 and the infant mortality rate is 12 per 1000 live births [9, 10].

The Panamanian Healthcare System

The Panamanian healthcare system is generally considered to be very affordable. There are three healthcare systems in Panama, two of which are run by the government. They are public hospitals run by the Ministry of Health, social security hospitals, and the private system. The same physicians work in both government-run and private hospitals. Outside of the Panama City, obtaining good-quality healthcare can be difficult. While the government provides health insurance to citizens and permanent residents, those who can afford it generally prefer to purchase additional private insurance. Most drugs are much cheaper than in the USA and can be purchased without a prescription. Many of the physicians who serve the Panamanian hospitals have trained abroad, often in the USA, and private hospitals are often affiliated with major institutions in the USA. While people from the west may consider the costs of healthcare in Panama to be low, it should be kept in mind that the average wages in Panama are quite low. Healthcare tourism is popular due to lower costs, availability of US-trained medical workforce, and the availability of spas and rehabilitation facilities [66, 67]. Life expectancy in Panama is 79 and the infant mortality rate is 10 per 1000 live births [9, 10].

The Cuban Healthcare System

As previously mentioned, the Cuban healthcare system is praised by many who believe that for a relatively poor country, Cuba is able to provide excellent healthcare to all its citizens. The fact that the life expectancy in Cuba is around 79 and the infant mortality rate is 4 adds value to those claims [9, 10]. The origins of the Cuban healthcare system date back to the socialist revolution of 1959. To reduce overall healthcare spending, Cuba has focused heavily on disease prevention and primary care. The doctor-to-patient ratio in Cuba also surpasses that of many highly developed countries. The salaries of doctors in Cuba are low, well below 100 USD per month, and many report that the infrastructure is crumbling. The government spends between 300 and 400 USD per person each year on healthcare but gains billions from its overseas medical missions. As Cuban doctors spend a lot of time participating in medical missions in developing countries, many argue that their lack of exposure to medicine in the developed countries may be impairing the modernization of their hospitals. The problem is not just the infrastructure and lack of international influence. Many essential medicines and pieces of equipment are in extremely short supply. Foreigners or Cubans living abroad are required to purchase health insurance with the option to do so upon arrival [68, 69].

The Brazilian Healthcare System

Healthcare in Brazil is a constitutionally guaranteed right, provided by both government-run and private institutions. All legal residents, including foreigners, can obtain free healthcare at government-run clinics and hospitals. All the medical services, including prescription drugs, are provided free of charge through the public healthcare system. Approximately 20–30% of the population use private health insurance since private hospitals tend to be better and the wait times are generally shorter. The quality of healthcare in rural areas may also be lacking in quality and quantity as most of the services and hospitals are located in cities. The overall costs of healthcare, even private, are significantly lower than in the USA. A family of four can purchase private health insurance for under 300 USD. Even those with private health insurance can still access the public healthcare system if they wish. Overall, it is believed that the quality of healthcare in Brazil is good and there are many state-of-the-art medical facilities available. Brazil spends around 8% of its GDP on healthcare [70]. Life expectancy in Brazil is 74 and the infant mortality rate is around 18 per 1000 live births [9, 10].

The Argentinian Healthcare System

The Argentinian healthcare system is divided into public, private, and social security systems. The public system is funded through regular contributions from employees and employers. The minimum level of coverage is guaranteed to all and people with preexisting conditions are covered. It is generally thought that the quality of healthcare in Argentina is good. Most of the medical services are free of charge and only some medications and chronic conditions require copays. The waiting lists can be long, especially for nonurgent and elective procedures. Around 10% of the wealthiest residents in Argentina also have private health insurance for additional benefits. The Argentinian private health insurance system is among the best in Latin America. The standards in larger metropolitan areas, such as Buenos Aires, are generally far higher than in more rural parts of the country. Basic private plans cost as little as 50 USD per month. Many of the physicians in Argentina have trained overseas, in Western countries. Buenos Aires also has British, German, Swiss, and Italian hospitals. In general, healthcare costs are often as little as 30% of those one would pay for the same services in the USA [71]. The life expectancy in Argentina is 77 and the infant mortality rate is around 10 per 1000 live births [9, 10].

The Colombian Healthcare System

The World Health Organization rated the Colombian healthcare system better than those of the USA and Canada. Colombia is also home to up to 40% of the best hospitals in Latin America. There are one public and a number of private health insurance plans. Public healthcare is available to residents who pay a monthly premium of around 12.5% of their gross earnings. Very poor and homeless people are covered by a separate free government-subsidized system. Those who can afford it are also able to purchase private insurance in addition to the public plan. People older than

60 are generally unable to enrol in private plans. Some of the perks of private health insurance plans are the ability to choose one's own physicians, the ability to see specialists without being previously referred to them, private hospital rooms, and some other comfort-enhancing benefits. The copayments in the public system are low for US standards. Even those who choose to pay out of pocket usually pay only around 50 USD for specialist consultations. Many medications in Colombia do not require prescriptions. Medical tourism to Colombia is becoming increasingly popular among the US adults, even for dental works which can be thousands of dollars cheaper than in the USA [72]. Life expectancy in Colombia is 76 and the infant mortality rate is around 14 per 1000 live births [9, 10].

The Venezuelan Healthcare System

Little can be said about Venezuela without triggering a political debate in the USA as the opinions on the desired US approach to its relationship with Venezuela could not be further apart. As a socialist country, Venezuela on paper guarantees healthcare to all citizens. Once upon a time, Venezuela was thought as a country with an excellent healthcare system, especially when compared to the neighboring countries. Today, many reports point to the system collapsing and people being unable to access healthcare when in need. Medicines, surgical equipment, and even the electricity are reported to be in short supply in many hospitals nationwide. The infectious diseases, including malaria, have been on the rise. Further increases in international, mainly American sanctions are likely to lead to further deterioration of the quality of healthcare in Venezuela [73, 74]. Life expectancy is 76 and the infant mortality rate is around 12 per 1000 live births [9, 10]. If the reports of crumbling infrastructure, poor sanitation, and lack of basic supplies are correct, those numbers are likely to deteriorate in the future.

Healthcare Systems of Japan, South Korea, Singapore, the United Arab Emirates, Australia, and New Zealand

Wealthy Nations Outside of North America and Europe

No analysis of global healthcare systems would be complete without looking at the systems in some of the richest countries in the world outside of North America and Europe. They are generally located in Asia and Oceania. All of these countries have high standards of living, long life expectancies, and low infant mortality rates. Their healthcare systems differ significantly as do their political and economic systems.

Healthcare in Japan

Japan is widely considered to be one of the most developed countries in the world, famous for some of the greatest technological advancements of the modern times. Japan is also the country with the highest life expectancy in the world (except Monaco) and the largest number of people who have lived for more than 110 years [3, 9]. Hospitals and clinics in Japan are equipped with state-of-the-art equipment and highly knowledgeable workforce. Japanese scientists are among the most respected worldwide. Generally speaking, healthcare in Japan is provided free of charge for citizens and foreigners [3]. Health insurance contributions are deducted from salaries automatically based on income. The patients generally pay 30% of the healthcare costs [3]. Private insurance is supplementary. There are monthly out-of-pocket maximums to prevent people from going bankrupt over healthcare bills [3]. The salaries of physicians in Japan are lower than in the USA and comparable to those in Western European countries. A potential problem for the Japanese healthcare system is the relative shortage of physicians when compared to most of the Western countries [31].

Healthcare in South Korea

Just like Japan, South Korea also has a healthy and long-living population despite spending only 8% of its GDP on healthcare [75, 76]. The healthcare system is universal and accessible to both citizens and foreigners who have lived in the country for more than 6 months [75]. Over the past 30 years, it has grown from a relatively poor and understaffed service to a highly advanced system that provides excellent care to the population. It is funded through a combination of subsidies by the government, external contributions, and, interestingly, tobacco surcharges [75]. The individual contributions are dependent on the earnings and people who earn more also contribute more to the system. Overall, the quality of healthcare is excellent although there are significant differences between urban and rural areas of the country and wait times can be lengthy [75]. Private facilities exist and are mostly found in urban areas. Some medications and procedures associated with chronic conditions, such as cancers, are often not covered and can be expensive [75]. Overall, patients pay around 20% of their healthcare costs out of pocket [75]. The exact amounts people pay are still significantly lower than in the USA and many other Western countries. Private insurance usually covers the copays and any medications or treatments not covered through the public system [75].

Healthcare in Singapore

The city-state of Singapore, known for extreme cleanliness, harsh legal ramifications for anyone breaking the law, and some of the most advanced technology in the world, also has an excellent healthcare system and long life expectancy. Oftentimes,

US politicians have used Singaporean system as the healthcare model that could be followed in the USA. It offers universal healthcare coverage to all citizens through a combination of government subsidies, which come mainly from tax revenue and private individual savings [3]. Everything is administered at the national level. The government pays for 80% of the total cost of care in public hospitals and clinics [3]. On top of that, there is a mandatory medical savings program to which individuals contribute a percentage of their salary. All the contributions and withdrawals are tax-exempt [3]. There is also an additional low-cost catastrophic insurance plan that covers major or prolonged illnesses that would be too expensive to be covered from the medical savings account [3]. There are also a number of options for purchasing private health insurance. The government has set up a separate safety net for the poor which helps them cover 100% of the healthcare costs [3]. The primary care is generally administered by private providers in a network of general practitioners [3]. There are numerous hospitals that offer specialist services and after-hours care [3]. Most of the hospitals are public and divided into groups based on the scope of care they provide [3]. It should be noted that the healthcare spending per capita in Singapore is significant but physicians themselves earn high salaries [3].

Healthcare in the United Arab Emirates

The United Arab Emirates (UAE) is a country that has seen significant development over the last few decades and is now one of the wealthiest countries in the world. It is also considered one of the most efficient healthcare systems in the world. It is also known for medical tourism. Both public and private facilities exist [77]. The public system is funded through taxes. For UAE nationals, accessing healthcare through public hospitals is inexpensive [77]. Expats are generally required to pay for any medical treatments [77]. There are many new state-of-the-art medical facilities and at the moment, private facilities outnumber the public ones. There are differences between the individual emirates as residents of Dubai and Abu Dhabi are required to purchase health insurance, while residents of some other emirates are not [77]. English is commonly spoken and most of the medical staff is foreign-trained [77]. Finding a doctor is easy and usually done online. Being married is a requirement to give birth [77]. Overall, the costs of healthcare in the UAE are high in part because of the widespread private healthcare system and the tendency of residents to seek specialist treatment without using general practitioners as gatekeepers [77]. Many pharmacies are open 24 hours a day [77]. Some report that mental healthcare is a weaker spot of the system and that there may be some stigma associated with mental illnesses [77]. Interestingly, the total healthcare expenditure was only 3.4% of the GDP in 2018 [78].

Healthcare in Australia

The Australian healthcare system is also widely seen as one of the most successful in the world as Australians enjoy some of the best life expectancy and quality of life in the world. It is also one of the most comprehensive healthcare systems around the world. There are two major components of the system: the public and the private system [3]. The public system consists of public hospitals, community-based facilities, and affiliated organizations [3]. It is accessible for free or at low cost through a tax-funded insurance program, Medicare [3]. The private system consists of private hospitals, specialist health, and pharmacies [3]. There are a number of ways people pay for care through the private system, including out-of-pocket payments and additional private insurance. Most of the time, general practitioners serve as gatekeepers [3]. Emergency care is generally provided at public hospitals [3]. Those who choose to undergo nonurgent treatment at public hospitals tend to face longer wait times compared to those who get the same services through the private system. Such system can sometimes become expensive for patients who require many specialist visits. Around half the Australian population has private health insurance in addition to Medicare. Out-of-pocket costs on medications are capped [3]. Out-of-hours care is also easily accessible. The total health expenditure is around 10% of the Australian GDP [3].

Healthcare in New Zealand

There is no question that the healthcare system in New Zealand also provides the population with high-quality healthcare. It is also a mix of a public and private system that compliments each other. All permanent residents have access to a range of public health services that are funded through taxes [3]. Nonresidents pay the full price of all services in the public sector [3]. Private insurance is offered by a number of different insurers. It is usually used to cover the services where the patient would be required to pay some of the cost [3]. It can also be used to gain faster access to nonurgent treatments. Most of the standard medical needs of the population are covered through the public system, including inpatient and outpatient management, prescription drugs, preventive services, mental healthcare, dental care for children, long-term care, hospice care, and disability support services [3]. General practitioner visits generally require copays [3]. There are multiple safety nets available to those who cannot afford the copays. General practitioners act as gatekeepers to specialist services [3]. They also organize after-hours care. Since the after-hours GP care can be more expensive than regular GP care, many patients choose to forego it and seek help in emergency departments [3]. Most of the hospitals are public, although private hospitals exist. The total healthcare spending in New Zealand is under 10% of its GDP with close to 80% of it going to the public sector [3].

The Electronic Medical Records

The term "electronic medical records" (EMRs) refers to digital versions of patient charts. Considering the vast amounts of data reported in each patient chart, there is no doubt that the use of computer databases simplifies the process of searching for the necessary information, makes it easier to do any required calculations, and facilitates communication between healthcare providers. They may also decrease many of the administrative costs. Potential issues include the risks of electronic failures and data breaches. EMRs are increasingly used in the Western health systems, such as those of the USA and Europe. In the USA, most hospitals have adopted some form of EMR, although the lack of system centralization and the existence of healthcare networks makes it more challenging to set up a functional EMR system compared to countries with single-payer healthcare systems [79–82].

References

1. World Bank Country and Lending Groups – World Bank Data Help Desk [Internet]. [cited 2020 May 26]. Available from: https://datahelpdesk.worldbank.org/knowledgebase/articles/906519
2. De Lew N, Greenberg G, Kinchen K. A layman's guide to the U.S. health care system. Health Care Financ Rev. 1992;14(1):151–69.
3. Mossialos E, Djordjevic A, Osborn R, Sarnak D, editors. International profiles of health care systems. New York: The Commonwealth Fund; 2017.
4. What's Medicare?|Medicare [Internet]. [cited 2020 May 27]. Available from: https://www.medicare.gov/what-medicare-covers/your-medicare-coverage-choices/whats-medicare
5. Military.com. VA Health Care: Cost and Co-payments [Internet]. Military.com. [cited 2020 May 30]. Available from: https://www.military.com/benefits/veterans-health-care/va-health-care-cost-and-copayments.html
6. PatientEngagementHIT. VA Sees Improvements in Patient Satisfaction, Care Access [Internet]. PatientEngagementHIT. 2019 [cited 2020 May 30]. Available from: https://patientengagementhit.com/news/va-sees-improvements-in-patient-satisfaction-care-access
7. Where 2020 Democrats stand on Medicare-for-all and other health-care issues [Internet]. Washington Post. [cited 2020 May 30]. Available from: https://www.washingtonpost.com/graphics/politics/policy-2020/medicare-for-all/
8. Trump Is Trying Hard To Thwart Obamacare. How's That Going? [Internet]. NPR.org. [cited 2020 May 30]. Available from: https://www.npr.org/sections/health-shots/2019/10/14/768731628/trump-is-trying-hard-to-thwart-obamacare-hows-that-going
9. The World Factbook — Central Intelligence Agency [Internet]. [cited 2020 May 30]. Available from: https://www.cia.gov/library/publications/the-world-factbook/rankorder/2102rank.html
10. The World Factbook — Central Intelligence Agency [Internet]. [cited 2020 May 30]. Available from: https://www.cia.gov/library/publications/the-world-factbook/rankorder/2091rank.html
11. How does the quality of the U.S. healthcare system compare to other countries? [Internet]. Peterson-KFF Health System Tracker. [cited 2020 May 30]. Available from: https://www.healthsystemtracker.org/chart-collection/quality-u-s-healthcare-system-compare-countries/
12. Hartman M, Martin AB, Benson J, Catlin A. The National Health Expenditure Accounts Team. National Health Care Spending in 2018: growth driven by accelerations in Medicare and private insurance spending: US health care spending increased 4.6 percent to reach $3.6 trillion in 2018, a faster growth rate than that of 4.2 percent in 2017 but the same rate as in 2016. Health Affairs. 2020;39(1):8–17.
13. US healthcare spending to hit $6.2 trillion by 2028; growth set to outpace GDP|S&P Global Market Intelligence [Internet]. [cited 2020 May 31]. Available from: https://www.spglobal.com/marketintelligence/en/news-insights/latest-news-headlines/us-healthcare-spending-to-hit-6-2-trillion-by-2028-growth-set-to-outpace-gdp-57739003
14. Cylus J, Hartman M, Washington B, Andrews K, Catlin A. Pronounced gender and age differences are evident in personal health care spending per person. Health Affairs. 2011;30(1):153–60. https://doi.org/10.1377/hlthaff.2010.0216.

15. Health Care Expenditures per Capita by State of Residence [Internet]. KFF. 2017 [cited 2020 May 31]. Available from: https://www.kff.org/other/state-indicator/health-spending-per-capita/

16. Current health expenditure (% of GDP)|Data [Internet]. [cited 2020 May 31]. Available from: https://data.worldbank.org/indicator/SH.XPD.CHEX.GD.ZS

17. Hankin A. How U.S. Healthcare Costs Compare to Other Countries [Internet]. Investopedia. [cited 2020 May 31]. Available from: https://www.investopedia.com/articles/personal-finance/072116/us-healthcare-costs-compared-other-countries.asp1.

18. Do Medical Bills Really Bankrupt America's Families? [Internet]. The Balance. [cited 2020 May 31]. Available from: https://www.thebalance.com/medical-bankruptcy-statistics-4154729

19. 41% of Americans would be able to cover $1,000 emergency with savings [Internet]. [cited 2020 May 31]. Available from: https://www.cnbc.com/2020/01/21/41-percent-of-americans-would-be-able-to-cover-1000-dollar-emergency-with-savings.html

20. Health Insurance Costs, Premiums, Deductibles, Co-Pays & Co-Insurance [Internet]. Debt.org. [cited 2020 May 31]. Available from: https://www.debt.org/medical/health-insurance-premiums/

21. How Much Does Individual Health Insurance Cost? – eHealth Insurance [Internet]. [cited 2020 May 31]. Available from: https://www.ehealthinsurance.com/resources/individual-and-family/how-much-does-individual-health-insurance-cost

22. Too many choices, high costs and bureaucracy: British expats grade American healthcare system "a pain in the arse" [Internet]. the Guardian. 2015 [cited 2020 May 31]. Available from: http://www.theguardian.com/money/2015/jan/12/us-healthcare-system-leaves-brits-baffled-enraged

23. NHE Fact Sheet|CMS [Internet]. [cited 2020 May 31]. Available from: https://www.cms.gov/Research-Statistics-Data-and-Systems/Statistics-Trends-and-Reports/NationalHealthExpendData/NHE-Fact-Sheet

24. 6 Reasons Healthcare Is So Expensive in the U.S. [Internet]. Investopedia. [cited 2020 May 31]. Available from: https://www.investopedia.com/articles/personal-finance/080615/6-reasons-healthcare-so-expensive-us.asp

25. Katz J, Quealy K, Sanger-Katz M. Would 'Medicare for All' Save Billions or Cost Billions? The New York Times [Internet]. 2019 Apr 10 [cited 2020 May 31]; Available from: https://www.nytimes.com/interactive/2019/04/10/upshot/medicare-for-all-bernie-sanders-cost-estimates.html

26. Active Physicians with a U.S. Doctor of Medicine (U.S. MD) Degree by Specialty, 2015 [Internet]. AAMC. [cited 2020 May 31]. Available from: https://www.aamc.org/data-reports/workforce/interactive-data/active-physicians-us-doctor-medicine-us-md-degree-specialty-20151.

27. Number of actively licensed physicians increased 12% since 2010 [Internet]. Healthcare Dive. [cited 2020 Jun 2]. Available from: https://www.healthcaredive.com/news/number-of-actively-licensed-physicians-increased-12-since-2010/447700/

28. AACN Fact Sheet – Nursing [Internet]. [cited 2020 Jun 2]. Available from: https://www.aacnnursing.org/News-Information/Fact-Sheets/Nursing-Fact-Sheet

29. Research Shows Shortage of More than 100,000 Doctors by 2030 [Internet]. AAMC. [cited 2020 Jun 2]. Available from: https://www.aamc.org/news-insights/research-shows-shortage-more-100000-doctors-2030

30. The US can't keep up with demand for health care workers [Internet]. [cited 2020 Jun 2]. Available from: https://money.cnn.com/2018/05/04/news/economy/health-care-workers-shortage/index.html

31. Physicians (per 1,000 people)|Data [Internet]. [cited 2020 Jun 2]. Available from: https://data.worldbank.org/indicator/SH.MED.PHYS.ZS

32. New report reveals alarming shortage of country doctors [Internet]. the Guardian. 2019 [cited 2020 Jun 2]. Available from: http://www.theguardian.com/society/2019/oct/13/nhs-consultant-shortage-rural-coastal-areas

33. NHS staff shortage: How many doctors and nurses come from abroad? – BBC News [Internet]. [cited 2020 Jun 2]. Available from: https://www.bbc.com/news/world-48205445

34. EU may need rules to stop doctors emigrating – German minister – Reuters [Internet]. [cited 2020 Jun 2]. Available from: https://uk.reuters.com/article/uk-eu-migration-germany-idUKKCN1P70GV

35. Romania's brain drain: Half of Romania's doctors left the country between 2009 and 2015|Romania Insider [Internet]. [cited 2020 Jun 2]. Available from: https://www.romania-insider.com/romanias-brain-drain-half-of-romanias-doctors-left-the-country-between-2009-and-2015

36. Janick AJ. IMGs Continue to Show Gains in 2019 Match [Internet]. ECFMG News. 2019 [cited 2020 Jun 2]. Available from: https://www.ecfmg.org/news/2019/03/15/imgs-continue-to-show-gains-in-2019-match/

37. Resources: Data – ECFMG J-1 Visa Sponsorship [Internet]. ECFMG. [cited 2020 Jun 2]. Available from: https://www.ecfmg.org/resources/data-sponsorship.html

38. U.S. medical school enrollment rises 30% [Internet]. AAMC. [cited 2020 Jun 2]. Available from: https://www.aamc.org/news-insights/us-medical-school-enrollment-rises-30

39. Medscape Residents Salary & Debt Report 2018 [Internet]. Medscape. [cited 2020 Jun 2]. Available from: //www.medscape.com/slideshow/2018-residents-salary-debt-report-6010044

40. Medscape Residents Salary & Debt Report 2018 [Internet]. Medscape. [cited 2020 Jun 2]. Available from: //www.medscape.com/slideshow/2018-residents-salary-debt-report-6010044

41. Llewellyn A. Resident Doctors Salary Australia: Pay Rates & Titles Explained. [Internet]. https://advancemed.com.au/. [cited 2020 Jun 2]. Available from: https://advancemed.com.au/blog/resident-doctor-pay/

42. Medicine salary: What medical professions earn [Internet]. [cited 2020 Jun 2]. Available from: https://www.academics.com/guide/medicine-salary-germany

43. Scavone F. Pay scales for junior doctors in England [Internet]. The British Medical Association is the trade union and professional body for doctors in the UK. [cited 2020 Jun 2]. Available from: https://www.bma.org.uk/pay-and-contracts/pay/junior-doctors-pay-scales/pay-scales-for-junior-doctors-in-england

44. Doctors' salaries exceed expectations [Internet]. SWI swissinfo.ch. [cited 2020 Jun 2]. Available from: https://www.swissinfo.ch/eng/society/healthy-income-_doctors%2D%2Dsalaries-exceed-expectations/44505806

45. Medscape Physician Compensation Report 2019 [Internet]. [cited 2020 Jun 2]. Available from: https://www.medscape.com/slideshow/2019-compensation-overview-6011286#2

46. Scavone F. Pay scales for consultants in England [Internet]. The British Medical Association is the trade union and professional body for doctors in the UK. [cited 2020 Jun 2]. Available from: https://www.bma.org.uk/pay-and-contracts/pay/consultants-pay-scales/pay-scales-for-consultants-in-england

47. Surgeon and Doctor Salary in Australia [Internet]. HealthStaff Recruitment. [cited 2020 Jun 2]. Available from: https://www.healthstaffrecruitment.com.au/news/doctor-salaries-in-australia-what-should-i-expect/

48. People TCFT. Nurse Salaries: Which US States Pay RNs the Best (2019 Updated) [Internet]. Nightingale College. 2019 [cited 2020 Jun 2]. Available from: https://nightingale.edu/blog/nurse-salary-by-state/

49. Adult nurse job profile|Prospects.ac.uk [Internet]. [cited 2020 Jun 2]. Available from: https://www.prospects.ac.uk/job-profiles/adult-nurse

50. Average UK salary by profession: check if you earn more or less than your colleagues [Internet]. [cited 2020 Jun 2]. Available from: https://www.telegraph.co.uk/money/special-reports/average-uk-salary-profession-check-earn-less-colleagues/

51. Nurse Salary – What do nurses earn? – HealthTimes [Internet]. [cited 2020 Jun 2]. Available from: https://healthtimes.com.au/hub/nursing-careers/6/guidance/nc1/what-do-nurses-earn/605/

52. Are you one of the "everyday Australians" politicians refer to? – ABC News [Internet]. [cited 2020 Jun 2]. Available from: https://www.abc.net.au/news/2019-12-30/are-you-one-of-the-average-australians-politicians-refer-to/11831700

53. Working conditions and salary of a nurse in Germany [Internet]. Morkel Pflegevermittlung. [cited 2020 Jun 3]. Available from: https://morkel-medpersonal.com/en/working-conditions-and-salary/

54. Canada's Health Care System [Internet]. Canada.ca. [cited 30 May 2020]. Available from: https://www.canada.ca/en/health-canada/services/health-care-system/reports-publications/ health-care-system/canada.html#a1
55. Milestones: universal policies [Internet]. Cpha.ca. 2020 [cited 30 May 2020]. Available from: https://www.cpha.ca/milestones-universal-policies
56. Allin S, Rudoler D. Canada: International Health Care System Profiles [Internet]. International. commonwealthfund.org. [cited 30 May 2020]. Available from: https://international.common-wealthfund.org/countries/canada/
57. Canadian Institute for Health Information. National Health Expenditure Trends, 1975 to 2019 [Internet]. 2020. Available from: https://www.cihi.ca/en/ national-health-expenditure-trends-1975-to-2019
58. How Much Does Canada Spend on Health Care? [Internet]. Effective Public Healthcare Panacea Project. 2020 [cited 30 May 2020]. Available from: https://www.ephpp.ca/ healthcare-funding-policy-in-canada/
59. Canadian Institute for Health Information. Age-Adjusted Public Spending per Person [Internet]. 2017. Available from: https://yourhealthsystem.cihi.ca/hsp/inbrief?lang=en#!/ indicators/014/age-adjusted-public-spending-per-person/;mapC1;mapLevel2;/
60. What OHIP Covers [Internet]. Ontario.ca. 2020 [cited 30 May 2020]. Available from: https:// www.ontario.ca/page/what-ohip-covers
61. Canadian Institute for Health Information. Physicians in Canada, 2018 [Internet]. 2020. Available from: https://www.cihi.ca/en/physicians-in-canada
62. Barua B, Jacques D. Comparing performance of universal healthcare countries, 2018 [Internet]. Fraser Institute: Vancouver; 2018. Available from: https://www.fraserinstitute.org/stud-ies/comparing-performance-of-universal-health-care-countries-2018?utm_source=Media-Releases&utm_campaign=Comparing-Performance-of-Universal-Health-Care-Countries-2018&utm_medium=Media&utm_content=Learn_More&utm_term=700
63. NHS statistics, facts and figures – NHS Confederation [Internet]. [cited 2020 May 31]. Available from: https://www.nhsconfed.org/resources/key-statistics-on-the-nhs
64. Healthcare in Mexico – International Living Countries [Internet]. International Living. [cited 2020 Jun 3]. Available from: https://internationalliving.com/countries/mexico/health-care/
65. HealthManagement.org. Radiology Management, ICU Management, Healthcare IT, Cardiology Management, Executive Management [Internet]. HealthManagement. [cited 2020 Jun 3]. Available from: https://healthmanagement.org/c/icu/issuearticle/ the-mexican-healthcare-system
66. About the Panama Health Care System – 3 Parts [Internet]. Living In Panama – Advice & Information. 2013 [cited 2020 Jun 3]. Available from: http://livinginpanama.com/ living-in-panama/health-care-system/
67. Panama improves access to health care system [Internet]. Oxford Business Group. 2015 [cited 2020 Jun 3]. Available from: https://oxfordbusinessgroup.com/overview/ towards-universal-coverage-improving-access-further-integration-health-care-system
68. Campion EW, Morrissey S. A different model — medical care in Cuba. N Engl J Med. 2013;368(4):297–9.
69. Warner R. Is the Cuban healthcare system really as great as people claim? [Internet]. The Conversation. [cited 2020 Jun 3]. Available from: http://theconversation.com/ is-the-cuban-healthcare-system-really-as-great-as-people-claim-69526
70. Massuda A, Hone T, Leles FAG, de Castro MC, Atun R. The Brazilian health system at crossroads: progress, crisis and resilience. BMJ Glob Health. 2018;3(4):e000829. https://doi. org/10.1136/bmjgh-2018-000829.
71. Healthcare in Argentina: Public & Private Hospital Information [Internet]. International Living. [cited 2020 Jun 3]. Available from: https://internationalliving.com/countries/argentina/ health-care-in-argentina/
72. Healthcare in Colombia: Low Cost and High Quality [Internet]. International Living. [cited 2020 Jun 3]. Available from: https://internationalliving.com/countries/colombia/ healthcare-in-colombia/

73. Venezuela's Health Care System Ready To Collapse Amid Economic Crisis [Internet]. NPR.org. [cited 2020 Jun 3]. Available from: https://www.npr.org/2018/02/01/582469305/venezuelas-health-care-system-ready-to-collapse-amid-economic-crisis

74. Long G. Venezuela crisis: malaria spreads as economy implodes [Internet]. 2019 [cited 2020 Jun 3]. Available from: https://www.ft.com/content/d980c25a-4fbc-11e9-8f44-fe4a86c48b33

75. Guide to Health Insurance and Healthcare System in South Korea|InterNations GO [Internet]. [cited 2020 May 30]. Available from: https://www.internations.org/go/moving-to-south-korea/healthcare

76. South Korea: national health spending 2018 [Internet]. Statista. [cited 2020 May 30]. Available from: https://www.statista.com/statistics/647320/health-spending-south-korea/

77. Guide to Health Insurance and Healthcare System in the UAE|InterNations GO! [Internet]. [cited 2020 May 30]. Available from: https://www.internations.org/go/moving-to-the-uae/healthcare

78. Healthcare Resource Guide: United Arab Emirates [cited 2020 May 30]. Available from: https://2016.export.gov/industry/health/healthcareresourceguide/eg_main_108626.asp

79. What are Electronic Medical Records?|USF Health Online [Internet]. [cited 2020 Jun 23]. Available from: https://www.usfhealthonline.com/resources/key-concepts/what-are-electronic-medical-records-emr/

80. What are the differences between electronic medical records, electronic health records, and personal health records?|HealthIT.gov [Internet]. [cited 2020 Jun 23]. Available from: https://www.healthit.gov/faq/what-are-differences-between-electronic-medical-records-electronic-health-records-and-personal

81. PSNC. Electronic health records – local and national initiatives [Internet]. PSNC Main site. [cited 2020 Jun 23]. Available from: https://psnc.org.uk/contract-it/pharmacy-it/electronic-health-records/electronic-health-records-list/

82. Electronic Health Records Vulnerable to Security Breaches|Kidney News [Internet]. [cited 2020 Jun 23]. Available from: https://www.kidneynews.org/kidney-news/cover-story/electronic-health-records-vulnerable-to-security-breaches

Chapter 4
The Life of International Medical Graduates in the USA: A Psychiatrist's Perspective

Noorulain Aqeel

Background

According to a report published in the *Journal of Graduate Medical Education* in 2018, about 25% of all practicing physicians in the USA are IMGs who play a vital role in serving the community by maintaining high standards and quality of service [1]. This piece is an attempt at delineating the numerous yet intricate cultural and emotional barriers that many of us faced as IMGs. When I was asked to author this chapter, I was transported back to 1990, the year I first came to the USA, as a fresh medical graduate from Pakistan. I arrived in Chicago, IL, with very little knowledge of the country and its systems, and all I knew was that I wanted to pursue postgraduate training in the USA for the betterment of my career and the future of my family. Arriving with my wife, I anticipated early in my journey that things were not going to be easy for me. I will forever remain grateful to my aunt and uncle who welcomed us into their home back then and whose kindness goes unmeasured to date.

As an IMG, I not only had to blend into a new environment but also operate at the intersection of immigration and acculturation, while familiarizing myself with a new and advanced healthcare system.

The Struggle

The transition was not a simple one by any means, but I was not alone in my struggles. Most of my friends who had travelled to the USA with the same vision as mine were also struggling with similar adaptation challenges in a new and frantic norm. Of course, the hurdles that came their way and the influences they had on their lives

N. Aqeel (✉)
Napa State Hospital, Napa, CA, USA

varied according to each individual, yet the underlying nature of the hardship remained the same. After speaking with many IMGs who have now settled into their lives, and are now past most of the hurdles required to reach a point of comfort along with reviewing and analyzing the results from the survey I had them all take, made me realize that each person experienced those challenges differently and developed unique mechanisms to learn and grow from them; it was as if each person who endured these obstructions along the journey were equipped with lifelong lessons and attributes which are now necessary tools of survival.

Some of us were fortunate enough to have extended families who were already living/migrated in America and could provide crucial support at a time of immense uncertainty. These lucky individuals did not have to worry about accommodation or rent and were able to dedicate more time toward preparing their board exams, thus increasing their chances of getting a higher score.

In many cases, IMGs struggle to achieve financial independence. Many of us found ourselves negotiating for extra hours, trying to pick up extra shifts working as security guards at the mall, to delivering medicine for pharmacies, to even being a cashier at your local supermarket. We could not help but compare our current situations to our lives a few months earlier, where we were all practicing physicians back in our home countries. For instance, I had gone from working in the emergency department of a trauma center in Karachi to working in a diagnostic lab in Chicago within a matter of months. My experience in clinical pathology allowed me to secure a job in the medical field, which was probably less ego-dystonic than finding work unrelated to medicine, a fate that many IMGs had to come across. I found additional work on some weekends at a pharmacy delivering medications and providing support in sales. Naturally, working multiple jobs left me little time to focus on my primary goal, which was to pass my first board exam. I had to fit studying into every opportunity that became available; some customers at the checkout line marveled at the books spread out behind the cash register at the pharmacy as I rang up their items.

The Sacrifice

It became clear to me that the dedication required to prepare for the USMLE exam would mean that I would not be able to spend as much time with my wife and newborn son. After leaving the lab at the end of the day, I would head straight to the library. By the time that I got home, my son would already be asleep. Knowing there was no other way for me to hear his voice, I would often call home from a payphone at the library and listen to him even just cry for a few minutes before returning to my books; this would motivate me each time to grind harder.

A couple of years later, we moved to California where my schedule allowed me to study at the clubhouse in our apartment complex as I continued to dedicate as much time as possible toward preparing for the exam, all while balancing multiple jobs and learning how to navigate through unfamiliarity each step of the way. I remember my son and his mother walking over every evening from our apartment to the clubhouse with my tea. I would play with my son for a while but ultimately had to return to my books despite the intense desire to spend more time playing with him. I found it difficult to concentrate on my studies after these brief moments of profound emotion which often lead my mind to wander and drift toward thoughts of "what if." What if I don't get a competitive score on my exam, what if I don't ever get into residency?" These questions would haunt my daily routine, yet at the same time be my motivation to succeed, for the sake of my family; there was no turning back and going back to Pakistan empty handed.

Unfortunately I had to take the Step 1 exam more than once and clearly remember failing by just 1 point, each of my first two of my attempts. Everything that I had struggled so hard for shattered in those moments of failure. I had even sold my car to be able to pay the examination fee. Nothing had changed yet hours of work had gone to waste. I was full of self-doubt and could not help but question my potential.

The Fight with Fear

Another interesting phenomenon which most, if not all, IMGs experience is the paradox of fear. Life as a foreign resident is definitely challenging, and there were numerous obstacles one must overcome to survive in the world of medicine. What all these challenges seem to have in common is "fear" and "unpredictability." However, this very fear of failure drives one to do their very best. They are intensely aware of each sacrifice made and the amount of motivation required to move forward.

The Residency Match

I finally passed my board exams after a few attempts and moved on to the next hurdle at hand: applying into residency programs. The first time that I applied, I recall appearing for nine interviews and travelling to different states, but the result was not a celebratory one. While struggling to match into a program, I continued to volunteer at a research facility at the University of California, Irvine. The following year, I matched into a psychiatry residency program in New York City, affiliated with New York Medical College.

The Residency Challenges: Cultural Issues

It was no surprise that residency would bring a completely new set of challenges. A massive struggle for IMGs was to navigate dual learning curves as immigrants and as residents. While IMGs were expected to master the clinical practice of medicine in such a short period and play catchup with American medical graduates, the US system does not take into account the differences in medical knowledge IMGs may carry from their home countries. Residents from developing countries may have very different perceptions of and experiences with healthcare, so it was also expected that there might be a lag for clinical and social practices to be learned and digested.

Additionally, immigrants were challenged with a new culture of medicine in which they must adapt to the expectations of patients, colleagues, and supervisors and learn appropriate behavior and practices in the workplace, which may differ from certain policies and normalities from your respected country of origin [2].

A fitting example that comes to mind is an interaction I had early in my residency training in New York. I had just started as an intern in a hospital in Manhattan and had to admit a patient into the psychiatric service for new-onset psychosis and aggressive behavior to the nursing staff at his respective nursing home. Tired and exhausted, working on my seventh admission of the night, I walked into his room and asked him how he was doing; he looked at me and said, "Not so hot." His response seemed strange to me and made me more perplexed, since it was snowing outside. I thought that he might be complaining about the temperature in the room not being warm enough or being too cold. Immediately I approached the thermostat and started adjusting the temperature to help him feel more comfortable. That was when the patient exclaimed and almost yelled at me in his New York accent, "Man, what the hell you are doing!" I then realized that he was not talking about the temperature at all, but instead, he meant to say that he was not doing well. Over the years, I went through many experiences in which I misinterpreted the vocabulary used by local residents. I eventually became more familiar with new idioms and phrases reflective of the local culture and language, but not until I experienced a few more similar situations.

Another example of a culture shock experience was when I was once interviewing a patient who told me he was suffering from depression and anxiety at an outpatient follow-up visit. I asked him if there was anything going on in his life that might be contributing toward his depression; he took a second to gather his thoughts and then he started crying and told me "I fell off the wagon." I was puzzled and began asking him if he had forgotten to fasten some kind of seatbelt or if the wagon was moving too fast. Did he fall out of the door? Did he trip? I began looking at his knees and hands, scanning him for possible injuries, but found nothing. After a few moments of visible confusion on both of our faces, he explained that he drank alcohol for the first time after 10 years of sobriety.

Textbooks, too, highlighted these cultural differences. I recall reading a textbook of pathology by an American author during medical school that talked about uric acid crystals shaped like a football. Coming from a country where football is the term used for soccer, played with a round ball, I always wondered why the elliptical-shaped crystals were compared to a round (soccer) ball. It was years later while watching American football that I realized that the ball was elliptical shaped and, hence, the description of crystals in the books.

Other instances differentiated between the way IMGs and the local residents understood emotions and processed feelings. For instance, I remember trying to discharge a patient to a local shelter in New York City during my first year of training. As I took his history during admission, the patient mentioned that he had a brother who lived in an apartment in Manhattan. Coming from a collectivist culture, it made perfect sense to me for the patient to go to his brother in New York City. Without giving it another thought, I asked him, "Why would you rather go to a shelter when your brother lives in New York City?" For me, it was an obvious question, but the patient looked at me in complete disbelief and replied, "Doc, what does he have to do with me? I need to go back to the shelter, why do I have to go to him?" While I may belong to a country, where family members are very involved in each other's lives and living with extended families is a norm, my patient came from an individualistic culture in which moving out of parents' house at the age of 18 is an understood and expected thing to happen.

Apart from interactions with patients, interactions in the workplace posed their own set of challenges. Just a few days into my internship in a new culture, I found that the professional practices I learned back home did not always conform to cultural norms in the USA. In Pakistan, whenever a teacher or instructor entered the room, it was customary to stand as a sign of respect. Hence, every time my attending physician entered the room, I would quickly stand up. I'm sure she had come across her fair share of diverse cultural norms from dealing with many IMGs in training, and after a couple of instances of noticing my behavior, she told me that she appreciated and valued my cultural practice and asked me not to stand up every time she entered the room and reassured that no one would take it as disrespect if I stayed seated.

These cultural barriers naturally extend into academia as well. In a survey that I conducted prior to writing this chapter, a fellow IMG recounted his experience while taking an exam. He received a question in which a patient had quit an addiction "cold turkey." After finishing the exam, he expressed his frustration to his fellow examinees and how the choices in the answers were completely unexpected. He had interpreted the question as pertaining to some type of gastrointestinal infection, but none of the given choices had anything to do with food poisoning or frozen turkey. As you can imagine, he was confused and, as a result, was going down on the wrong path to answer this question.

As my time in America progressed, so did my curiosity. I stumbled across a concept known as a "meme." Today, a meme refers to a specific Internet phenomenon, but originally, a "meme" was a component of culture, passed on to others via cultural exchange. Nowadays the power of the Internet has propelled the transfer of information from person to person in a matter of seconds.

To understand this better, let us compare it to the building blocks of genetics, i.e., the gene. The difference is that a gene passes from one individual to another to continue the thread of life. Memes pass from one human being to another by nongenetic means, by simple act of imitation. This imitation generally catalyzes the further spread of culture. If humans grew up, away from civilization, their natural instincts might be well developed but their cultural identity would not. They would be unable to grasp the concept of language or speech and would be a stranger to literature, religion, law, and science. These disciplines and concepts are forwarded or exchanged through a cultural phenomenon and not just genetically.

Other Challenges: Paving the Way for Future Generations

A popular issue for IMGs, which is beyond the scope of this chapter, is that of the process immigration itself, which is the biggest challenge of them all. Some IMGs have had to serve in underdeveloped areas of the USA in order to qualify for immigrant status. Moreover, the process itself is long and tiresome. Additionally, in order to adapt to the US healthcare system, one has to unlearn some legal, ethical, and clinical aspects, which we learned in medical school and clinical rotation. Thus, foreign students coming to the USA and those going to foreign countries from the USA, both, have their own set of challenges to overcome in their journey of being international medical graduates.

My first child was born in Chicago and raised in California. He went to further his education experience by pursuing medical school in Pakistan. An amazing nostalgic feeling rushed through my mind, but this time my son was leaving the USA and entering a new country and culture to pursue medicine.

Through my son's journey as an international student, I have not only been able to compare his experiences with my own but also witness him enjoy his time in Pakistan. While I was flustered by the changes that came with me moving to a new country, my son seemed to flourish in his new environment. Not only did he have extended family to fall back on, but Karachi also exposed him to a newfound freedom. For instance, his perception of travelling the streets changed while he lived in Karachi, a city with the population of more than 25 million. He experienced a lifestyle and culture that was exciting, spontaneous, and definitely more adventurous. Jaywalking had a thrill of its own, as did travelling in rickshaws and grabbing a cup of chai at 3 am with a side of a kabob roll fresh off the grill. Local street foods opened up an even bigger world of possibilities, not only enhancing his approach to cultural delicacies but also enhancing his palate as well. The longer he spent in Pakistan, the more accustomed he became to the local slang and vocabulary.

Living in Pakistan also made him more street smart. He learned to bargain, negotiate, and interact with local vendors without feeling like an outsider. Most importantly, he had the opportunity to experiment, take chances, grow, and be able to adopt a different culture.

After spending 5 years in Pakistan, my son returned to the USA as an IMG, but for him there were no cultural-linguistic barriers, no worries about finding a place to live, or the guilt of leaving his family. For him, the process simply meant returning home. That is not to say that applying for residency did not pose any challenges for him. He was born in the USA, received college education, completed requirements for admission and went overseas, and came back as a foreign medical graduate. In addition, he automatically had some less advantage against those who attended medical school in the USA.

Conclusion

My life story depicts the scenarios and the situations that most of IMGs face up to some extent: the challenges of moving to a new country and learning a new culture, the stress of applying for a residency position, and the inevitable thought of returning home empty handed. However, with determination, dedication, and hard work and of course with the blessing of God, any goal can be achieved. Surely, IMGs can beat these challenges if they are willing to face the pain associated with this process. In the journey of recognitions and discovery, I realized how important it is to enjoy the moment, to appreciate the blessings, and to acknowledge them.

Polish-British writer Joseph Conrad once said, "The world little knows or cares about the storm through which you have had to pass. It asks only if you brought the ship safely to port." There is nothing easy about this journey, but there is relief in knowing that we are not alone on it. We are all drops of water making our way into the ocean, carrying our languages, our cultures, our beliefs in one direction and contributing toward a greater vision. Our struggle to fit and blend in makes us realize that while culture is a melting pot, it does not have a standard recipe. It leaves room for each of us to bring our own legacy and ingredients to produce a result that is bigger than the individual elements.

In a poem titled *Fear*, Khalil Gibran illustrates the risk it takes to leave everything behind and merge into something much bigger than our individual entities. A river is beautiful and vast on its own, but going into the ocean, it feels so much smaller, so insignificant. The river needs to take the risk of entering the ocean, because only then will fear vanish. It is then the river realizes that it is not risking its existence and disappearing into the ocean, but rewarded, as it becomes the ocean.

References

1. Ahmed A, Hwang W, Thomas C, Deville C. International Medical Graduates in the US physician workforce and graduate medical education: current and historical trends. J Grad Med Educ. 2018;10(2):214–8.
2. Chen PG, Curry LA, Bernheim SM, Berg D, Gozu A, Nunez-Smith M. Professional challenges of non-U.S.-born international medical graduates and recommendations for support during residency training. Acad Med. 2011;86(11):1383–8.

Dr. Noorulain Aqeel is an attending psychiatrist at Napa State Hospital, Napa, California. He is a graduate from Sindh Medical College from Karachi, Pakistan, and has completed his residency in General Psychiatry. He then went on to pursue a fellowship in Geriatric Psychiatry from Brown University School of Medicine. He is board certified in General Psychiatry, Addiction Medicine, and Geriatric Psychiatry and has also taken special interest in subspecialties to include Consultation and Liaison Psychiatry (Psychosomatic Medicine) and Psychodermatology. Dr. Aqeel also serves as an associate professor of Psychiatry at the California Northstate University College of Medicine and Touro University School of Osteopathic Medicine, California.

Chapter 5
The Triangle of Residency

Hassaan Tohid

Introduction

It has already been discussed in other chapters of this book how international medical graduates (IMGs) apply for the United States (US) clinical residency positions each year and the hurdles and constraints they face during the process.

In this chapter, I will highlight what I call "The Big Three" and "The Triangle of Residency" (see Fig. 5.1). This triangle of residency includes the three essential things that every IMG should have on his/her curriculum vitae (CV) to be more competitive for the residency match. I have noticed during my teaching and mentoring career that these three essential things serve to be decisive factors in IMG residency match applications. These three things are the United States Medical Licensing Examination (USMLE) [1], any US clinical experience they may have, and last of all, research experience or publications [2]. If any of these factors are missing, applicants greatly reduce their chances of matching. This is common knowledge and most IMGs are already aware of it. However, what many IMGs do not know is how to surpass these targets, how to pass the USMLEs, how to get clinical experience, and how research opportunities are found.

Not knowing these technicalities and details will seriously hamper their chances of getting a residency match. Having enough clinical experience gives them the idea of how things work in the US and it also gives them an opportunity to earn some reasonable letters of recommendation (LoRs) to apply for a residency match. The healthcare system in the US is different from many other countries; therefore, the residency directors are expecting IMGs to gain some US experience before applying for the match. This is not an unreasonable expectation considering IMGs need to learn the culture, customs, language (which is the biggest problem for many

H. Tohid (✉)
California Institute of Behavioral Neurosciences and Psychology, Fairfield, CA, USA

© Springer Nature Switzerland AG 2021   89
H. Tohid, H. Maibach (eds.), *International Medical Graduates in the United States*, https://doi.org/10.1007/978-3-030-62249-7_5

Fig. 5.1 The triangle of residency, which includes USMLE, US clinical experience, and research experience or publications

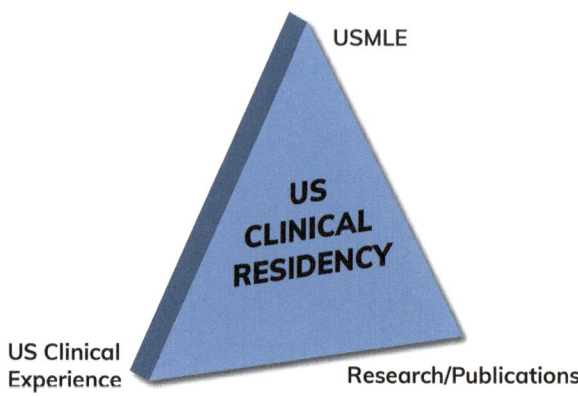

IMGs), and at the same time the US healthcare system and revise their medical knowledge.

The research experience not only enhances their knowledge about the subject but also gives them some publications (if they are lucky). Getting research experience is also essential in getting some letters of recommendation and some contacts that can help them get some interviews and learn about the research world. The research world can also open doors for them in other domains such as the academic world and possibly even obtain jobs as scientists. Therefore, getting research experience can help them secure their career by finding alternate paths in case they change their mind, or they do not match into a residency program. Having publications can help them get jobs as research assistants or coordinators and can also help them start an alternate career as a teacher in academia. Many IMGs are aware of the importance of research and the options it provides them for their career. However, they do not actually know how to find such positions and how to publish papers.

In this chapter, I will highlight some points on US clinical experience, USMLEs, and research experience.

United States Medical Licensing Examination (USMLE)

The one thing that now almost all IMGs unanimously are aware of is the need of passing the USMLE to be eligible for the US residency match, regardless of their specialty. As discussed previously, the USMLE is a three-step exam. It is a computer-based exam and is taken in a Prometric center designed to conduct the USMLE online. Step 1 of USMLEs is a basic science exam, while Step 2 is a clinical knowledge (CK) exam. Step 2 is also divided into clinical knowledge (CK) and clinical skill (CS) [1, 3]. However, due to COVID-19, the Step 2 CS is suspended for a few months as of August 2020 and is replaced with an English language test known as occupational english test (OET). After Step 1 and Step 2 are passed, the students are educational commission for foreign medical graduates (ECFMG) certified and are usually eligible for the US residency (due to COVID-19 a pathway system has been introduced for the IMGs to apply for US residency without CS; this arrangement seems temporary until the pandemic is under control). Once the students are ECFMG certified, they are eligible for the Step 3 exam, which is a 2-day exam.

The IMGs ideally should start preparing for these exams during medical school just like many American medical students. If they prepare for the exams during their medical school education, it will save them a lot of time and it will be easier because of already being in the momentum of studies. However, many IMGs do not consider it as an easy task to take the USMLEs during medical school because of various reasons such as the difference of the curriculum and focus. They prepare either for their medical school exams or for the USMLEs. Therefore, doing both at the same time can be a daunting task. They may take the exams as soon as they graduate or prepare for a year after graduating and then take the exam, whatever suits them. However, the more they delay, the older the year of graduation becomes, which makes it more challenging for the IMGs to match. With every year they delay, the chances of matching reduce. Thus, IMGs should be careful about deciding when to take the exam and how long they should delay the exam post-graduation.

The test itself is considered by many as one of the toughest professional exams and stressful for IMGs [4, 5]. To prepare for the exam IMGs must remember not to re-invent the wheel. Utilizing the resources used by other IMGs who successfully passed the exam should be the key approach in taking it. They should ask their seniors or find successful candidates who passed the exam, on social media. The most commonly used books to pass the Step 1 USMLE are Kaplan Lecture Notes, the Step 1 First Aid Book, and UWorld Question Bank and/or Kaplan QBank. For Step 2, Kaplan Lecture Notes and UWorld/Kaplan Question Bank are commonly used. For the CS exam, most students use First Aid or Kaplan core case books and other similar resources such as UW. As time passes, the exam will inevitably be modified and so will the resources to study. As of 2020, the resources mentioned above are most commonly used. Therefore, the IMGs should keep the approach of always being aware of the current trends and what other successful candidates do.

The information on how to enroll for the exam and the cost is available on the ECFMG website. Students planning to enroll should get the information from authentic websites rather than believing on word of mouth.

Before students can appear for the exam, they need to fill out the form 186 for their credential's confirmation. This is required by the ECFMG to verify the student's identity diploma/degree of a foreign medical graduate. Although the form is not needed per se to appear for the exam, it is needed for complete transparency of information. It remains valid indefinitely [6].

US Clinical Experience

International medical graduates come from different countries around the world with different healthcare systems, different cultures, and different ways of medical practice. Therefore, not only do many residency programs require them to get some

US clinical experience, but also it is needed at the time as well. During the clinical experience, the IMGs can learn how doctors practice in the US and how things actually work in the country, including the patient's behavior, fellow doctors' behavior, the administration, the billing system, the diagnostic procedures (which were not always readily available in their own countries), and many other details that are useful for them to acclimatize with the US system.

The ideal time for the IMGs to start US clinical rotations varies. Some students do their clinical rotations when they are medical students, while some wait until they graduate. If they do get accepted for clinical rotations, they travel to the US besides completing the pre-requisites of the hospital or the university program they applied for. The process could be daunting for most IMGs due to the financial burden associated with the process, yet many IMGs give it a try. The clinical rotations they do during their medical school times are commonly known as "Electives," while the same clinical rotation, if done after graduation, is called either "Observership" or "Externship."

The IMGs who usually want to start their clinical rotations after graduation then come to the US to start their rotation. They usually prepare for the USMLEs and do their clinical rotation at the same time. It is obviously challenging, but these hardworking IMGs do it anyway in order to be more competitive for the residency match. They understand that without US clinical experience, the chances of them matching are very slim.

One of the great challenges these IMGs often face is how to find US clinical experience. Many of their seniors and social media peers do tell them the importance of US clinical experience, but very few of the IMGs are aware of how to find such positions. There are several ways IMGs can find proper clinical rotations in the US.

Internet Search

By far the most common way to look for US clinical experience is by simply googling it. By just typing the keywords "US clinical expression for IMGs" in the Google search bar can give various options and a lot of information on available opportunities for clinical experience.

Personal Connections

It is a well-known way of finding opportunities of clinical experience. Asking one's peers, friends, seniors, classmates, and family is a very useful and time-proven way of finding such opportunities. There are various organizations that help IMGs in finding these placements.

Contacting Hospitals and Programs

The students can also contact the programs directly by just making a phone call or simply sending an email of inquiry. The key to this approach is to overcome the feelings of shyness and just take action. Many IMGs are pleasantly surprised by the immediate yes many receive after following this approach. The best way that works in the favor of IMGs is the law of averages. The law of averages almost always gives them the one yes they are looking for. In my personal experience showing up physically and asking for the opportunity is the most powerful way of getting it.

Almost all the states in the US have such opportunities available and simply just asking works every time. Therefore, IMGs should keep looking and never give up, because finding clinical experience is not an option, it is a compulsory requirement for the residency match.

Types of Clinical Experience

There are various types of clinical experience available for IMGs. The following are the most common types of clinical experience in the US:

1. Electives
2. Externships (hands-on clinical experience)
3. Volunteer work
4. Observerships
5. Others

Electives

When IMGs do a few weeks or months of clinical rotations in the United States before graduation, it is known as electives. The opportunities of electives are found by following any of the approaches or all the approaches mentioned above [7].

Externships

This is a hands-on experience and difficult to find in comparison to an observership. Yet, it is possible to find. In some states such as California, the hands-on clinical experience for IMGs is not possible, but many other states do provide this opportunity.

Volunteering

Volunteering at a private organization is illegal in the US; however, IMGs can volunteer at a public hospital or university. Volunteering can be simply assisting in nature or like a scrub job. The IMGs can also work in the rehabilitation or drug addiction treatment facilities as a volunteer. These organizations are usually non-profit and always welcome volunteers. These kinds of volunteer positions cannot just give them an additional point to mention on their CV, but can also provide them with clinical experience. It can be like hitting two birds with one stone.

For psychiatry applicants especially, these volunteer positions at substance use treatment programs can be ideal to also learn counseling and get clinical experience at the same time.

Thus, there are so many volunteer opportunities that can help IMGs get some clinical experience of different varieties. IMGs should look for such opportunities especially if it relates to their own field of choice.

Observership

Another useful clinical experience is observership. During observership, as the name suggests, the IMGs can only observe but do not get hands-on clinical experience. Of course, it is normal to assume that hands-on experience is worth more than observerships, but it is also true that something is better than nothing. Observerships can also help the IMGs get some useful letters of recommendation (LoRs).

Other Opportunities

Anyone working as a respiratory therapist assistant, counselor, sleep technologist, speech pathologist or assistant, or similar jobs can not only just work and make money (if he/she has legal status to work in the US) but also can show this as clinical experience on his/her CV. There are plenty of jobs like these, and IMGs can find them by properly searching for them.

Some clinical jobs that can be counted as clinical experience are as follows:

- Psychologist
- Counselors (drug addiction)
- Family therapists
- Parole agents
- Probation officers
- Speech pathologist
- Respiratory therapist
- Clinical research coordinator or assistant
- Medical scribe
- Sleep technologist, and so on.

Some of these clinical jobs are regulated, which means proper certification from the appropriate board is needed. If IMGs have a plan for alternate careers or they want to first gain some clinical experience and then later apply for the US residency match, then they can follow this approach. They can have a professional job as a clinician and get some clinical experience, and at the same time save some money and prepare for the USMLEs and residency match. This is a slow process, but this option does exist. It may take an IMG 4–5 years to be certified first, get a job, then get some clinical experience, and make money. While making money, they can prepare for the exam, and at the same time, if they feel that they do not need residency and are happy to be in a particular field, then it is up to them as well.

How Can They Make the Most Out of It?

In order to make the most out of the clinical rotations, the IMGs must develop certain qualities. The following are some of the key qualities IMGs can develop:

Responsibility

The first thing that IMGs should do is to take absolute responsibility for their careers. When they are responsible, they will likely make the most of their US clinical experience.

Respect of Time

I would like to mention a real story of an IMG. He got his observership in his desired specialty and thought, that is it. He thought he would get the LoR and would have US clinical experience to show on his CV. However, he did not take his observership seriously and was almost always 15–30 minutes late to his shifts at the hospital. The supervising physician expressed his dissatisfaction over this behavior, yet the student continued to be tardy to his shifts. As a result, the supervisor later did not issue an LoR for him. The supervisor probably thought that the LoR would harm this candidate more if they mentioned the level of his sincerity and responsibility. Therefore, being on time is the key to show your seriousness about the profession. It also is a sign of respect to everyone to be on time.

Improve Listening

It is imperative that IMGs become better listeners. They should always take notes and not interrupt the supervisor or other seniors who are with them. By being bad listeners, IMGs can severely hamper their chances of impressing anyone and earning great LoRs. They should also keep in mind that if the hospital they are associated with as an observer happens to be a residency program, then they also severely inhibit their chances of getting an interview from that program. Many IMGs think that if they just find observership at an accredited residency program, they will match. That is far from the truth. Though it is true that the chances of getting an interview at the same hospital are high, these chances depend upon the performance of the students. If they do not impress anyone and keep interrupting others instead of listening, then the chances of getting an interview reduce tremendously.

Grooming

IMGs should consider everyday as an interview day while observing at a hospital. They should keep in mind that their every movement counts. Grooming well will raise their chances of being liked and respected. Remember, getting an interview is directly related to likability.

Be a Learner

The IMGs should understand that their learning does not stop at Step 3 of USMLE. A good doctor is a life-long learner. The supervisors will respect and like the students more if they show good attitude toward learning. IMGs should have a bedside book related to their specialty such as Oxford or handbooks and keep reading and refreshing their knowledge of the books.

Positive Mental Attitude

This is by far one of the most important qualities IMGs should develop (if they do not have it already). It is rightly said by the famous coach and trainer Zig Ziglar that "it is not the aptitude but your attitude that decides your altitude." The IMGs must work on improving their attitude and learn more and more about being positive, because there is always room for improvement. There are plenty of books available on attitude that one can read and improve their personal and professional attitude.

There is so much negativity around that maintaining a positive attitude all the time is almost impossible. Therefore, continuous practice of improving one's attitude could help students tremendously.

Expense Needed to Get US Clinical Experience

It is indeed an expensive process for most IMGs, especially if they do not have family or friends in the US or they are a non-US citizen. It is easier for IMGs to find rotations near their home; however, not everyone is that lucky. Most IMGs travel farther to acquire this experience. They have to take care of living expenses, food, utilities, travel, and the fee of the hospital (if there is any), or the organization that is arranging the US clinical experience for them. The overall expense could be easily between 3000 and 5000 USD for just 1 month of rotation as of 2020. Some lucky students get it cheaper if they find rotations near their home and with contacts, but again this is difficult and not all IMGs can find these opportunities with minimal or almost no cost at all. Therefore, proper financial planning is essential to start the whole journey of USMLE.

I had a privilege to interview Jonathan Bernad, the Founder and CEO of American Clinical Experience (ACE), an organization that provides opportunities of US clinical experience. In the interview, Jon addressed some important points. The interview is as follows:

#1: "What should IMGs do to get US clinical experience?"

If a trainee is still in medical school, it is possible to apply directly to hospitals for electives. The first thing is to ask your medical school if they have any programs in place coordinated directly between the school and the hospital. There are also some hospitals that will take applications directly and process them without any school affiliation being necessary. Aside from that, it is common to tap into one's personal network of friends and family to be connected to a rotation possibility. The solution I know best is to hire an agency that has its own pre-existing relationships in place with doctors and hospitals.

#2: "Why has United States clinical experience (USCE) become a mandatory requirement?"

Well, with any job application, the employer wants to see that the applicant has some relevant experience in order to show they can handle the job in question. Because the job of a first-year resident involves taking care of patients in a US hospital setting, the program director wants to be reassured that the incoming resident can contribute as a team player to make everyone's job easier and not to be a distraction to make everyone's job harder. If someone is unfamiliar with the US system and has never been inside a US hospital, then obviously the person might take longer to adapt. As the healthcare system is different from country to country, the best type of experience to demonstrate in your CV and LoRs will be experiences with US doctors and US healthcare systems.

#3: "What strategies should IMGs use to find experiences?"

This is similar to question #1: asking your school for any programs that already exist, applying widely directly to hospitals, tapping into your personal network of friends/family members, and lastly hiring a known agency that can coordinate on your behalf.

#4: "What can IMGs do to get a strong LoR during a rotation?"

Trainees should always demonstrate the accreditation council for graduate medical education (ACGME) core competencies as these are valuable statements to later have in your LoR. Practically speaking I would say to put your phones away, be nice and professional to everyone (the entire staff – especially anyone who reports directly to the doctor or who might assist in creating or uploading the LoRs as sometimes doctors will have assistants who help on that). Always show up on time, dress appropriately, and do all of the little things correctly. Also, it is a good idea to send a picture of yourself later on when reminding the doctor to write and upload the LoR into electronic residency application service (ERAS). If possible, I suggest going one step further and visiting the doctor again during application or interview season. When face-to-face, and telling the doctor you have an interview next week at a specific hospital, the doctor is more likely to make a phone call to the program on your behalf, as you are fresh on his or her mind.

Research Experience/Publications

The third and the last corner of "The Triangle of Residency" is the research experience or publications. Many residency programs require IMGs to have some publications. Some specialties require more publications than other; however, they all unanimously see publications as an important factor in deciding to call a student for an interview. A research experience with no publication in the end is naturally considered less valuable than a research experience with publications. The factor that IMGs should be aware of is that learning to write papers is essential, and it is evident by a publication as a first author. If a student has a publication as a first author, it is considered extremely valuable. The IMGs should know the following points while finding the research experience.

What Kind of Experience It Was?

If the student was just one of the authors among a group of authors, then naturally it is less valuable on the CV. The students should also understand the study design pyramid before deciding the type of research experience. For example, writing and publishing a letter to an editor is a publication, but it is considered weaker evidence as compared to a student who writes and publishes a systematic review or a clinical trial. Therefore, study design selection is very important. Many residency directors do understand that it is not always possible for a young graduate to publish tons of articles in top journals, but they do expect at least some publications in reasonably good, indexed journals.

Where Was the Article Published?

Some IMGs believe that research experience with no publication is also considered valuable. Though I do not deny it, but I want to make a point here that in the United States, if anything is not written and documented, it means it is not done. That is the usual perception. Therefore, research experience with publications is seen with more delight and importance than a research experience without publications. Therefore, the students must learn to write and take responsibility of the project so they can finish the manuscript on their own as the first author.

The second challenge is, where is it published. The recent times have seen a bombardment of fake/fraudulent/and predatory journals. Thus, the students should check if the publisher of the journal they choose is not among the list of predatory journals. To check whether the journals are on the list, one can Google "Beall's list of predatory journals." The students should refer to Beall's list and check and confirm if the journal they have selected is from a reliable publisher.

Usually, to avoid being trapped by the predatory journals, the students should look at websites like Scimagojr or Springer for reliable journals list. Moreover, the indexing is also important in this regard. Usually the publications indexed in PubMed, PubMed Central, and Medline are seen more favorably in comparison to the articles published in other indexing. Other reliable indexing are Scopus, EMBASE, EBSCO, Web of Science, and so on.

Importance of Writing a First-Author Paper

The IMGs should strive to get a first-author publication. Usually the lab projects are run by senior professors who have grants to run the projects. Therefore, becoming a first author in that project is not feasible, especially when other students are involved as well. Obviously only one person can be a first author. Therefore, the IMGs should be proactive, and try to write some review articles such as traditional and systematic reviews to get a first-author publication. Waiting for an opportunity to get a first-author paper just wastes more time; therefore, taking action and leading one's own project is the key to get a first-author paper. Of course, it is not possible without learning to write; therefore, the students should be open to learn how to write and publish. There are plenty of courses available that teach how to write and publish. We at the California Institute of Behavioral Neurosciences and Psychology (CIBNP) initiated writing and publishing training, and successfully helped IMGs become published authors in a reasonably short span of time. In this training program, the IMGs get a chance to write and publish their first-author review article (systematic or traditional review) while learning side by side.

The students must remember that having a publication as the first author is considered way more important than other publications, but the publications as second author, third author, and so forth are also worth a lot. It is the thought that having something is better than nothing. Moreover, a low-quality publication as the first author versus a high-quality publication in a renowned PubMed indexed journal will be looked at differently. Using common sense is always the best approach.

Be Careful

The IMGs must be careful about shady publication practices. Some people sell publications where the students do not work or contribute in anyway whatsoever on the articles and just pay to have their names in publications. Buying one's names in publications is more harmful than good for various reasons. The main reason is that there are no shortcuts in life. What students usually think is the easy way actually turns out to be the hard way. Because the program directors may ask relevant questions pertaining to the project and not working hard and buying one's way to publications can expose them. Moreover, in order to get into the fellowship programs, having publications is a plus point. Thus, if a student never learned to write, it will be apparent to the directors that he/she lied about his/her publication. Recovering from such a loss of respect and trust is very difficult, it can be detrimental for one's career.

The IMGs must also remember that all these means of buying publications turn out to be scams and they charge them a handsome amount of money. Then, in the end, the paper, it is just published in a predatory journal. Thus, being careful and being a person of integrity is the key to success.

When Should They Start Finding Research Opportunities?

There is no ideal time to start looking for such opportunities. If students can get an opportunity in their medical school times, then it is a good start. Managing time with studies could be challenging, but it can be done by proper management. Many medical schools around the world also provide opportunities for conducting some kind of research. However, the students can also find research electives and be a part of some research projects in the United States. This process is expensive, yet possible and many students do it. If they are lucky, they may get some publications during this time. However, if the students feel that they are really busy and do not have time, then they may wait until they graduate to find such opportunities. They should also keep in mind that the more they delay the less publications they may get.

How to Find It?

The approach to find such opportunities is exactly the same as finding clinical rotations. The students can use personal connections or directly contacting the research labs or scientists who are conducting projects. They may also contact different university's human resources department or student affairs to collect more information about how they can go about it. The key to remember is that if they remain persistent, they can find such opportunities. Applying and contacting various places at the same time is the key. The students should not wait for one place to reject their application, or request and keep applying. One more strategy they must adopt is to do continuous follow-up. Following up with the scientist, lab manager, or HR of a university will help and do wonders, proving they are serious about finding such opportunities. Many students are reluctant to approach directly and following up because of being shy. The shyness will just do more harm than good. They should be confident and persistent enough to find a desired position.

How to Learn to Write?

Once IMGs find such positions, they should strive to learn to write papers on their own so that they can obtain an authorship, and at the same time, they should try to write some kind of manuscript to get a first-author publication. There are plenty of courses available nowadays to teach IMGs how to write. This information is easily available on the internet. There are plenty of books also available on this subject that may help the students improve their writing skills. However, most students who have not written anything before in their careers should try to enroll in an online or offline course to learn how to properly write so they can become independent writers. Research writing is not difficult if one is determined and motivated enough to do whatever it takes to succeed.

Types of Research Experience

Most common types of research experience are

1. In-person experience
2. Online research training with publication opportunity

In-person Experience

This is the most commonly known research experience where the students assist a professor/scientist who has grants and is running a research project in a lab or clinical setting. There are several types of studies the students can participate in. The following are the list of some study designs that IMGs can be a part of in an in-person research experience:

1. Clinical Trials or Experiments:

   The clinical trials are the experimental studies also known as "Interventional Studies" where a researcher intervenes or manipulates the environment and then observes, follows up, and studies the effects of that intervention. The clinical trials are of two main types: randomized control trial or non-randomized control trial (quasi-experiment). These opportunities are easily found by searching different well-known university websites. Another way to find such opportunities is by typing on Google "Clinical Trials Near Me?" The IMGs will be pleasantly surprised by the number of search results showing some clinical trials being conducted near them; they can directly call them or just visit them and request to be a volunteer. If they have legal status to work in the US, then they may apply to work as an employee and get paid while getting research experience.

2. Observational Studies:

   Another broad category of study design is observational studies. There are various kinds such as cohort studies, case-control studies, cross-sectional studies, longitudinal studies, and case series. These opportunities are also available if the students look at renowned university program's websites and contact the lab director or manager directly.

3. Other Opportunities:

   The other designs are case studies, animal studies, or in vitro studies. All of these are considered weak evidence on a study design pyramid, but they can still help IMGs get some publications. The IMGs applying for residency match should also keep in mind that any publication helps, and the residency directors know that it is not always possible for everyone to find clinical trial experience. Therefore, their effort of working on any project and getting publications will be looked at with admiration.

Remote or Online Research/Publication Opportunities

Now students can learn to write and publish papers sitting in the comfort of their home. The CIBNP remote research writing and publishing program (Be a Published Author Program) is an example. In these opportunities the students can actually learn and write the strongest research evidence on study design pyramid such as systematic reviews/meta-analysis, or case studies, traditional reviews, letter to the editor, and so on [8].

Expense

Finding research positions even as a volunteer can be an expensive process. The IMGs must plan wisely and calculate the expenses for traveling, living, utilities, and others. However, the remote opportunities are far more economical than in-person opportunities. If IMGs want in-person opportunities, then finding such opportunities near their home is the best way.

How to Make the Most Out of Research Opportunities?

The philosophy remains the same. The IMGs must show positive attitude, punctuality of time, discipline, good behavior, and great listening skills. However, to get strong LoRs and publications, the students must learn writing. Research writing is an essential task that all IMGs must learn; if they do so, the chances of getting first-author publications increase tremendously. The principal investigators (the supervising scientists) will be very likely to use the skills by IMGs and will be happy to add their names in research papers. On the other hand, if the opportunity is remote, they should learn to write, so they can lead a project of higher research evidence such as a systematic review.

Once the rotation or research experience is over, staying connected with the supervisor and other team members is very important.

Conclusion

It is an open secret that IMGs applying for the US residency match each year need to focus on other things besides high scores. Of course, if the scores are unusually high such as 270 plus (which is very rare), then the students may get plenty of interviews. However, under normal circumstances, with normal USMLE scores such as 230 to 240 (remember the Step 1 scoring system will be eliminated after 2021), the students must show more valuable experience on their CVs such as US clinical experience and research experience (US or non-US), ideally with publications.

Finding US clinical experience and research opportunities are daunting tasks. However, with proper planning and determination, it is possible. The IMGs must look for such opportunities and make the most out of them by taking them seriously. The triangle of residency is "USMLEs, US clinical experience, and research opportunities with publications." The letters of recommendation are the end result of US clinical and research experiences. Therefore, running after letters is not a wise approach, but focusing on the triangle and performing one's best is the key to success.

Some IMGs think that they need strong LoRs. This is the wrong thing to focus on because the LoRs are earned with your performance. The letters of recommendation are the end result or effect of a "cause," and the cause is performing well during these clinical and research positions or opportunities. Thus, focusing on the cause is the best approach, and the effect will happen on its own.

Acknowledgments I am thankful to Jonathan Bernad from ACE for taking out time for this interview.

Conflict of Interest Dr. Hassaan Tohid is the founder and CEO of California Institute of Behavioral Neurosciences and Psychology, an organization that helps IMGs with remote research.

References

1. USMLE Score Interpretation Guidelines. 2015 ed. Available from: https://www.usmle.org/pdfs/transcripts/USMLE_Step_Examination_Score_Interpretation_Guidelines.pdf
2. Rogers CR, Gutowski KA, Munoz-Del Rio A, Larson DL, Edwards M, Hansen JE, Lawrence WT, Stevenson TR, Bentz ML. Integrated plastic surgery residency applicant survey: characteristics of successful applicants and feedback about the interview process. Plast Reconstr Surg. 2009;123(5):1607–17.
3. US Medical Licensing Examination, 2019 Bulletin of Information. National Board of Medical Examiners. [cited 2018 Sep 15]. Available from: https://www.usmle.org/pdfs/bulletin/2019bulletin.pdf. [Ref list].
4. Sturesson L, Heiding A, Olsson D, Stenfors T. 'Did I pass the licensing exam? 'aspects influencing migrant physicians' results: a mixed methods study. BMJ Open. 2020;10(7):e038670. Published 2020 Jul 19. https://doi.org/10.1136/bmjopen-2020-038670.
5. Haist SA, Katsufrakis PJ, Dillon GF. The evolution of the United States Medical Licensing Examination (USMLE): enhancing assessment of practice-related competencies. JAMA. 2013;310(21):2245–6.
6. IWA Frequently Asked Questions (FAQ). ECFMG Education Commission of Foreign Medical Graduates. Available from https://iwa2.ecfmg.org/iwafaq.asp
7. Alsayid M, Jandali IS, Alahdab F. Trends in the performance of Syrian physicians in the National Resident Matching Program® between 2017 and 2019. Avicenna J Med. 2019;9(4):154–9. Published 2019 Oct 3. https://doi.org/10.4103/ajm.AJM_140_19.
8. California Institute of Behavioral Neurosciences and Psychology. Available from https://www.cibnp.com

Chapter 6
The Problems That an IMG Faces When Moving to the United States

Raguraj Chandradevan and Ian H. Rutkofsky

International medical graduates (IMGs) make up nearly one-quarter of the total graduate medical education (GME) physicians and fully licensed practicing physicians which encompass many specialties, including primary care, sub-specialties, and medical research [1, 2]. Though it is a hurdle for those with language barriers as well as cultural barriers to become prosperous in this route, we present this chapter with our own personal experience as well as the information we gathered from our peers. We have divided this chapter into different sections with different plans and approaches for an international medical graduate (IMG) to commence one's journey. With firsthand experience this chapter offers help to individuals to better facilitate this progression into the US healthcare system as functional doctors. We wholeheartedly believe this chapter and book will be useful for IMGs, and we anticipate our experience may better prepare all medical students abroad to become stronger applicants.

The healthcare system in the United States is considered one of the greatest systems worldwide with cutting-edge practices based on the principles and findings of evidence-based medicine [3, 4]. Many of the internationally trained doctors have relocated to the United States with the hope of practicing in an improved healthcare system that offers strict protocol and ultimately gain personal satisfaction in lifestyle, from work-life balance to the lucrative opportunity the practice of medicine provides to the US-trained doctors [5]. Being trained in a foreign country or working as a physician in a foreign country sometimes comes with many challenges to

R. Chandradevan (✉)
Graduate Medical Education-Internal Medicine, Northside Hospital Gwinnett, Lawrenceville, GA, USA
e-mail: raguraj.chandradevan@northside.com

I. H. Rutkofsky
Department of Psychiatry, HCA – Aventura Hospital and Medical Center, Aventura, FL, USA

Department of Research, CiBNP, Fairfield, CA, USA
e-mail: Ian.Rutkofsky@hcahealthcare.com

© Springer Nature Switzerland AG 2021   105
H. Tohid, H. Maibach (eds.), *International Medical Graduates in the United States*, https://doi.org/10.1007/978-3-030-62249-7_6

overcome, and one must acclimate to the new system and culture. Most IMGs experience economic, cultural, language, and emotional adjustments during this journey which is a unique experience for every individual as the United States attracts residency candidates from all over the world [6]. Thus, this chapter provides a more general idea about the direction to ensue to remain on track and ultimately become a successful candidate for US post-graduate medical training.

Indeed, medicine is the science and practice of establishing a proper diagnosis, prognosis, treatment, and prevention of disease [7]. It encompasses a variety of healthcare practices and includes diverse therapies. Medicine also frequently requires the integration of spiritual and cultural understanding, and therefore, one should be keen on religious and psychosocial beliefs of local culture. Getting to recognize cultural diversities and language, integrating into acceptance, and maintaining professionalism are all challenges, but are essential to depict for patient's trust. One of the most important successes of healthcare practice depends on the physician-patient relationship. We will be looking at the obstacles of the IMGs in the aspects of language proficiency in communication; understanding the slang terminology and accents; writing and processing; challenges in passing through the United States Medical Licensing Examination (USMLE), especially USMLE Step 2 Clinical Skills (CS); getting through the residency interviews; adapting to the new healthcare system; professional communication throughout residency with co-residents, faculty, and healthcare workers; and patient-centered interaction, and we will be looking at each aspect and how we can overcome each aspect. These experiences not only give an overview but also would make many graduates to prepare and anticipate what to expect during their journey in the USMLE pathway.

USMLE

International medical graduates must get through the USMLEs prior to participating in the match process. Residency positions have become more competitive year by year. Scores above 240 are highly preferred for most specialties, and an IMG should get this score on the first attempt to secure a position [8]. English competency is essential for the USMLE Step 1 and USMLE Step 2 Clinical Knowledge (CK) as well as Step 2 CS. There is no actual time limit for writing these exams as there is for US medical students, but taking these exams in a time frame (2–3 years postgraduation) is very important and one of the factors that will be looked at during the interview process [9]. In our experience, it is recommended to do the USMLE Step 1 initially and then go to the USMLE Step 2 CK and CS. Even though some medical graduates, as they finish the clinical training during the final years, prefer to do USMLE Step 2 CK first, it might have some barriers. Most of the basic science concepts and ethics learned in Step 1 would be repeated at least 10–15% during Step 2 CK. Also studying for the Step 1 gives a great fundamental knowledge for the Step 2 CK. This step-by-step process may help build from the Step 1 knowledge, and it is highly preferred to go in an orderly manner. The average time for USMLE

Steps 1 and 2 CK would be 4–6 months and Step 2 CS would be 2–3 months for international medical graduates. Step 3 examination is not mandatory for the residency application; however, if there is some extra time during the match process, it is advisable to do Step 3 as well. There are some components of Step 3 called computer-based case simulations (CCS), which could be more natural if we are doing a residency; however, there are plenty of resources and applications to try these stimulations. Most of the Step 2 CK concepts are repeated in Step 3 and would be beneficial for international medical graduates. Nevertheless, the Step 3 exam is expected in order to obtain an H1B visa, which would be required before the match date. (Please refer to the visa-related chapter in this book for further details.)

English competency, grammatical knowledge, and spoken proficiency would help in the USMLE exams in various ways. Having sufficient language familiarity will help one to grasp the medical knowledge from various resources: books, video lectures, or live lectures. This will help with the preparation of your medical exams as well as your interaction with patients. It is essential to understand and acquire the medical knowledge from the books and handouts, which are essential factors during the USMLE exam preparation; it allows faster reading and interpretation or understanding of board questions as well. English skills and test-taking skills can be acquired from late childhood, as many countries outside the United States teach English as a second language. Some medical schools outside the United States even teach medicine in the English language or their lectures and rounds are conducted in English. In some cases, board review books are used in other counties for their final medical exams. We also found that many countries have their own books and literature on medicine, but their education is provided in English; for example, China offers a medical curriculum in this option. The hurdle for the medical students from this country is they must first learn English and they have to mitigate the similar norm of medicine with this English knowledge and apply this technique to read well as most of the USMLE books are written in English and most of their lectures and tutorials are conducted in English. This also applies to the USMLE Step 2 CS examination as English competency, knowledge, and spoken English are assessed by the simulated patients. Mastering the cases and understanding the clinical entity, accent of the patients, and the conversation are very important during this exam, while for US graduates the aspect of this exam would be like a reflex as they do this on a routine basis during their clinical rotations.

Medical students who wish to pursue their career in the United States should start learning and understanding grammar no later than high school or early on during medical school. Once they familiarized well with the English language, they should start reading on a daily basis or looking over and reviewing USMLE books during medical school, and practicing USMLE questions will help continuous reading toward the USMLE path after graduating from medical school. It might be hard to initiate this during medical school, but taking an attempt to review the books and question pool is highly advisable. Even to get the concepts of clinical pearls, some of the Step 2 CK and Step 3 question banks and books can be used for the final exams in some of the international medical schools. One of the other aspects of the USMLE board exam is the USMLE score, which is the most important factor in obtaining a residency spot. But second to scores, attempting the board exams in a timely manner will win the trust of the program director to rank them, as they believe they will be successful in their pursued board exams on their specialties. There are mean scores on the USMLE Steps 1 and 2 CK exam expected to apply for each specialty. These details can be found in the National Resident Matching Program (NRMP) residency match data for the recent year. It is important to make adequate efforts to achieve this score to be comfortable in applying these specialties.

Spending time on the board exams and utilizing adequate time and also making smart goals each week aid in finishing the exam in a timely manner. It is important to make a calendar and use logbooks to best plan which sources you are using in your USMLE preparation. Often tutorial classes would help to expedite taking the USMLE Step 1 and Step 2 CK and CS exams. A number of institutions both inside and outside the United States conduct online and live classes for the USMLE preparations. Some international medical graduates may feel that these classes are costly. But spending money on these classes and resources are worthwhile for getting sufficient scores. At the end of the day, it does not matter how we get a score; what only matters is the scores on this exam and achievements in a timely manner to advance and secure a position. So, it is advisable to spend on these classes as an investment. Sometimes, having friends from US medical schools, joining the forums and Facebook groups, and contacting seniors and residents who succeed in the USMLE exam would help to get advice to shine in the exams. In regard to the USMLE Step 1 and Step 2 CK, they are particularly online exams; hence, exceeding in the books, clinical concepts, and question pools and familiarizing well with the system will help. For USMLE Step 2 CS, it is important to learn information in communication, language proficiency, and present to the standardized patients about the medical knowledge and English knowledge in addition to the history, physical, and diagnosis we enter into the system. USMLE books consist of specific questions for each complaint and how to conduct the exam out there. They are the most useful. Practicing these words again and again as well as talking and recording and listening to the same recording would also help to correct your own pronunciation. It is also advisable to attend live classes conducted by many institutions for USMLE Step 2 CS specifically as it would help very well for international medical graduates. If medical graduates did US clinical rotations, that also would help to familiarize the system and handling of patients. Some of the myths exist on the exam centers for USMLE Step 2 CS; however, all the centers are standardized, and we do not feel any discrepancy in taking exams in one center to another. These are very important strategies to follow as the USMLE step exams open up the door for the opportunity to obtain residency interviews.

As the saying goes, when international medical graduates score well on the USMLE exams or have about ten interviews, the chance of matching to a residency is quite likely [10]. Getting plenty of interviews is key to secure a position. It is a distinct milestone and life-changing step. The journey often leads to difficult times, with days and nights without sleep, and many stressful and emotional situations may arise. It is not easy! It is best to utilize mentors and resources from your medical school as IMGs are on our own. We have to find our peer groups and study groups and manage to take the exam in a reasonable amount of time. The residency application process may at times feel as if you are all alone. There are plenty of resources out there, and finding a balance in selecting the right pathway for the individual is critical as it is often hard to back down or change your path once you begin this journey. It is very important to make good friends who are also motivated and are supportive of this effort which can help you maintain a motivated attitude. Equally important is to have some activities to help relax. Having a hobby or caring for pets will keep your spirits active. Having enough financial support is also necessary. Even though there are plenty of opportunities to work as a medical assistant or research assistant in some universities while doing the exams, it may depend on how we organize our time, visa status, and personal competency.

Externships and Observerships

Every international medical graduate will have his/her unique struggles and difficulties. It will take an average of 2 years of your time to get to know the system, understand the system, and find out the trend of the USMLE, residency application process, interviews, and health system. During this time, it is extremely important to have exposure to the US health system. There are plenty of programs in the United States that offer 4–6 weeks of international medical student electives. This will be the best opportunity for medical students if they have goals of continuing medical education. Even though its expensive to get some clinical externship, it might help a lot during the process of application. By doing an externship will convince program directors, we are familiar with the system and to obtain a letter of recommendation, in which three US letters are likely to help with your application. Medical observerships are available in several hospitals; however, there may be limited direct patient care which might not give enough value during the residency interview. So, it is highly important to find an elective during the medical student period or a hands-on externship. An internship in a medical institution or a combination with observerships and externships may help to better understand the healthcare system, residency structure, and communication skills. Having an average of 2–6 months of this experience would significantly impact the residency application. During the electives, medical graduates can get to know the system, take a history, perform physical exams, and develop a plan. Being friendly with residents, other medicals students, and other healthcare workers, and taking good care of patients are necessary during this rotation. It is also important to have a clear presentation to the attendings during the rounds and answer the questions while regarding. These characters and behaviors will give opportunities to obtain the letter of recommendation from the attending physicians and program director. At times, many international medical graduates have performed well during these rotations and successfully secured a position in the same institutions, hence the nickname "Audition rotation" [11].

Residency Interviews

The next step after applying to residency is obtaining the residency interviews. Preparation is critical for a good interview [12]. Once you have been invited to a program, consider yourself as equal to others you meet on interview day; although you may be at a disadvantage compared to an American medical graduate (AMG), having a well-rounded CV with research, US clinical rotations, and great USMLE scores can put you at the top of the rank list if your interview day goes well. Communication skills, kindness, interest, and sincerity can go a long way to help you perform well during the interview. Most international graduates experience interviews for residency as the first job interview; in contrast, many US graduates may have experienced ample interviews from their high school or college internships. During the interview process, there are certain questions commonly asked which often challenge the character of the individual. We recommend that international medical graduates get to understand the US culture and the geography at the place you obtained the interview, including the demographics about the patient population. Also, one must not forget to project the knowledge you have learned about the faculty and institutional leadership. You can usually find all this information by google search or the program website. Spending some time to find this information would be incredibly valuable. There are plenty of ways to get adapted to the culture and customs in the United States. Watching television, TV series, dramas, and films may help a lot of people to get to know American rituals. Having friends through multiple ways and get to know them and their tradition as well as joining some of the forums and small groups might help. Get to know how to communicate and improve the English spoken proficiency, and try to understand slang terminally, which would help during any challenging questions during the interview day or even while you are examining patients. Discussing with residents the night before the interview at the interview dinner is a good way to learn more about the program, and when discussing the program during your interview day, you can address some of the details you have learned about the program. Discussing ties to the area may also be helpful. But foremost, everyone should have a well-prepared answer for the questions like "tell me about yourself," "why do you like the specialty," "why do you like about our program," "what makes you a good candidate," and "what can you contribute to our program." At the end of the interview session, program leadership often will ask questions. One question they will ask you is "Do you have any questions?" It is necessary to have a meaningful question to ask each of them. This will definitely resemble your interest and curiousness about their program.

Interview preparation can be done through several ways. First, write down the possible questions that can be asked during an interview. We can prepare the answers for the questions and memorize them. Memorizing common questions and rehearsing answers should allow you to sound very natural and thought out. Attempt this by recording the answers and replaying them or rehearsing them over and over again. We can practice these answers with some of our friends or utilize boot camps or take classes by specialists regarding interview preparation. Learning from a coach would also benefit by way of direct guidance to boost the interview skills. Different programs have different styles which can differ from state to state. From day to day there may be a lot of variables or themes, but having a good framework will better prepare you for the most common questions, and you should always remark with non-judgmental comments. Indeed conversations with the residents and healthcare workers are also essential manners to follow during the day. After two or three interviews, the interview trial will begin to feel easier, as you get into the flow of things. Once the interview day is concluded, following up with the program faculty by writing thank you letters or sending holiday cards may be helpful to prove your interest.

The pathway and preparation during residency is certainly a challenge. The USMLE, externships, and interviews are among many efforts stowed upon this path to residency, but one must know the real struggle begins with residency itself. It is going to be a unique and memorable journey. It is very important to be friendly with everyone, receptive to feedback, and form constrictive criticism. Caring and empathy toward others is valued in every circumstance. Residency is a learning process. You will meet and make new friends. From every day on you will take care of patients from different creeds, cultures, languages, and religions. We all have to keep in mind that the purpose of being in the medical profession is to provide a healthier life or to save lives. Residency will allow you to learn while taking care of patients, through this remarkable experience, and every patient will teach you something new, and you may actually learn more from them than they have received from you.

We are going to divide the residency section into several challenges like language and communication barriers with co-residents and healthcare workers, to understanding differences in healthcare settings to technological difficulties, electronic health records, documentation, patient's satisfaction, to interpersonal and communications skills with patients, to advanced competencies, scholarly activity, and wellness. We will also discuss how to maintain a life balance such as spending time with friends and relaxing during residency.

Language and Communication

First, if we look at language and communication with various medical professionals as well as patients, we will find that the English accent and language are different from state to state. This can sometimes impair or create frustration during communication as well as during healthcare delivery [13]. For example, in the southern part of the United States, people often speak with different accents which might be difficult to understand at such times for international medical graduates [14]. It is very important to ask relevant questions and get as much history as possible without a need of repeating the same questions many times. It is also important to listen to the answers while listening to their conversation, noting the necessary information and appropriately directing the interview to get the correct diagnosis without cutting their answers short. A pertinent history from a patient or from their relatives is necessary to make the correct diagnosis and appropriate treatment plan. At times collateral information may be needed to be obtained from family or a language line may be used to translate. However, the best way to learn language, accents, and cultural values are to listen to the local and national news, and watch English films and TV series. Most of the documentaries, Netflix series, and other radios will help you to get familiar with the English accent, local terminologies, slang words, cultural basis, and patterns of questions. Sometimes reading newspapers, magazines, story books, or online media might help with language and grammar. It is also very appropriate to have friends who speak English as their first language, and you should try not to shy away from participating in social events. Engaging in English will help you to get the language pattern down and ease your communication in a short time frame. English conversations at home with friends will ease communication skills and improve the social friendliness. There are also some teaching modules out there that can be utilized during the time of residency to enhance and improve the language, interpersonal, and communication skills. Some residency programs even offer these modules and courses for their residents to improve those skills.

Electronic Health Records

Next, we will look into the medical system and electronic health records [15], and how they could create a barrier for IMGs. The US health system may be completely or partially different from the system where most international graduates have trained. The healthcare sector in the United States is mostly private-based as well as insurance-based [16]. Many aspects of medicine can be learned with time, but having a general idea about how to navigate the system and electronic health records would help to jumpstart residency training. Most of the US graduates are trained in the US system during third and fourth years of medical school clerkships, and they are aware of the systems and have a general idea of this process. Learning these systems in clinical training such as externships would help international graduates start residency without any hesitancy or issues. When we start residency, residents and faculty expect all the interns to be at the level of competence toward these computer systems. Therefore, it would be helpful for international graduates if they do clerkships or externships in a program that will allow them to get familiarized with the electronic health record system.

Understanding the essence of keeping medical records and coordination of care, and establishing familiarity with multiple healthcare electronic health systems allow for better monitoring and handling healthcare regimens through the electronic systems. Using electronic records may be challenging, but ultimately, documentation is better organized and better regulated via healthcare delivery with the use of technology. For some IMGs the use of the technologies in the healthcare setting may be a new entity [17]. Meanwhile practice would allow to better understand multiple aspects of teamwork with nurses, social workers, and different specialties and team dynamics during residency. This will smoothly transition the start of residency. There will also be opportunities for international medical graduates to work as research interns or associates in university medical centers. There are several opportunities in research institutions to contribute especially to obtain data from the patient chart and contribute some participation in healthcare. This will help to familiarize the system and get used to the electronic health records system to gather data for research purposes and get a keen understanding of data entry, storage, and systems in clinical research. Indeed, getting to know residents, fellows, attendings, and professors during research may provide a doorway for residency and open up a career in the same institution. In addition, research experience would help to formulate research projects during residency.

Scholarly Activities

We will now look at scholarly activities during residency as well as prior to the residency application. English language, punctuations, and grammar might be difficult to handle for international graduates as a second language. This is very important when it comes to an abstract presentation, poster presentation, or oral presentation. We would highly suggest having a native English-speaking person to have a look at the draft and go through and provide the edits. For oral presentations, it is important to record the speech and play it again and again, to become a more proficient speaker. As mentioned above, outside from patient care and clinical practice, we have limited time for scholarly activities and research. More opportunities to publish research will come during residency, but having prior training in research would really help to write and formulate a case series or case report, or systematic review, and working with a motivated team of residents at your residency program is an effective way to publish articles and present at conferences. Having scholarly activity during residency is important as it will provide a unique opportunity literature to improve your medical knowledge, contribute to the medical world, and build your application for fellowship [18].

As we have breaded our look into the important aspect of this section, we realize the importance of genuine patient care, communication and language, and message delivery. The ultimate goal of residency is to better prepare medical graduates to become fully trained physicians. English as a second language creates some degree of barrier for direct patient care. Most patient's native language is English, and therefore, it is important to recognize the patterns and specific questions we can use or apply to elicit the patient's history. It is also very important to know the social and current world and local happenings and practical knowledge in the United States to hold a deep conversation during the patient interaction. It is also important to have general conversation outside medicine and become friendly with patients as well as to mix with their conversations. Knowing social situations helps patients feel more relaxed and may contribute to establish a better patient-physician relationship [19]. We can read newspapers, watch television, and listen to radios to improve these skills. Patients would like to get advice from their cultural norms; for example, when we talk about a diet for an American, it is important to deliver a diet pattern that is practiced in their culture. When we talk about a specific sports or hobbies or wellness activities, it is very important to know and recognize the views of these activities in their pattern rather than just our simple focus. Resembling the great qualities, empathy and show enthusiasm as patients should get the feel that the physicians care and advocacte [20]. It is also very important to recognize some slang words when having a conversation with the patients. It will maintain a flow of conversation and the patient would like to keep you as their primary care provider and continue their care under your service.

In this chapter we have mentioned many different struggles that international medical graduates will likely face as they rise near residency and become a physician in the United States. We also outlined the circumstances and expressed various struggles IMGs face. One thing to keep in mind during the journey is you are not alone, and many international medical graduates have made it through this struggle and have reached their goal. If you work hard, success and wisdom will follow one day. This chapter in addition to other chapters in this book was designed to guide IMGs along the journey to becoming a physician in America.

References

1. Ahmed AA, Hwang WT, Thomas CR Jr, Deville C Jr. International medical graduates in the US physician workforce and graduate medical education: current and historical trends. J Grad Med Educ. 2018;10(2):214–8.
2. Ranasinghe PD. International medical graduates in the US physician workforce. J Am Osteopath Assoc. 2015;115(4):236–41.
3. Simoes E. Health information technology advances health care delivery and enhances research. Mo Med. 2015;112(1):37–40.
4. Durrani H. Healthcare and healthcare systems: inspiring progress and future prospects. Mhealth. 2016;2:3.
5. Parsi K. International medical graduates and global migration of physicians: fairness, equity, and justice. Medscape J Med. 2008;10(12):284.
6. Kehoe A, McLachlan J, Metcalf J, Forrest S, Carter M, Illing J. Supporting international medical graduates' transition to their host-country: realist synthesis. Med Educ. 2016;50(10):1015–32.
7. Croft P, Altman DG, Deeks JJ, Dunn KM, Hay AD, Hemingway H, et al. The science of clinical practice: disease diagnosis or patient prognosis? Evidence about "what is likely to happen" should shape clinical practice. BMC Med. 2015;13:20.
8. Mittal VK, Lax EA. Hurdles in US surgical training for international medical graduates. Indian J Surg. 2016;78(4):257–8.
9. Puscas L. Viewpoint from a program director they can't all walk on water. J Grad Med Educ. 2016;8(3):314–6.
10. Liang M, Curtin LS, Signer MM, Savoia MC. Understanding the interview and ranking behaviors of unmatched international medical students and graduates in the 2013 main residency match. J Grad Med Educ. 2015;7(4):610–6.

11. Saeed F, Majeed MH, Kousar N. Easing international medical graduates' entry into US training. J Grad Med Educ. 2011;3(2):269.
12. Hariton E, Bortoletto P, Ayogu N. Residency interviews in the 21st century. J Grad Med Educ. 2016;8(3):322–4.
13. Baquiran CLC, Nicoladis E. A doctor's foreign accent affects perceptions of competence. Health Commun. 2020;35(6):726–30.
14. Clopper CG, Levi SV, Pisoni DB. Perceptual similarity of regional dialects of American English. J Acoust Soc Am. 2006;119(1):566–74.
15. Evans RS. Electronic health records: then, now, and in the future. Yearb Med Inform. 2016;Suppl 1:S48–61.
16. Ridic G, Gleason S, Ridic O. Comparisons of health care systems in the United States, Germany and Canada. Mater Sociomed. 2012;24(2):112–20.
17. Ajami S, Bagheri-Tadi T. Barriers for adopting Electronic Health Records (EHRs) by physicians. Acta Inform Med. 2013;21(2):129–34.
18. Bourgeois JA, Hategan A, Azzam A. Competency-based medical education and scholarship: creating an active academic culture during residency. Perspect Med Educ. 2015;4(5):254–8.
19. Verlinde E, De Laender N, De Maesschalck S, Deveugele M, Willems S. The social gradient in doctor-patient communication. Int J Equity Health. 2012;11:12.
20. Lauer AK, Lauer DA. The good doctor: more than medical knowledge & surgical skill. Ann Eye Sci. 2017;2

Chapter 7
Cultural Barriers

Bindu Pillai

General

Immigration of International Medical Graduates (IMGs) was encouraged in the United States during the late 1960s after the Medicare and Medicaid federal programs were passed. Prior to these programs, there were noticeable gaps in healthcare, especially in the rural and inner cities. By the early 1970s, over 33% of physicians were International Medical Graduates. Many worked in the inner cities and rural areas and served in the primary care specialties [1]. IMGs make up a significant distribution of physicians in training and working in the United States. These physicians are those that graduated from medical schools outside of the United States. Currently, 25–30% of the physician workforce are IMGs, and one in four physicians are IMGs [2]. According to an Educational Commission of Foreign Medical Graduates (ECFMG) 2019 report, the top four countries to be ECFMG certified were India, Pakistan, Canada, and China. In addition, more than 100 languages are spoken by IMGs [3]. These individuals undergo medical education different from the US model of education [4]. Though they play an important role in healthcare, many face unique challenges [5, 6]. IMGs from certain ethnic or racial backgrounds may find it hard to build a rapport with their patients because of their cultural differences [7]. IMGs are faced with language and cultural barriers when providing patient care. These challenges exist throughout the length of their medical career [6].

B. Pillai (✉)
Laguardia Community College, Long Island City, NY, USA
e-mail: bpillai@lagcc.cuny.edu

© Springer Nature Switzerland AG 2021   117
H. Tohid, H. Maibach (eds.), *International Medical Graduates in the United States*, https://doi.org/10.1007/978-3-030-62249-7_7

Language Barriers

Communication is an activity that can differ across cultures [8]. Any IMG seeking to practice in the United States is assessed for his/her fluency in the English language. This is done through the TOEFL and/or the Step 2 Clinical Skills assessment (CS). Although these assessments are done, this does not reduce the barriers that exist with language. Research has shown that one of the first barriers IMGs encounter is language. A review done in 2012 indicated that 82% of the physicians that were in psychiatry fields stated that English was a second language [9]. Therefore, language barriers are seen in physicians from countries whose primary language is not English [10].

Language barriers are barriers to communication which can result in a misunderstanding or misinterpretation. If a language barrier exists, this can lead to patient not adhering to management modalities. IMGs will have a hard time gathering patients' medical history because of language barriers. Many feel their questions could be misunderstood or not in a way a patient can understand [4]. Language barriers become frustrating for patients and physicians and can lead to patients complaining, seeking compensation for malpractice, and being unsatisfied [11].

Language Barrier Situations

Studies on a group of IMGs reported that they faced difficulties when it came to sarcasm, idioms, accents, regional dialects, voice inflection, colloquialisms, and body language [2, 4]. One IMG reported in a study that "meetings" were difficult to understand [1]. Many IMGs are trained in countries that use British English. Certain medical terms are pronounced differently than in the United States. In addition, IMGs have struggled with medical slang, abbreviations, and acronyms. Many names for diseases differ in other countries [12].

Tone of voice can also become an issue or a barrier. Certain cultures or countries use a high-pitched voice during conversation, and these cues may get confusing for an IMG [1]. Physicians from cultures that have strict rules about eye contact felt it was a challenge to look at the eyes of patient of the opposite sex [12]. Any IMG or non-IMG also struggle with "other" languages. If a patient speaks a language other than English, such as Spanish, this complicates the already existing barrier. IMGs struggle with family members "translating," which then further complicates the situation. Using a professional interpreter may help, but still becomes complicated [13]. In addition, not every healthcare setting will have an interpreter readily available. Unfamiliar accents could be too strong to patients, and this will cause a strain in the physician–patient relationship [12].

Nonverbal and Casual Communication

Nonverbal cues vary between cultures and include posture, tone of voice, touch, gestures, personal space, and facial expressions. Gestures such as hugs or kisses by certain cultures may make an IMG uncomfortable. This is especially the case with an IMG that may be from a country where gestures such as these are considered inappropriate. These cues of communication could present as a challenge and culture shock to some [14]. About 80% of nonverbal cues may be provided during a physician–patient encounter [13]. Understanding these cues is essential in managing the conversation. A handful of patients that come in to speak with their physicians also want to "small talk." Small talk is important to a patient as they feel the physician respects them and values their life in general. IMGs may feel uncomfortable in small talk or casual conversations. They are more comfortable with providing medical information that is readily available. Evading "small talk" could appear as if the physician is detached [13, 15]. In a study where physician interviews were conducted, it was reported that IMGs felt that their authoritative or direct communication strategies appeared ineffective with patients [12].

Individual Versus Family System

Many IMGs come to the United States leaving their extended families behind. Many of these physicians are from close-knit families. Leaving a family behind can cause interferences in an IMG's professional life [10, 15]. Physicians who are raised in households outside the Western culture may not have the same childhood experiences as the West. An individual from India does not experience the childhood as one from the United States. Many outside Western cultures have been raised by a large extended family. Individuals in Western cultures have seen or have experienced living with divorced parents, dating, or even going to daycare. Americans are unaware of the values and beliefs that immigrants from India have been taught, and this holds true vice versa [10].

Types of Societies

The type of society an individual is raised will often determine their personality. Individuals from a sociocentric or collectivist culture identify with "kinship." They are loyal to their community or group. IMGs from these cultures value group/family decisions and interdependence and are concerned about the well-being of others. These societies exist in Japan, China, India, and Pakistan [16, 17]. Studies have shown that the Chinese are ranked highest in the collectivist society [16].

Egocentric or individualistic cultures are those seen in Western societies such as the United States, the United Kingdom, Canada, and Australia. The ties between these societies are not as strong as compared to the sociocentric groups. These societies focus on the individual's autonomy and believe "every man is for himself." These cultures exhibit emotional independence, the need for privacy, financial security, and self-realization [16, 17]. Studies have shown that the United States ranks the highest in self-centered societies [16]. An IMG coming from a collectivist society such as India would face issues in the individualistic society of the United States. They would not be able to fathom the cultural difference [17]. According to a cross-cultural study conducted in 2001, it was found that people from countries with a collectivistic culture have lower levels of mental illness [18].

Examples

IMGs who are in practice have come across patients from both individualistic and collectivistic societies. Patients from a collectivistic society will come in with their loved ones for "moral" support. On behalf of the patient, family members answer to many medical history questions. IMGs from collectivistic cultures tend to give the family and friends information on the disease and prognosis of the patient. This is a norm in many collectivistic countries. Due to malpractice and Health Insurance Portability and Accountability Act (HIPAA) laws in the United States, this is not acceptable nor is it practiced. Patients from an individualistic society tend to be different and value privacy and confidentiality in their care. They are solely responsible and exhibit autonomy in their care [16, 17].

Religious Barriers

Religion is defined as the beliefs and worshipping of a higher power. In addition, religious groups have certain practices and rituals that are sacred to them [19]. Many people feel religion influences their health and behavior and is used as a coping mechanism [20, 21]. A 2001 study reported that over 90% of people from the United States believe in a higher power. Of these individuals, many pray weekly or attend religious services. About 58% of them reported that religion is "important" to them [21].

When religion is involved, it may cause a barrier for IMGs. These barriers can be at the patient level or provider level. An IMG coming from a religious background may treat their patients based on their beliefs. It is important to be culturally competent when we are faced with diverse religions. Being culturally competent can help an IMG deliver the best care to their patients [20, 21]. This will result in meeting the cultural, religious, and social needs of the patients [22]. Many centuries ago, the role of medicine was one that tended to the mind, body, and spirit.

Barriers at the Patient Level

Spiritual beliefs have been a controversy within the medical community for a long time. Barriers in healthcare because of religion can start with the patient [23]. Religion is an important aspect in an individual's life. Women from Islamic faiths value their modesty and privacy. One of the fastest growing religions is Islam, with more than 1.5 billion followers [20]. Patients coming from a Middle Eastern country to the US healthcare system will prefer a physician of the same gender or need a female chaperone. In addition, women will have either their spouse or a female family member during the physician–patient encounter. IMGs from a country not familiar to these cultures may perceive this as a barrier. Treating the patient becomes a barrier especially if the who is a woman feels embarrassed and may in turn withhold information that is pertinent to their treatment. In some cases, men are considered head of household and interact with the physician on behalf of the woman. This barrier can result in lack of treatment or care [20]. Some patients may display symptoms and may have different beliefs about these symptoms that could result in a missed diagnosis. Denying a patients' religion or spiritual beliefs may greatly influence the well-being of the patients [24]. IMGs who provide low level of care and hold stereotyped attitudes of their patients are doing a disservice to their profession.

Barriers at the Provider Level

In a 2017 study, it was reported that 29% of physicians stated that religion or spiritual beliefs influenced them to be a physician and influenced their daily practices of medicine [25]. It is important that IMGs do not stereotype. One must not think one religion is superior to another. Islamic men who are IMGs may have issues in looking at the eyes of a female patient. IMGs also may not "treat" their patients based on their beliefs or practices. Many IMGs from non-Western cultures may hold certain beliefs in abortion or premarital sex. These beliefs may hinder or become a barrier in treating patients [20]. In one study, IMGs felt that they lacked the knowledge and training to care for the opposite sex and felt unfamiliar with common disease conditions in them [12].

Cultural Daily Routine Differences

A 2011 study found 108 IMGs faced difficulties in acculturation and poor social support [26]. There are many cultural differences between Western and non-Western countries. Some IMGs come from a country where doctors are not questioned and are "godlike" [27]. Many IMGs come in to the United States not having an understanding of the hospital system or medical documentation. Many countries have not adopted a proper workflow or even electronic health record systems. IMGs feel they are not trained in these and the psychosocial aspects of patients [27, 28]. IMGs and their work ethics differ from that of Western cultures. Studies have shown that Asian and African cultures emphasize tradition and collectivism. These cultures are inclined to be introverts [29]. These traits are usually good when it comes to work ethics, but it can be misunderstood. American or Western cultures tend to be less introverted and more extroverted [29]. IMGs practicing in the United States feel as there is a loss of autonomy compared to their home country. Many are not comfortable with a shared decision-making approach and are unaware of lower hierarchical structures in healthcare settings [2, 27, 30].

Male doctors from the Middle East have a difficult time working in a healthcare team. This could be because of the unfamiliarity of the role of other healthcare professionals [31]. The authority of a female supervisor has been challenging for some male IMGs, and this could negatively reflect on the care provided to patients [12, 15]. IMGs from a collectivistic culture are familiar with the culture and understand when family members are involved with the patients' medical care [20]. IMG physicians may have a hard time understanding the social or cultural morals in the United States. IMGs may not have experienced youth sexuality, premarital relationships, and lesbian, gay, bisexual, and transgender relationships. It is important that IMGs refrain from acting strangely in front of people that fit these categories [15]. Some IMGs have felt that asking about a patient's sexuality is being intrusive. IMGs may not be trained in talking or assessing patients about suicide [12, 15].

Acculturation

Acculturation is a process by which a member of one culture adapts to another culture. This process is a multidimensional process that includes a cultural and psychological change. At first, moving from one country to another can cause stress to IMGs and anybody in that situation. Acculturation includes adjusting to work settings, new languages, or a different healthcare system [10, 32]. IMGs from Asia or the Middle East may face a "culture shock" [17]. Female IMGs have different needs or issues than their male counterparts. They may leave behind a spouse or children. They may have "home" expectations such as raising a family that may clash with their "professional" expectations [30]. IMGs may either lose their own culture or adopt both cultures as their new norm [17]. Ultimately, the IMG will orient themselves to the new culture [10].

Conclusion

In conclusion, any individual leaving their country of origin will be faced with difficulties when adjusting to a new place. IMGs are likely to face barriers before, during, and after residency. These barriers can include communication, religion, teamworking, and the understanding of the healthcare setting hierarchical structure. Many healthcare systems have established interventions that include language skills courses, shadowing opportunities, orientations, "buddy" programs, and web-based resources. IMGs can be greatly assisted in aspects that touch on communication and the physician–patient relationship. If IMGs do not adjust to their environment or healthcare system, their lives can be affected both personally and professionally. IMGs are valuable in a healthcare setting and bring a variety of experiences into their profession.

References

1. Laird LD, Abu-Ras W, Senzai F. Cultural citizenship and belonging: Muslim International Medical Graduates in the USA. J Muslim Minority Affairs. 2013;33(3):356–70. https://doi.org/10.1080/13602004.2013.863075.
2. Chen PG, Nunez-Smith M, Bernheim SM, Berg D, Gozu A, Curry LA. Professional experiences of International Medical Graduates practicing primary care in the United States. J Gen Intern Med. 2010;25(9):947–53. https://doi.org/10.1007/s11606-010-1401-2.
3. Educational Commission for Foreign Medical Graduates. 2019 ECFMG certification report. Available from: https://ecfmg.org/resources/data-certification.html
4. Jain P, Krieger JL. Moving beyond the language barrier: the communication strategies used by International Medical Graduates in intercultural medical encounters. Patient Educ Couns. 2011;84(1):98–104. https://doi.org/10.1016/j.pec.2010.06.022.
5. Chen PG, Curry LA, Bernheim SM, Berg D, Gozu A, Nunez-Smith M. Professional challenges of non-U.S.-born International Medical Graduates and recommendations for support during residency training. Acad Med. 2011;86(11):1383–8. https://doi.org/10.1097/ACM.0b013e31823035e1.
6. Rao NR, Kramer M, Saunders R, et al. An annotated bibliography of professional literature on International Medical Graduates. Acad Psychiatry. 2007;31:68–83. https://doi.org/10.1176/appi.ap.31.1.68.
7. Fiscella K, Frankel R, Fiscella K, Frankel R. Overcoming cultural barriers: International Medical Graduates in the United States. JAMA. 2000;283(13):1751. https://doi.org/10.1001/jama.283.13.1751-JMS0405-6-1.
8. Dorgan K, Lang F, Floyd M, Kemp E. International medical graduate–patient communication: a qualitative analysis of perceived barriers. Acad Med. 2009;84:1567–75. https://doi.org/10.1097/ACM.0b013e3181baf5b1.
9. Boulet JR, Cassimatis EG, Opalek A. The role of international medical graduate psychiatrists in the United States healthcare system. Acad Psychiatry. 2012;36:293–9. https://doi.org/10.1176/appi.ap.11040060.
10. Selvadurai R. Problems faced by international students in American colleges and universities. Commun Rev. 1998;16:153. http://search.ebscohost.com.rpa.laguardia.edu:2048/login.aspx?direct=true&db=a9h&AN=5809246&site=ehost-live. Accessed 1 Mar 2020.
11. McMahon GT. Coming to America "â€" International Medical Graduates in the United States. N Engl J Med. 2004;350(24):2435–7. https://doi.org/10.1056/NEJMp038221.
12. Triscott JAC, Szafran O, Waugh EH, Torti JMI, Barton M. Cultural transition of international medical graduate residents into family practice in Canada. Int J Med Educ. 2016;7:132–41. https://doi.org/10.5116/ijme.570d.6f2c.
13. Partida Y. Language barriers and the patient encounter. Virtual Mentor. 2007;9(8):566–71. https://doi.org/10.1001/virtualmentor.2007.9.8.msoc1-0708.
14. Remland MS, Jones TS, Brinkman H. Interpersonal distance, body orientation, and touch: effects of culture, gender, and age. J Soc Psychol. 1995;135(3):281–97. https://doi.org/10.1080/00224545.1995.9713958.

15. Hamarneh A. Lack of language skills and knowledge of local culture in International Medical Graduates: implications for the NHS. Hosp Pract. 2015;43(4):208–11. https://doi.org/10.108 0/21548331.2015.1075349.
16. Darwish A-FE, Huber GL. Individualism vs collectivism in different cultures: a cross-cultural study. Intercult Educ. 2003;14(1):47. https://doi.org/10.1080/1467598032000044647.
17. Kalra G, Bhugra DK, Shah N. Identifying and addressing stresses in International Medical Graduates. Acad Psychiatry. 2012;36:323–9. https://doi.org/10.1176/appi.ap.11040085
18. Maercker A. Association of cross-cultural differences in psychiatric morbidity with cultural values: a secondary data analysis. Ger J Psychiatry. 2001;4(1):84–93.
19. Ayvaci E. Religious barriers to mental healthcare. Am J Psychiatry Resident's J. 2016;11(7):11–3.
20. Tackett S, Young JH, Putman S, Wiener C, Deruggiero K, Bayram JD. Barriers to healthcare among Muslim women: a narrative review of the literature. Women's Stud Int Forum. 2018;69:190–4. https://doi.org/10.1016/j.wsif.2018.02.009.
21. Hebert RS, Jenckes MW, Ford DE, et al. Patient perspectives on spirituality and the patient-physician relationship. JGIM. 2001;16(10):685–92. https://doi.org/10.1111/j.1525-1497.2001.01034.x.
22. Swihart DL, Martin RL. Cultural religious competence in clinical practice. [Updated 2019 May 29]. In: StatPearls [Internet]. Treasure Island: StatPearls Publishing; 2020. Available from: https://www.ncbi.nlm.nih.gov/books/NBK493216/.
23. Astrow AB, Sulmasy DP. Spirituality and the patient-physician relationship. JAMA. 2004;291(23):2884. https://doi.org/10.1001/jama.291.23.2884.
24. Scheppers E, Van Dongen E, Dekker J, Geertzen J, Dekker J. Potential barriers to the use of health services among ethnic minorities: a review. Fam Pract. 2006;23(3):325–48. https://doi.org/10.1093/fampra/cmi113.
25. Robinson K, Cheng M-R, Hansen P, Gray R. Religious and spiritual beliefs of physicians. J Relig Health. 2017;56(1):205–25. https://doi.org/10.1007/s10943-016-0233-8.
26. Atri A, Matorin A, Ruiz P. Integration of International Medical Graduates in U.S. psychiatry: the role of acculturation and social support. Acad Psychiatry. 2011;35:21–6. https://doi.org/10.1176/appi.ap.35.1.21.
27. Michalski K, Motschall E, Vach W, Boeker M, Farhan N. Dealing with foreign cultural paradigms: a systematic review on intercultural challenges of International Medical Graduates. PLoS One. 2017;12(7):1–20. https://doi.org/10.1371/journal.pone.0181330.
28. Kirmayer LJ, Sockalingam S, KP-L F, et al. International Medical Graduates in psychiatry: cultural issues in training and continuing professional development. Can J Psychiatr. 2018;63(4):258–80. https://doi.org/10.1177/0706743717752913.
29. Chon A. Asia and America: how cultural differences create behavioral (2014). Social Impact Research Experience (SIRE). 26. http://repository.upenn.edu/sire/26
30. Kehoe A, McLachlan J, Metcalf J, Forrest S, Carter M, Illing J. Supporting International Medical Graduates' transition to their host-country: realist synthesis. Med Educ. 2016;50(10):1015–32. https://doi.org/10.1111/medu.13071.
31. Huijskens EGW, Hooshiaran A, Scherpbier A, Van Der Horst F. Barriers and facilitating factors in the professional careers of International Medical Graduates. Med Educ. 2010;44(8):795–804. https://doi.org/10.1111/j.1365-2923.2010.03706.x.
32. Sam DL, Berry JW. Acculturation: when individuals and groups of different cultural backgrounds meet. Perspect Psychol Sci. 2010;5(4):472–81. https://doi.org/10.1177/1745691610373075.

Chapter 8
Nobody Knows You: Become Somebody from Nobody by Establishing a Professional Network

Dong Hyang Kwon, Bilal Haider Malik, and Ian H. Rutkofsky

What Is Networking?

Networking may sound like a nebulous concept especially to those whose culture does not emphasize on the practice of networking. Networking is "developing and maintaining relationships" with individuals. Simply put, it often begins with an exchange of contact with the intention of getting to know each other and become known by the others. Networking can be largely divided into social and professional.

Social networking is about building friendships and bonding with the intention of having fun and distraction, and enjoying the company. Professional networking is more goal-oriented with the intention of sharing information and finding opportunities for advancing one's career. However, the line can start to blur as many professional networkings can be done during a social networking environment in both casual and formal settings. This chapter will focus on a professional networking setting.

D. H. Kwon (✉)
Department of Pathology, MedStar Georgetown University Hospital, Washington, DC, USA

B. H. Malik
CiBNP, Fairfield, CA, USA

Institute of Behavioral Neurosciences and Psychology, Fairfield, CA, USA

Internal Medicine, Research, California Institute of Behavioral Neurosciences & Psychology, Sacramento, CA, USA

I. H. Rutkofsky
Department of Psychiatry, HCA – Aventura Hospital and Medical Center, Aventura, FL, USA

Department of Research, CiBNP, Fairfield, CA, USA
e-mail: ian.rutkofsky@Hcahealthcare.com

© Springer Nature Switzerland AG 2021
H. Tohid, H. Maibach (eds.), *International Medical Graduates in the United States*, https://doi.org/10.1007/978-3-030-62249-7_8

Why Network?

In the United States (US), there is a famous quote, saying: "it's not what you know, but who you know." Although this is an overly simplified statement to be taken as literal, this goes to show the importance of connecting with others.

First, professional networking is the single most efficient tool to get you connected to key personnel who can find you an opportunity for career advancement, share new information, and provide you with support [1]. Many readers are interested in successfully completing the United States Medical Licensing Examination (USMLE) and matching into a residency program. Study shows that those who network tend to advance in career more often than those who do not. For those who are interested in matching, networking may serve as an important tool to find an observership opportunity or to receive an interview.

Second, successful networking may be a reflection of having important qualities that make you a successful residency candidate. According to the 2018 National Resident Matching Program (NRMP) Program Director Survey, program directors highly valued "interaction with faculty and housestaff" and "interpersonal skills" for candidate selection [2], which are all valuable assets for someone working in a high-stress environment. Similarly, the Accreditation Council for Graduate Medical Education (ACGME) that accredits all graduate medical training programs (residency and fellowship) introduced the six core competencies that are expected to be acquired by the training physicians by the time they become independent, and two of which included "interpersonal and communication skills" and "professionalism" [3]. Those who navigate the network successfully have great communication skills and professionalism, highly sought-after qualities for residency applicants. At the same time, networking is a great way to practice those qualities and improve emotional intelligence.

Third, networking is one way to explore one's identity and find the group of like-minded people with similar goals. When international medical graduate (IMGs) arrive in a new country, networking helps to meet new professionals in the similar field and share information.

Hopefully by now, you are convinced that networking is something that cannot be ignored. The journey to the medical profession in the United States requires a tremendous amount of work. Networking alone will not allow someone to pass the board or obtain a residency position; however, networking may be regarded as a "booster" that can enhance one's ability to achieve a goal. Main recipe to success is endurance and persistence, while a sprinkle of networking is a flavor-enhancer.

Where Can IMGs Network?

There are various venues to find appropriate settings for professional networking. For our purpose, the network can be largely divided into traditional networking and modern networking. Traditional networking involves meeting people face-to-face and participating in various activities in person. Modern networking, as the name implies, has emerged in recent years and involves Internet-based connection. Here are examples of opportunities that IMGs can employ to expand professional networks.

Traditional Networking

Rotation, Externship, and Observership

Rotation, externship, and observership all in essence refer to medical education focused on clinical experiences. Many IMGs are already taking advantage of these opportunities, and this is probably the easiest and most effective way to build a professional network. These clinical experiences are a perfect venue for networking, where one can meet mentors and show skill sets that may not necessarily be apparent in the curriculum vitae (CV), in addition to gaining US clinical experiences. Another advantage of clinical experiences is finding mentors who can write excellent letters of recommendation for residency application.

Rotation or clerkship is provided by the medical schools for those who are currently enrolled. Most of the Caribbean schools have a built-in US clinical rotation that allows them to be exposed to the US clinical practice and also to establish relationships with the hospital. Medical students may consider an elective rotation in a hospital with residency program, which can serve as an "audition rotation."

The terms externship and observership are usually reserved for those who have completed their medical school but wish to gain additional clinical experiences outside of one's medical school. Externship emulates internship with a lot more clinical privileges, while observation does provide clinical privileges. Some program directors may regard observership and externship to be similar, and the terms may be used interchangeably. However, externship puts a heavier emphasis on direct patient care and may be regarded to be better experiences overall. Externship positions are often limited and more popular due to the hands-on nature.

US medical students have their own application service to apply for elective/away rotation. However, IMGs must set up the clinical experiences independently. The hospital policy differs greatly, and the best way to explore clinical opportunities is to visit the hospital website or email the program coordinator and program director. Please note that some rotations may require a payment, and it is up to the discretion of the hospital policy. If possible, it will be most beneficial to find a hospital with residency programs to increase the chance of receiving an interview.

During the rotation, it is imperative to be punctual, stay interested, and ask relevant questions. Ask the preceptors and attending faculty for research opportunities. It is also important to be polite and pleasant to everyone, including staff and residents, as their opinions will be highly considered. Remember that every day should be considered like an interview day and strive to be the type of person that everyone wants to work with.

Volunteer Work

Volunteer work is a non-paid position often requiring short- to long-term commitment. To obtain a position, directly contacting the hospital or organizations is recommended. Keep in mind that these volunteer works may not always be clinically oriented and the organization may be hesitant to grant permission to work in a clinical setting. Non-US citizens or permanent residents may be denied due to their immigration status, as background check is rigorous, and prefer someone who is based in America.

Research Position (Paid/Non-paid)

Research position usually requires a longer commitment and may not come easily if you do not have any "network," but is a great way to show your commitments and get to know your mentor and colleagues at a personal level. Clerkship, observation, and externship are great ways to obtain a research opportunity. You can inquire about these positions. Unless you have a PhD and had prior experience in the lab, most of the positions will require you to go through chart review and organize data. Some formal research positions with one- or two-year commitment may be a paid position and may involve you in the clinical arena with patients or tissue samples.

Majority of these positions are unpaid, and it is saddening to see that long work hours are not financially compensated. However, the advantage of research experiences includes publication and building the CV. This is also a great period to be combined with studying for the USMLE in order to reduce the number of "gaps." In the future, when you are applying for residency, board exam, and license, you will be asked to explain the "gaps" that you have had, and it looks a lot more favorable if you had been active apart from studying. Therefore, a research position can serve to fill the gap. Another advantage is that you will get to know the mentors at a personal level due to frequent contact, and they are more likely to go extra miles for you. Since they know you at a personal level, they can help connect with other key personnel, write letters of recommendation, or possibly pick up the phone for an extra interview.

In certain situations, a non-paid research position can become a paid position if the mentor finds you to be a hard-worker and would like to compensate you for the work you have performed.

Study Institution

California Institute of Behavioral Neurosciences & Psychology (CIBNP) is an example of an online-based institute that offers various courses to help IMGs to become successful candidates. The most notable course is an online group class that teaches how to publish papers with an end goal of multiple publications. Joining group courses like this will help you stay motivated and receive direct guidance. Publication is one of the most efficient ways to increase the credentials in the CV.

Conferences and Society Meetings

All the major specialty fields are represented by professional associations and societies that hold regional to national/international meetings. The major purpose of these meetings is to present abstracts (poster or platform), to obtain Continuing Medical Education (CME) credits, and to network and reunite with the colleagues. If you have a research project or two, ask the mentors if you can submit your abstract to one of the meetings. If the abstract is accepted (either poster or platform), it is a great honor to include it in your CV and also have a good reason to attend the meeting.

These meetings often have fellowship fairs, social events, or other resident-centered sessions that may be attended. Find the major society of the field of your interest and try to attend one of these meetings. You will find many program directors, coordinators, and residents. It is important not to be overly enthusiastic or aggressive in finding a residency position. A simple acquaintance and salutation is sufficient for them to remember who you are and will be appreciated. You can introduce yourself to program director and express your interest. Do not forget to bring a copy of your most updated CV and appear professional. Registration fee may be required.

Professional Subspecialty Associations

Being a member means you can receive some educational benefits and stay up-to-date in the field of interest. In the Electronic Residency Application Service® (ERAS®)application, there is a separate section that asks you to write the association member you are part of. Joining this can show your commitment and demonstrate interest in the field. Most often, the fees are minimal to none as a trainee. By no means, this is a comprehensive list, but it provides a list of most popular societies. There are international, national, regional, and local societies that support various functions and meetings and host educational seminars. One may consider also joining a local group if there is a particular area that he or she would like to work in (9).

Family Medicine
- American Academy of Family Physicians (AAFP)
- Society of Teachers of Family Medicine (STFM)
- Association of Departments of Family Medicine (ADFM)
- North American Primary Care Research Group (NAPCRG)

Internal Medicine and Subspecialties
- American College of Physicians
- American Medical Association
- American Society of Internal Medicine
- Alliance of Academic Internal Medicine
- Society of General Internal Medicine
- Alliance for Academic Internal Medicine

- American Academy of Hospice and Palliative Medicine
- American Geriatrics Society
- American Academy of Sleep Medicine
- American Association of Clinical Endocrinologists
- American College of Cardiology
- American Heart Association
- American Society of Nuclear Cardiology
- American Society of Echocardiography
- American College of Gastroenterology
- American Gastroenterological Association
- American Society of Gastrointestinal Endoscopy
- Endocrine Society
- American College of Rheumatology
- American Society of Clinical Oncology
- American Society of Hematology
- American Society of Nephrology
- National Kidney Foundation
- American Society of Transplantation
- American Thoracic Society
- Infectious Diseases Society of America
- Society of Critical Care Medicine

Obstetrics and Gynecology
- American College of Obstetricians and Gynecologists
- American Gynecological and Obstetrical Society
- American Association of Obstetricians and Gynecologists Foundation
- Central Association of Obstetricians and Gynecologists
- Infectious Diseases Society for Obstetrics and Gynecology
- American Pregnancy Association

Neurology
- American Academy of Neurology
- American Neurological Association
- Child Neurology Society

Pathology
- College of American Pathologist
- United States and Canadian Academy of Pathology
- American Society of Clinical Pathology
- International Academy of Pathology

Pediatric
- American Academy of Pediatrics
- Academic Pediatric Association
- American Pediatric Society

Psychiatry
- American Psychiatric Association
- American Academy of Child and Adolescent Psychiatry (AACAP)
- American Association for Geriatric Psychiatry
- The American College of Neuropsychopharmacology
- The American Foundation for Suicide Prevention (AFSP)
- Association of Women Psychiatrists "A Voice for Women in Psychiatry"

Surgery and Subspecialty
- American College of Surgeons
- American Association for the Surgery of Trauma
- American Hepato-Pancreato-Biliary Association
- American Laryngological Association
- American Society for Surgery of the Hand
- American Society for Metabolic and Bariatric Surgery
- American Society of Breast Surgeons
- American Society for Reconstructive Microsurgery
- American Society of Transplant Surgeons
- Association of Women Surgeons
- Association for Academic Surgery
- American Society for General Surgeons
- Association for Surgical Education
- International Society for Heart and Lung Transplantation
- Orthopedic Trauma Association
- Society for Surgery of the Alimentary Tract
- Society of American Gastrointestinal Endoscopic Surgeons
- Society of Critical Care Medicine
- Society of Gynecologic Surgeons
- Society of Laparoendoscopic Surgeons
- Society of Surgical Oncology
- Surgical Infection Society
- Women in Neurosurgery
- Women in Thoracic Surgery

Radiology
- American College of Radiology
- Radiological Society of North America

Ethnic Physician Association

Apart from the professional association, there are numerous ethnically oriented associations that one can become part of. Refer to Chap. 16 for a comprehensive list.

Religion Communities

In addition to the medical and professional communities, joining religious communities is also a great way to find support and expand networks. Many universities or hospitals offer religious services, and joining these services may be a great way to connect with professionals within the community.

Modern Networking Setting

The Internet and social media have changed the way people connect in modern society. Social media allows a convenient way to disseminate information and communicate without geographic barriers. In addition, social media provides an alternative training environment and has revolutionized medical education. Among the over 150 million users in the United States are medical professionals, health organizations, and other stakeholders. Many health organizations and health care professionals are encouraged to actively engage in social media to disseminate information quickly, create direct contacts with other professionals or patients, and improve the public image. Therefore, readers must understand that social media will play a significant role in expanding both professional and social networks by participating. In this section, select popular social media platforms will be introduced and explore effective ways to engage in platforms. First and foremost, here are three fundamental basic rules and recommendations for best practices to maximize the benefits of social media.

Social Media Platform
- LinkedIn: https://www.linkedin.com/ LinkedIn is first introduced in 2002 and has over 630 million registered users as of 2019. This is probably the top business and employment-oriented platform out of all other social media, as LinkedIn is mainly used for professional networking. The basic function is that the users create profiles to showcase one's education, work experiences, and publications in a format that is very akin to curriculum vitae (CV). The advantage of the website is that the content can be controlled by the user and the website allows you to import contact lists and connect with other on professional grounds. LinkedIn is also a popular place for job recruiters to scout future employees. To maximize the benefit of LinkedIn, be involved in professional groups that engage in regular online conversations. Update the profiles regularly and showcase the recent work experiences. Creating a LinkedIn website is highly recommended for professionals at any stage of their career.
- Doximity: https://www.doximity.com Doximity was founded in 2011 and is one of the largest social media networks of medical professions. One in four American doctors have used the mobile app, and it was listed as a top five app by the American College of Physicians. This platform provides various features including messaging systems (Health Insurance Portability and Accountability Act

[HIPPA] compliant fax/email/text) with the patients and physicians and personalized medical news. Similar to LinkedIn, the user can update the profiles and can link up their websites and Twitter account. The website can also automatically update the profile on behalf based on the publicly available information, such as licensure and certification. One of the most interesting features is "residency navigator" that helps residency applicants learn about the program based on information collected from the user-submitted evaluations and US residency database.

- ResearchGate: https://www.researchgate.net/login ResearchGate was established in 2008, and as the name implies, it provides more research-specific functions. This European-based platform is one of the largest sites for academics with heavier emphasis on science. The platform allows users to upload PDF copies of the publications and download available articles directly from the authors, as if it is an "open-access." The users can receive notifications on new publications from the peers and receive statistics on impact score. One caveat of uploading the PDFs is the copyright policy by the publishers. Otherwise, this is a great way to showcase one's own research and also be connected with individuals with similar interest. It is unlikely to receive requests for collaborative work, but ResearchGate creates a positive public image for the Match applicants, especially if the name is searched on the website and the ResearchGate is one of the top sites shown.

- Twitter: https://twitter.com/ Twitter was first introduced in 2006 and provides a "microblogging" platform, where the basic premise is for registered users to post (or *tweet)* a short, 140-character text that instantly updates information [4, 5]. The users can *follow* other users to receive updated notification or be followed by *followers.* The easiest and best way to network via Twitter is to *follow* an organization or prominent people of the field. Medical professionals will often share interesting cases and study material. Users may "retweet" or share the information to increase the exposure and gain more attention. All in all, Twitter is best used for being informed, rather than starting a discussion, unless the user is already well-established in the field. Some of the important organizations to be followed by international graduates would include Educational Commission for Foreign Medical (ECFMG) for IMG and ECFMG J 1 sponsorship to be informed of changes in policies. Hashtag (#) is often used to categorize the conversation so that when searched by the hashtag sign, all the relevant tweets can be pulled up. For instance, you may tweet about something you learned in preparation of USMLE, you may wish to use #usmle in order for your tweet to be grouped with other similar contents and can be easily identified when other users are searching for similar tweets.

- Facebook: facebook.com Facebook was first founded in 2004 and is one of the most popular social networking platforms. Increasingly, Facebook is being used for professional development by creating a page or professional Facebook site. One efficient way to use Facebook is to join a group and stay up-to-date on important information such as USMLE or Visa policies for many IMGs. One may find study groups and find a supportive community to stay focused on the goal. Facebook is also used for open learning resources for medical education.

As will be discussed later in this chapter, it is necessary to set boundaries when using Facebook for both professional and social networks. Professionals should keep the Facebook page appropriate and contents must not be offensive. Be cautious when taking advice from group chats, as they may reflect personal opinions rather than facts. Facebook has an advantage that it has many groups that you can join. Research groups to VISA-related groups.

Overcoming Cultural Differences in Networking

Medical graduates spend an incredible amount of time acquiring medical knowledge, but so little time is vested in professional networking. They express discomfort and embarrassment in approaching strangers. Building confidence and positive attitude will be further discussed in the next chapter. This section recognizes barriers arising from the inter-cultural variability and highlights some of the important aspects to be considered by international/foreign medical graduates. In order to have a successful network, it is important to integrate into the American culture and acknowledge the differences and find a way to bridge the gap.

- *Mindset*: As it was alluded to in the introduction, IMGs express various negative emotions associated with networking, including embarrassment and guilt. Some may feel guilty for asking for opportunities as they assume they appear to be calculative or manipulative. Some may be concerned that they are burdening the others. Conscious efforts should be made to overcome these negative feelings and recalibrate their perceptions, which are shaped by the upbringing, values, and beliefs. In general, it is expected and acceptable to ask for assistance.
- *Eye contact*: Eye contact and touching are considered to be an effective tool to communicate during the clinical practice [6]. In some cultures, however, eye contact is regarded as rude. In America, establishing good eye contact will be perceived as attentive and confident. Meanwhile, a long stare will cause discomfort and an elicit feeling of hostility; therefore, a balance is required. Avoiding eye contact can imply submissive nature or lack of confidence. A general rule is to maintain eye contacts for about 4–5 seconds, then glance to the side and come back. When you are actively listening, try to maintain eye contact for two-thirds of the time, while when you are speaking, maintain eye contact for one-half of the time [7].
- *Hierarchy of the role*: In certain cultures, the hierarchy of social class, gender roles, and age is more pronounced than what is tolerated in America. America has undergone myriads of revolution that calls for independence, equality, and freedom. During the conversation, it is important not to impose these hierarchical mannerisms during non-verbal and verbal communication regardless of the gender or age.

Etiquettes of Conversational Networking

Communication and professionalism are high in priority in American culture and medical programs. Some studies have suggested that communication skills are not prioritized in developing countries where shortage of staff and clinical skills take precedent [8]. Here are a few tips to follow to initiate a conversation:

- The first step is to know the motivation and the purpose of establishing the relationship. Is it simply getting to know someone new? Do you already know the person you wish to reach out and you are trying to introduce yourself? Are you looking for an opportunity? Once you have a clear picture of what you want to get out of the conversation, the networking can be easy.
- The initial step of successful networking is establishing a good impression. You can draw someone's attention and greet with a pleasant smile and a handshake. When introducing yourself, pronounce your name clearly and slowly. Also reveal your function at the meeting (e.g., visitor and speaker) or organization (e.g., researcher, observer, and rotator) so that the others "know" who you are and ready to connect with you. Try to make an effort to remember people's names. If you call them by their name, they will feel the desire to call you by your name and remember you better.
- When you have started a conversation and acquainted yourself with the stranger, instead of going around the bush, it is most effective to directly express your intention earlier in the conversation or direct the conversation in a way that you can comfortably segway into revealing your intention. Once the initial contacts have been exchanged and the motivation has been shared.
- Interpersonal and communication refer to both verbal and non-verbal interactions with others. Practice speaking as clearly and naturally as you can during the conversations. Be polite and pleasant to reflect on your excellent interpersonal skills. Be an active listener and use agreeable gestures (e.g., nodding and eye contact) to maintain the interest level. Understand that not everyone is interested in meeting people or having a conversation. It is important to gauge their level of interest by being aware of the social cues and observing people's body language. Do they need to go somewhere else? Are they interested in sharing information? Are they feeling comfortable/uncomfortable? Professionalism has many subcomponents, but largely encompasses integrity and accountability, cultural competency, code of conduct, and humanism [3].
- During professional networking, maintain a comfortable physical distance and use professional language. Acknowledge that America is a diverse country with different backgrounds and be sensitive on the topics and body language used during the conversation. In certain cultures, it will not be appropriate to ask personal questions such as age, marriage status, or income. It is best to avoid conflicting topics such as religion or politics during the initial encounter. It is important to maintain the boundaries and understand what are acceptable topics to discuss.

- In a group conversation, speak loudly and confidently. Keep your stories short and follow the conversation with the flow. Some may feel compelled to jump into the conversation before allowing someone to speak and that can be very disruptive. Some also may want to share a story and they tend to hold on to that one topic you want to say, it is best to pay attention to the current conversation and jump in as needed. If you are thinking of the opportunity to say that one thing you want to say or missed a chance to say, the conversation may have already moved on and you may not be part of it.
- After creating the network, maintaining the connection with occasional friendly holiday or birthday wishes is important. Nowadays, social media allows an easier way to maintain the relationship. Utilize it wisely so that you are not overcommunicating.

Etiquettes of Online Networking

Many people, especially of the newer generations, nowadays, neglect etiquettes while using social media. One possible explanation is the lack of face-to-face interaction that gives an impression of being "unseen" or "hidden" behind the screen. However, for this *very* reason, extra attention needs to be paid particularly to etiquettes. Most of the online communication takes place without non-verbal cues. The absence of body language, facial expression, and tone of voice is a perfect setup for misunderstanding. Here are rules and recommendations for international medical graduates to avoid problems:

- *Create a good public image*: Social media operates under a virtual network of community, which is becoming a powerful source of information. Patients are increasingly depending on the online ratings and physician reviews before choosing to see a doctor. Damaged public image is very difficult to restore. It is recommended to choose a well-groomed, professional profile picture. It may be worthwhile to invest in a photography session, which can be found at a reasonable price (i.e., shopping mall or online). For those who are participating in the MATCH, use the same photo as the profile picture, for a quick recognition.
- *Be cognizant of what you post*: Although American is known for "Freedom of Speech," it is wise to avoid posting controversial contents for mutual respect and also for maintaining a good public image. In general, any discussion involving politics and religion should be avoided. America is a country with a diverse cultural background. Differences in opinions should be respected, but posting such contents can potentially invoke negative feelings by those who disagree. Particularly during the Match season, it is wise to minimize posting opinions altogether, as it is difficult to know who will come across the posts. Offensive or explicit contents and languages should never be used in any type of language. Remember that what is posted online will stay online forever.

- *Not everyone shares the same humor*: Unless the message is sent privately, posting on the social media invites all levels of social groups to view the posts. What may appear to be funny to one person may be offensive to others. Especially when the posts are made out of non-verbal context, the posts can be misinterpreted. It is best to be conservative with humor and learn to draw a boundary. If there is a strong desire to share the humor targeted toward certain groups, consider using a private messaging function to avoid any conflicts. Beware that humor is not shared universally.
- *Do not violate HIPPA*: The Health Insurance Portability and Accountability Act of 1996 (HIPAA) is a bill mandating that Personally Identifiable Information must be protected from fraud and theft. The consequence of HIPAA violations will be serious, including penalty and compromising ability to practice. Do not post any information that can potentially identify the patient, including but not limited to name, date of birth, or face. Be careful when uploading pictures from the modern devices. Automatic timestamp function and GPS location can potentially be used to identify the patients.
- *Let us not be creepy*: Although social media is used to establish networks, it should be used appropriately. Aggressive networking tactics such as multiple messaging or connection requests should be avoided, as they can make people feel uncomfortable or violated. For those who are participating in the Match, sending Facebook friend requests or private messages to the residency program-related personnel (program directors, coordinators, residents, and staff) will be considered inappropriate and perceived negatively. Facebook friend request is best reserved for close peers or colleagues, while LinkedIn and ResearchGate may be more appropriate for acquaintances and strangers at a professional level.

Conclusion

This chapter discussed various venues to expand professional networks from traditional to modern methods. In general, it is best to be judicious and conservative with social media during the Match season and use it mainly to be informed on the latest update. Later in the career, social media can serve as a great way to expand the professional network. In this chapter, we provided resources that can be used to create professional networks and optimize your chance to succeed. The next chapter will discuss further on self-image and confidence that will be crucial in developing social skills to successfully navigate through the journey.

References

1. De Janasz SC, Sullivan SE, Whiting V. Mentor networks and career success: lessons for turbulent times. Acad Manag Perspect. 2003;17(4):78–91.

2. 2018 Match result by Program Director https://mk0nrmp3oyqui6wqfm.kinstacdn.com/wp-content/uploads/2018/07/NRMP-2018-Program-Director-Survey-for-WWW.pdf
3. Ludwig https://www.acgme.org/Portals/0/PDFs/Milestones/ProfessionalismPediatrics.pdf
4. Karger DR, Quan D. What would it mean to blog on the semantic web? In: McIlraith SA, Plexousakis D, van Harmelen F, editors. The semantic web – ISWC 2004, LNCS 3298. Berlin: Springer-Verlag; 2004. pp. 214–228.
5. Marwick AE, Boyd D. I tweet honestly, I tweet passionately: Twitter users, context collapse, and the imagined audience. New Media Soc. 2010;13(1):114–33. https://doi.org/10.1177/1461444810365313.
6. Marcinowicz L, Konstantynowicz J, Godlewski C. Patients' perceptions of GP non-verbal communication: a qualitative study. Br J Gen Pract. 2010;60(571):83–7. [PMC free article] [PubMed] [Google Scholar].
7. https://www.canr.msu.edu/news/eye_contact_dont_make_these_mistakes
8. Haveliwala YA. Problems of foreign born psychiatrists. Psychiatry Q. 1979;51:307–11.

Chapter 9
"Confidence, Self-Image, Self-Esteem"

Ian H. Rutkofsky, Dong Hyang Kwon, and Bilal Haider Malik

Introduction

First and foremost, let us take a moment to be mindful – mindful that you must already have a level of confidence above many others who have dreamed big. Your dream of becoming a physician takes an incredible amount of confidence to fulfill, as many people with big dreams do not have the motivation or courage to follow through with their dreams.

This being said, becoming a physician is not only one of the most honorable professions one can aspire to become, but it is also one of the most tedious processes that require sacrifices and an incredible amount of confidence. When chasing your goal of becoming a physician, you must reflect on your abilities and desire to prove to yourself that you are capable of saving one's life, to be selfless and put your patient's first!

So, before we begin to discuss confidence and what it takes to become a physician in the US medical system, I want you to be aware that you already have what it

I. H. Rutkofsky (✉)
Department of Psychiatry, HCA – Aventura Hospital and Medical Center, Aventura, FL, USA

Department of Research, CiBNP, Fairfield, CA, USA
e-mail: ian.rutkofsky@Hcahealthcare.com

D. H. Kwon
Georgetown University, Washington, DC, USA

Department of Pathology, MedStar Georgetown University Hospital, Washington, DC, USA

B. H. Malik
CiBNP, Fairfield, CA, USA

Institute of Behavioral Neurosciences and Psychology, Fairfield, CA, USA

Internal Medicine, Research, California Institute of Behavioral Neurosciences & Psychology, Sacramento, CA, USA

© Springer Nature Switzerland AG 2021
H. Tohid, H. Maibach (eds.), *International Medical Graduates in the United States*, https://doi.org/10.1007/978-3-030-62249-7_9

takes to get there. The truth of the matter is that the United States Medical Licensing Exam (USMLE) process and the US MATCH process may be one of the most difficult medical education achievements and accomplishments in the world. This being said it is important for you to stay confident, keep your composure, portray yourself with dignity and strong character, and keep a positive self-image and self-esteem.

In this chapter we will discuss confidence, self-esteem, and self-image, and go over some solutions to keeping a confident image of yourself. Additionally, we will discuss how to present yourself when facing some challenging and important matters including the residency interview or preparing for the USMLEs and entering the US MATCH process.

Discussion

What does it mean to be confident?

Before we begin try to answer the question. Start by writing down four answers that may make you feel more confident:

1. _____
2. _____
3. _____
4. _____

By writing down ways that make you feel confident, you are working on your self-image and ultimately your self-esteem. We will discuss all these terms in more detail, but first we will define the meaning of confidence.

Confidence

Confidence is defined in many ways, but most importantly, being confident means one's capacity to believe in oneself and one's abilities. In many cases this may also include maintaining one's hope and trust during life's challenges or relationships.

Listed below are four ways that may allow you to feel more confident. Please take a moment to compare and reflect on what you have written above and relate to what has been listed below.

Four ways to increase your confidence:

1. *Believing in yourself and your ability and never blaming yourself for prior failures.*
2. *Reflecting on past challenges in your life that you have overcome and reflecting on goals you have already accomplished.*
3. *Changing your mindset about yourself and image and keeping your mind positive. (For every negative thought you may have about yourself, you must write down on paper in ink two positive thoughts about yourself.)*
4. *Do not be overly critical of yourself. Create healthy habits including exercise and proper diet, and monitor progress rather than dwell on what can be improved.*

Now, that we have discussed a few ideas about what may make us more confident, let us expand on these four important confidence boosters and begin overcoming any self-image or self-esteem issues you may harbor.

Self-Image

Self-image is related to one's concern about their view of their self, abilities, appearance, and personality. Having a sense of pride in the way you look, dress, or act is important in reflecting one's day-to-day interactions. Defining who you are, your style, and your comfort is important. The popular term "swagger" is an urban-modern term that reflects the way one conduct's themselves or how one exudes self-confidence through a personalized style. Finding who you are and working on your insecurities is the best way to begin. So begin with evaluating your appearance; it is okay to reinvent yourself from time to time. Try a new hairstyle, purchase a new outfit, or rewrite your workout plan. You can use free apps like Instagram or Pinterest or search for videos on YouTube. Ultimately, if you feel you look cool, then you will exude confidence and create good image of your-self.

Please take a moment as this is an appropriate time to now reflect on yourself. In some cases one may display traits of low self-esteem or self-image and may not be aware of them. Other people may notice these traits about you before you even develop a sense of your own self-esteem. Thus, it is important to be mindful of your daily actions and be aware of the characteristics of your self-esteem.

Characteristics of Low Self-Esteem

Low self-esteem is characterized by a lack of confidence and usually a sense of feeling negative about oneself. People with low self-esteem often feel unloved or incompetent. Many people with low self-esteem eventually develop symptoms of depression, anxiety, and irritable mood. One may try to avoid social situations due to feelings of inadequacy, and others may try to be the life of the party and attempt to gain praise and attention from others. Note: attention-seeking behaviors secondary to low self-esteem are generally done in non-conservative fashion, either through seduction (sexual) attention or by trying to impress others with material objects. But as a side note, just because people have fine taste in material objects, this does not necessarily mean you have poor self-esteem.

Common personality traits and characteristics associated with low self-esteem
1. *Blaming yourself*
2. *Expecting the worst or negative outcomes*
3. *Underestimating yourself*
4. *Being too critical of yourself*

Now, if we reflect on these four common personality traits of low self-esteem and how they relate to confidence, we can compare the four important confidence boosters discussed earlier in this chapter to overcome any self-esteem issues. Note that the four confidence boosters listed earlier are directly related to the four common personality traits listed to be associated with low self-esteem. Please notice below, listed 1–4, how they relate to each other:

1. *Blaming yourself:* Start believing in yourself and your ability and never blame yourself!

    Do not blame yourself, try to improve, learn from past mistakes, and most importantly believe in yourself. Many people in this world who have achieved have likely had failures along the way. Remember this quote by Denzel Washington, "If you don't fail, you're not even trying!"

2. *Expecting the worst of negative outcomes*: Remember reflecting on past challenges in your life that you have overcome or reflecting on goals you have already accomplished. Try to recall a past exam in medical school that you did well on. Do you remember working hard and the feeling you felt when you received a passing score? Now pat yourself on the back and think about more success is yet to come. Recalling positive events from the past is the best reinforcement to prevent catastrophizing and to stay motivated. You will continue to achieve and with each achievement develop more confidence.

3. *Underestimating yourself:* Changing your mindset about yourself and keeping your mind positive. Do not confuse confidence with arrogance. They are not similar. You can appear confident and genuine at the same time. The power of positive thinking allows you to focus on the good things that make you who you are as an individual. Again, we cannot express enough how important it is that every time you have negative thoughts about yourself, you must remember to write down on paper two or more positive thoughts about yourself.

4. *Being overly critical of yourself.* Rather than dwell on things you do not like about yourself, create *healthy habits* including an exercise routine and proper diet, and monitor progress in your life. This can also help you to improve yourself overall and result in a positive self-image.

Healthy Habits

Exercise

Exercise and fitness has been proven to boost one's mood, memory, and self-esteem. It is important to have a daily exercise routine. Remember that a balanced life keeps your mind fit too. Exercise can improve the self-esteem not only in adults but also in children [1]. It is important to start these habits early and teach them to our young ones. Resistance training such as weight lifting is important for maintaining your muscle mass and increasing your Basal Metabolic Rate. Weight training is an anaerobic exercise. Cardiovascular exercise such as jogging on the treadmill or elliptical can be either anaerobic or aerobic depending on how high your heart rate is during your cardiovascular exercise. It is important to warm up your muscles before doing weight training. You can do this either by slow, 10-minute jog or stretching. Many suggest a 10-minute jog on the treadmill is a good warm-up prior to lifting weights. After lifting weights, you can then directly return to the cardiovascular routine and exercise at your target heart rate. A graph measuring your age and target heart rate is often provided on the machine. Listed below is a chart of the target heart rate between ages 20 and 55 years old. To find out more about target heart rate, consider the following link: https://www.pennmedicine.org/updates/blogs/heart-and-vascular-blog/2018/march/exercise-target-heart-rate

Age (years)	Beats per minute (BPM)
20	130–160
30	124–152
35	120–148
40	117–144
45	114–140
50	111–136
55	107–132

Chart modified from the original from penmedicin.org

Diet

Keeping a healthy diet has been scientifically proven to not only keep you healthy and live longer but also maintain proper brain chemistry and improve your mood and anxiety. There are many popular diets endorsed by celebrities. From the low-carb, whole-food diet, the Atkins diet, the South Beach diet, the Ketogenic diet, or the Paleo diet, one may have a difficult time finding a proper diet. Some individuals keep diets based on their ethical or religious beliefs such as animal activists who maintain a vegan diet or Hindus most of whom are vegetarian or Jews and Muslims who refrain from eating pork and eat Kosher or Halal foods respectively. The important thing is that with any diet, one must eat proper nutrients; however, keeping on a diet that will contribute to keeping tone and your waistline thin can make you feel and look great. Food and indulgence can also make us feel great, but with quick regret. So when you indulge in a great meal, remember to eat a balanced diet and not to overeat. Try to maintain a diet; keeping a planned diet has been known to improve your self-esteem and self-image.

Sleep

When we are stressed, we tend to stay up late at night and worry about a thing in our life. While staying up late to get more accomplished is sometimes unpreventable, it is important to keep proper sleep hygiene and attempt to go to sleep and wake up at similar times each day. Many individuals find they feel most refreshed and relaxed with approximately 7 hours of sleep each night. Dreaming occurs in the stage of sleep known as Rapid eye movement sleep (REM sleep), and dreaming is thought to help you better cope with some of those things that are on your mind that are keeping you pondering. Missing even one night of proper rest can leave you feeling anxious the following day. Anxiety and nervousness related to sleep deprivation can lower your confidence and self-esteem and affect your performance and judgment. It is therefore important to balance your life with a proper sleep regimen. Some individuals experience recurrent nightmares, especially if a traumatic event may have occurred. These nightmares may be at random, but if a traumatic event has occurred and you are replaying the event over and over and suffering from nightmares related to this event, there is a high likelihood that these symptoms are caused by either acute stress disorder (ASD) or post-traumatic stress disorder (PTSD). If you are experiencing bad dreams at night or have not been able to fall asleep at night, you can talk to your doctor about medications that may help, such as trazodone or zolpidem for insomnia or prazosin, a competitive alpha-1 adrenergic receptor blocker, for nightmares. Proper sleep hygiene should always be attempted first before starting medication to achieve better sleep. The following is an example of how to improve sleep hygiene according to sleepfoundation.com. A more detailed list can be found on sleepfoundation.org.

Limit daytime naps to less than 30 minutes.
Avoid stimulants such as caffeine and nicotine in the evening.
Do as little as 10 minutes of aerobic exercise each day; however, nighttime exercise may stimulate you. It differs from person to person.
Avoid fatty or spicy meals, citrus fruits, and carbonated drinks at bedtime.
Get natural light during the day and keep your room dark at bedtime. Avoid watching TV or laptops before sleep.
Keep a relaxing bedtime routine.
Keep your room at comfortable temperature and invest in a comfortable bed.

Prayer, Meditation, and/or Mindfulness

While many readers may consider themselves as agnostic or just stray away from theology, there are some important benefits of prayer or meditation to mention. Self-confidence can be delivered in prayer by developing a faith that good things will happen to you and that a higher power is there to support you; thus, for many individuals, spirituality can lead to a more meaningful life. Scientifically, both prayer and meditation are characteristically very similar when it comes to the neurophysiologic response in the prefrontal cortex and the posterior cingulate cortex. Additionally, prayer, meditation, and mindfulness produce alpha waves (8–12 Hz) on electroencephalogram (EEG). Increased alpha waves are said to be related to your brain's ability to lower stress, feel calmer, and reduce nervousness, which is important to maintain one's daily life and enhance one's self-confidence.

Indeed, there are endless reasons why one may develop low confidence or low self-esteem. We have discussed some of the most common personality traits associated with low self-esteem and poor confidence, and we have discussed how to improve your self-image, but now we will discuss one of the most important barriers to improving one's confidence, self-esteem, and self-image. This barrier is otherwise known as the "inner critic."

Your Inner Critic

"The inner critic" is the voice inside your head; it is your mind and is a concept used in psychology and psychotherapy, similar to the Freudian superego [2]. The inner critic often functions as a reward or punishment censor; it can reinforce positive things you have accomplished or it may say that you are wrong. At times your inner critic may even be derogatory, and ultimately, you may start to believe you are inadequate, worthless, and guilty. It is important to differentiate the inner critic from psychosis, as the inner critic is one's thoughts or one's voice; for example, when you have a negative mindset, your inner critic may say in your voice, "You're dumb," "You're too fat," "Everyone hates you," or "You're worthless." You may even remember other people telling you this before and hear their voice in your head. This is different from experiencing psychosis. People who are experiencing psychosis may be told the same derogatory statements, but they are hearing auditory hallucinations such as other people's voices in the room when no one else is present in the room.

Several self-help books have been published about the inner critic to help overcome these challenges. Please note that if you are hearing voices that are not your own or you have thoughts of self-harm, suicidal ideations, or homicidal ideations, please go to the nearest emergency department or call your doctor today. You may also call 911 for police or the emergency dispatch. Law enforcement can bring you to the hospital for a psychiatric evaluation. There is no legal ramification for seeking psychiatric help if you believe you may be a risk to yourself or others.

Furthermore, these inner voices or negative thoughts about oneself destroy one's self-esteem. To overcome low self-esteem, you must challenge these negative thoughts and defend yourself from your inner critic.

Self-help techniques to let go of your inner critic

Give to others who are in need.
Know yourself.
Know your strengths and weaknesses.
Acknowledge your achievements.
Never compare yourself to others.
Balance your work/life with proper diet, exercise, and sleep.
Limit your interaction with negative people.
Surround yourself with positive people.
Reinvent yourself.
Discover a spiritual outlet.
Respect yourself.

Keeping confident while pursuing a residency in the USA is essential. The process is rigorous, and as an international medical graduate (IMG), you must perform exceptionally well on the USMLEs to be invited for an interview. You must also perform well on those interviews to be ranked and to ultimately MATCH into a residency training program in the USA.

It is a big step: the United States Medical Licensing Exam (USMLE)

The USMLE will be discussed in more detail in other chapters, but there are some important factors related to exam taking and confidence. IMGs are required to take the USMLE Step 1, Step 2 Clinical Knowledge (CK), and Step 2 Clinical Skills (CS) to MATCH into residency and to become Educational Commission for Foreign Medical Graduates (ECFMG) Certified. Many candidates are opting to also take the USMLE Step 3 before entering into the MATCH although it is not required for the MATCH. This may also become more common after the USMLE Step 1 becomes a pass/fail exam in 2022. Please refer to USMLE program announces upcoming policy changes at https://usmle.org/announcements/

The USMLE Step 1

Of course, there are many sources for you to learn from. Once you find the books or lectures of your choice, the most important step to take in your preparation is to use practice questions! Around 75–80% of your study time should be invested in doing practice questions. Why is doing practice questions so important? It is important because practice makes perfect. The better you know the exam material, the more prepared you will feel and the more confident you will become. Doing practice questions allows for "active learning" rather than "passive learning." It also trains your brain to be confident in selecting answers and gives you a chance to simulate a timed exam. In 2022, the USMLE Step 1 will become a pass/fail exam. I understand this puts IMGs in a hard position. The new way toward achievement will be to engage more frequently in extracurricular activities, publish research manuscripts, and do very well on your Step 2 CK exam without failures or attempts on the USMLEs.

The USMLE Step 2 CK

The Step 2 CK exam is very similar to the USMLE Step 1 as far as preparation goes. Study preparation should also consist of approximately 75–80% of your study time invested in doing practice questions. The USMLE Step 2 CK is commonly noted to be less challenging compared to the USMLE Step 1. This is because the Step 1 exam is focused on basic science principles and pathology, while the USMLE CK exam is the more clinical-based exam and tests your clinical knowledge. Many

IMGs have been working in the clinical setting before attempting the exam, and many aspects of the exam may come second nature to you. However, just like USMLE Step 1, the exams are difficult. It is a must to show improvement from the USMLE Step 1 to the USMLE Step 2 CK. Residency programs are looking for consistency from exam to exam and want to see improvement. If you can prove that you are consistent with your exams, it shows that you can maintain a strong will to learn and are likely to continue to do well into residency. To stay consistent year after year from the time of medical school and into residency training, one must have a positive mind and good self-esteem; otherwise, you are bound to burnout. Burnout is a common phenomenon that many physicians suffer form. They lose a sense of desire to continue to work and usually develop signs of depression and some even have committed suicide. Performing poorly on Step 2 may show signs that you are already starting to burning out. After 2022 when the USMLE Step 1 becomes a pass/fail exam, the Step 2 CK is going to be a critical exam in the MATCH process and will be your chance to prove yourself and your competence.

The USMLE Step 2 CS

USMLE STEP 2 CS exam and the residency interview process can feel like a similar endeavor. They are very similar to each other. During your residency interviews, you will need to maintain a similar composure. In both cases, you will move from room to room and need to shake hands, maintain eye contact, and look confident. The patient interaction in the clinical skills exam is very similar to a real patient encounter; however, your patient is a trained actor. To do well on this exam, you should practice live cases with a partner. There is an online simulation you can download from the exam website to practice writing your notes. Use mnemonics to remember the questions you need to ask, and always portray yourself professionally and trustworthy.

USMLE Step 3

Many applicants are increasingly opting to take the USMLE Step 3 to become more competitive for residency placement. Others may be eager to write the exam before the MATCH to increase the chance of obtaining an H1B visa rather than a J1 visa. The J1 visa requires 2-year home return unless you can receive a waiver from your employer post-residency training. The H1B visa does not require a home return for employment but does however require the completion of Step 3 before starting residency. Taking and passing the USMLE Step 3 before interviews will also allow you to feel more confident about your applicant, knowing that you stand out with achievements that many other candidates on your interview day have yet to accomplish. If you have an attempt on a USMLE exam and did not pass on the first time, it is highly suggestive to pass the Step 3 exam before applying to residency. Note: The hardest thing to overcome is an attempt on a USMLE exam. If you have an attempt, you need to stand out consider taking the USMLE Step 3, publishing papers, and doing more externships in your specialty.

Why is a failed attempt on the USMLE so bad?

The reason why failing one of your USMLE exams is thought to be a huge obstacle to overcome is that the exam failure on the first attempt is thought to be in one's poor judgment. What this means is that if you have failed one of your exams on the first try, this may have been too having poor insight in your ability. Overconfidence in your abilities can make a program director nervous about your judgment with patient care. In some cases, you may have felt impulsive rather than patient with your studies and ready to get it over with. Surely, it is a long route, and a hard one, but if you take the time to do proper research, you will find consistent USMLE marks associated with the MATCH, per specialty. Take your time to do your research and to study and attempt to score on par with your colleges. Failing your USMLE exam may come off as if you are unable to analyze your limitations. Again, take the time to pass on the first attempt. It is better to take longer in your preparation than to fail the exam. If you have a failure on any USMLE exam, it is critical to improve on the second attempt. Depending on your financial situation, you should also consider passing the USMLE Step 3 first before entering the MATCH.

What can be done to overcome poor scores or attempts on the USMLE?

This is a question I frequently hear asked all the time. "What can be done to overcome poor scores or attempts on the USMLE?" Or "What can I do to get interviews next year?" Start by reviewing your CV or resume and attempt to strengthen it. As you review your CV or resume, compare it with others who you may know have already Matched into a residency training program. Remember it is important to make sure you appear well-rounded and stay active in your pursuit.

What can I do to develop a strong CV?

1. *US Clinical Experience (USCE)*

USCE is defined as experience working with patients conducted in the US medical system. There are two ways in which clinical training can be continued after medical school education. One of the routes is called an observership. An observership is similar to a medical school clinical rotation, but instead you observe. Here you will often take patient information and present the information along with a plan to the attending physician in charge, but you may not have hands-on experience during an observership. On the other hand, externships may become available, which will provide more hands-on training. Externships may require malpractice insurance depending on the location or hospital policy. Externships may allow you to treat the patient and document patient notes under supervision, much like a resident physician. Optimally, a combination of the two would justify your time as being well spent while applying for the residency MATCH.

It is important to stay clinically relevant post-medical school graduation. For IMGs, spending time in the US medical system at US hospitals as either an observer or extern is a great way to feel confident about your ability to adapt to the US workplace and feel comfortable with the US healthcare system. I recommend having at least a minimum of 4 months of USCE. There are a number of services available that can set up clinical training in different cities and states around the USA. Often times the rotations can be pricey, but no-cost rotations are sometimes offered. If you have the opportunity for an externship or observership at a clinical site that has an Accreditation Council for Graduate Medical Education (ACGME) residency program, this may in fact increase your chance of obtaining an interview there.

2. *Publications*

Writing and publishing manuscripts is an important way to impact your CV. California Institute of Behavioral Neurosciences and Psychology (CIBNP) is a premier online institute designed for helping IMGs learn how to write and publish manuscripts during their 8-week course. Each student co-authors with each other on multiple manuscripts while learning how to write one of their own and becoming a first name author. Having PubMed published papers strengthens your CV and builds self-confidence while contributing to the greater scientific community. In recent years, many residency programs, including university- or community-based, have started requiring applicants to have publications. Program ranking sometimes works on a point scale, where numerous publications can increase your points and lead to being ranked higher. Applying to residency without publications is sometimes looked at as an incomplete CV. I recommend every applicant applying to the US residency MATCH to have a minimum of two publications at the time of application; this may maximize the chance of Matching. For those who have poorer performance on the USMLE, this is an opportunity to impress those program directors who value research.

3. *Improving My CV with the USMLE STEP 3*

If you have an attempt on one of your USMLE exams or it has been over a year since you have passed the USMLE Step 2 CK, then taking the USMLE Step 3 should become one of your top three priorities along with USCE and publishing manuscripts. Passing the USMLE Step 3 will lift your spirits by knowing you have no more USMLEs ahead of you. This will take a lot of pressure off you and it will also catch many program directors' attention. Residency programs cannot promote residents beyond the Post Graduate Year (PGY)-2 year without obtaining a passing mark on the USMLE Step 3. Passing the USMLE Step 3 prior to applying will also eliminate any concern from a program that you may not pass the exam by the deadline. In addition, you will feel more competent and confident to make medical decisions as an intern after completion of the Step 3 exam.

4. *Certifications*

Remember to dedicate a section for relevant certifications on your CV. There are a number of ways of obtaining these certificates. From online universities to research institutes such as CIBNP, there are a number of platforms and workshops to choose from. When applying to residency, having unique certificates from a verity of learning platforms will highlight your interests and give character to your CV.

Recommended Paying Certifications in North America:

Gauge your interest. Some certifications can provide for a part-time job. Consider the following certifications in the healthcare industry:

- Emergency Medical Technician (EMT)-Basic
- Personal Fitness Trainer Certification
- Behavioral Technician Specialist (there are four levels of certification)
- Certified Phlebotomy Technician (CPT)
- Professional Coder
- Pharmacy Technician Professional
- Medical Assistant
- Medical Front Office Administration Specialist
- Patient Care Technician (PCT)

Recommended Online Learning Platforms with Certificates:

- Coursera
- California Institute of Behavioral Neurosciences and Psychology (CIBNP)
- Pluralsight
- LinkedIn Learning
- Udemy
- Udacity
- Khan Academy
- Codecademy
- edX
- Dataquest

5. *National Conferences*

Attending national conferences and joining professional organizations will allow for an opportunity to connect and meet with other medical professionals from across the country. Participating at national conferences will allow you to either attend public-speaking events or present your own work. Two ways to showcase your work and add remarkable experience to your CV are

- designing and presenting academic posters
- oral presentations

(Please refer to Chap. 8 for a list of organizations which hold annual meetings or to learn more about networking at various national conferences.)

6. *Volunteer*

You may feel it is prerequisite to volunteer. Volunteering offers the opportunity for you to be selfless – to provide your time to the community where you can make a difference to people in dire need of help. Volunteering also allows for developing new skills and experiences. There are many options and places for you to volunteer in North America.

Please consider volunteering at the following listings.
Your effort can truly make a difference in the community.

- Disaster relief efforts
- Homeless shelters
- Suicide hotlines
- Places of worship (such as temples, churches, synagogues, or mosques)
- Animal rescue shelters
- National parks
- Food pantries
- Habitat for humanity
- Local libraries
- Young Men's Christian Association (YMCA)
- Red Cross
- Retirement homes

Residency Interviews

Practice mock interviews. If there is one way to boost your confidence, it is looking the part and having your act down cold. Remember "Fake It Till You Make It," this is a well-known TED talk presented by Amy Cuddy in 2012. It is used for career readiness and confidence and is admired TED talk and workshop for enhancing self-confidence in the workplace.

Look the Part (Attire during the interview)

All right, so you now have your first interview and it is time to impress those who will be judging you, your character, and your every movement. It is very important to stay confident, and this means you must look the part, look rested, and be ready to serve your community. The interview process is formal and what this means is that you must wear your best suit. Your shirt should be a solid color with a classic button-down shirt. Your shoes should be polished leather and for women a closed toe flat or small heel are more professional and also more comfortable during the tour. The hospital tour may last over 1 hour.

Consider a solid color suit, either navy blue (preferred), gray, or black. For men, you must wear a necktie and women should have their hair and makeup done professionally and conservatively. The interview day is long; you will have a tour of the facility, meet the residents, and be interviewed by three to five people, often 15–45-minute meetings. When time is up you will hear a knock on the door and it will be time to end the conversation and say your closing remarks. One mistake we often make is appearing overly confident. Do not interview the interviewer; let them interview you. Practice your act! Know what to ask and what is appropriate. Show them that your confidence is real, avoid being aggressive, and do not act desperate. If you act desperate, it will not help you, but it will hurt you. If you act overly confident, either it appears as arrogant or that you are compensating for poor self-esteem. Being aggressive or desperate may also come off as being weak. You can avoid looking aggressive by not talking over other candidates, being courteous and friendly to everyone, even if you feel other interviewees are your competition.

The interview dinner

The interview dinner may be just as important as the interview itself. Depending on which program you are interviewing at, the feedback from the residents may be taken very seriously. This is because some programs emphasize the ability of your communication with your peers. Your co-residents will want to be your team members as well as your friend. They will ask themselves: Do I see myself working with this person? Do I see myself spending time outside of the hospital with this person? Would I like to invite this person to dinner to meet my family? Does this person have the right judgment to be a doctor and serve the community which I love? At the dinner, remember to act professionally and dress business casual, no jeans or shorts. This is your time to show you are committed to the field, the geographical area, and the program. It is also your time to show your true colors, be personable, and make friends. If you have been granted an interview, you have a good chance to MATCH if things go right at dinner and during the interview. One common misperception is that if you have a friend in the program and they help get you an interview, then it is a guarantee that you will MATCH. While connections may help you get the interview, the program will likely be even more critical about your application and make sure you have the profile they are looking for and that you are equally completive to other candidate's interviewing. People with low confidence about the MATCH often stand out and are not appreciated during the dinner. Always show respect to others at dinner and be friendly to other applicants.

Supplementary information

Remember you are not alone. Consider finding professional help with your CV or a counselor if you feel overwhelmed or lost. The MATCH process can certainly be difficult on one's ego and out self-esteem. Consider using self-help books; try attending professional and informative seminars/webinars, and continue reading books that can guide you in the right direction toward fulfillment. Keeping in touch with friends who share your same experience may help the process transition more smoothly. Making new contacts can be fun and helpful and can lead to lifelong friendships or relationships. Remember making new contacts can be through attending conventions, volunteering, or exploring social media networks. Additional information on "Making Contacts" (refer to Chap. 8) and "Social Media" (refer to Chap. 9) is given.

Is It Okay to Have a Plan B?

According to Shin and Milkman's (2016) publication, "How backup plans can harm," they discovered that there are consequences and risks of having a back-up plan or a "Plan B." They discovered that once you begin thinking about a fallback plan, your aspiration to attain your definitive goal declines [3]. It is natural to think, "What if I never MATCH?" This may be a reality. The MATCH process is highly competitive. But it is very important to engage in self-talk. Remember to tell yourself every day, "I will reach my goal," "I will improve my CV," and "I will have the most impressive CV on the interview day." This will help to improve your confidence and motivation to continue down this path. With all this being said, if you have expired all options and you can no longer bear the path to US residency, if you have failed time and time again to MATCH, Plan B should be considered. Four of the recommended paths for a back-up plan are as follows: (1) consider being a physician in another country; (2) apply to nursing school which can lead to Registered Nurse (RN) or Nurse Practitioner (NP); (3) apply to physician assistant (PA) program; (4) consider the "Assistant Physician" (AP) path which was authorized by the Missouri legislature in 2014 and fully implemented on January 1, 2017, to work as a provider. Even if you have decided on an alternate path or Plan B, continue to establish networks you can still apply again later.

Conclusion

In summary, individuals suffering from low self-esteem and poor self-image often have a sense of inadequacy and often feel rejection and disapproval from others, leading to sensitivity to rejection, depression, anxiety, and irritability, and eventually develop low confidence in themselves. Low confidence often causes individuals to become overly critical of themselves, blame themselves, and underestimate themselves, leading those to predict the worst possible outcome and ultimately limiting one's motivation to achieve. As physicians, we must work on our confidence as well as judgment. Often those with poor self-esteem behave immorally, overcompensate, or act dishonorably. Self-help tools provided are good practices to overcome your inner critic and learn how to value oneself in a positive light. The USMLE and MATCH process is a stressful time; if you feel you need professional help to overcome issues discussed in this chapter, both psychologists and psychiatrists are there to help you overcome these limitations, build your confidence, and get you on track to a prosperous future. Good luck to you all! Our communities here in the USA need you!

References

1. Ekeland E, Heian F, Hagen KB, Abbott JM, Nordheim L. Exercise to improve self-esteem in children and young people. Cochrane Database Syst Rev. 2004;1(1):1–52.
2. Elliott KJ. The inner critic as a key element in working with adults who have experienced childhood sexual abuse. Bull Menn Clin. 1999;63(2):240–53.
3. Shin J, Milkman KL. How backup plans can harm goal pursuit: the unexpected downside of being prepared for the future. Organ Behav Hum Decis Process. 2016;135:1–9.

Websites

https://www.pennmedicine.org/updates/blogs/heart-and-vascular-blog/2018/march/
   exercise-target-heart-rate
https://www.sleepfoundation.org/articles/sleep-hygiene
https://usmle.org/announcements/
https://www.moneycrashers.com/good-places-volunteer-opportunities-organizations/

Chapter 10
Restriction to Specific Fields

Arturo J. Rios-Diaz and Saïd C. Azoury

Introduction

International medical graduates are an essential component of the US workforce and are key to providing high-quality and accessible healthcare [1]. According to estimates from the Federation of State Medical Boards, the number of licensed physicians who were international medical graduates (IMGs) increased by 18% from 2010 to 2018 [2], reaching an astonishing figure of 226,556 licensed IMGs in 2018 [2] and effectively comprising nearly a quarter of licensed physicians in the USA [2, 3]. This upward trend is expected to continue as 2019 data from the National Resident Matching Program (NRMP, also known as The Match®) revealed the highest match rate to post-graduate year-1 (PGY-1) positions since 1990 for US citizen (59%) and since 1991 for non-US (58.6%) citizen IMGs matched to post-graduate year-1 (PGY-1) positions since 1991 and 1990, respectively [4]. The vast majority of these IMGs apply and match into primary care specialties such as internal medicine, family medicine, pediatrics, and psychiatry. However, IMGs face challenges when applying to non-primary care specialties such as surgical specialties, dermatology, interventional radiology among others due to several factors including competitiveness and even discrimination. This chapter aims to provide perspective on how competitive some specialties are for IMGs, the obstacles they may face when

A. J. Rios-Diaz (✉)
Department of Surgery, Thomas Jefferson University, Philadelphia, PA, USA

Division of Plastic Surgery, Department of Surgery, University of Pennsylvania, Philadelphia, PA, USA
e-mail: arturo.riosdiaz@jefferson.edu

S. C. Azoury
Division of Plastic Surgery, Department of Surgery, University of Pennsylvania, Philadelphia, PA, USA

© Springer Nature Switzerland AG 2021
H. Tohid, H. Maibach (eds.), *International Medical Graduates in the United States*, https://doi.org/10.1007/978-3-030-62249-7_10

applying to them with a special emphasis on plastic surgery, as well as potential solutions to overcome these barriers. We will focus mostly on non-US IMGs since they comprised the majority of IMGs and they are intrinsically different than US-IMGs.

Competitiveness Factors

Factors affecting and/or preventing IMGs from applying to certain specialties are multifactorial, but one of the main drivers is the competitiveness of those specialties. Competitiveness can be defined by several measures, some of which are more in control of the applicant (modifiable) such as the United States Medical Licensing Examination (USMLE) exams (also known and referred to as Steps), research, and clinical experience. Others are nonmodifiable such as the availability of positions and programs' willingness to consider IMGs applicants. We will dive into each of these and provide potential solutions for the IMG applicant.

Availability of Residency Spots

One of the main limitations that prevent IMGs, and any applicant, from being accepted into specific specialties is the availability of positions. This measure may be used to reflect overall competitiveness by calculating the ratio of available positions per applicant. For instance, Chen utilized NRMP data to evaluate positions available per US applicant and demonstrated that interventional radiology was the most competitive specialty in 2018 by this measure with only 0.66 positions per applicant, followed by orthopedic surgery (0.88), plastic surgery (0.92), urology (0.95), neurological surgery (0.96), and ophthalmology (0.96) [5]. Instead, pathology (2.68), internal medicine (2.32), and family medicine (2.22) were among the least competitive specialties [5]. Not surprisingly, this finding coincides with specialties in which some programs depend on a significant proportion of IMGs (>50%) to fill their PGY-1 spots and with specialties that tend to be more appealing to IMGs as demonstrated by the proportion of IMGs applying to them [6].

   In order to illustrate the differences in popularity and competitiveness, we extracted and reviewed data from the 2018 Match® [6] and compared the top and bottom five specialties by volume of non-US IMG applications and match rates (Table 10.1). We also conducted Pearson's correlations to assess the association of match rates and the ratio of non-US IMG applicants per position offered by specialty. There were 6786 non-US IMGs applying to 19 specialties, of which 3494 matched (51.5% match rate). Analyses of specialties by popularity among non-US IMGs revealed that internal medicine was by far the most popular specialty with 53.6% of applications, followed by family medicine (10%), pediatrics (7.2%), psychiatry (5.4%), and neurology (4.9%) with a total of 5510 applications, which

Table 10.1 Summary of positions, applicants, and match rates for the most and least competitive specialties for non-US IMGs

Specialty	Total positions offered	Total applicants	Ratio of applicants per position	Non-US IMG				
				Matched	Not matched	Total	Non-US IMG proportion (%)	Match rate (%)
Top five specialties by volume								
Internal Medicine	7916	10,032	1.27	2042	1593	3635	23.5	56.2
Family Medicine	3629	4402	1.21	267	412	679	6.1	39.3
Pediatrics	2858	3059	1.07	309	182	491	2.7	62.9
Psychiatry	1556	2383	1.53	131	239	370	3.5	35.4
Neurology	859	1070	1.25	180	155	335	2.3	53.7
Group total (average)	*16,818*	*20,946*	*(1.27)*	*2929*	*2581*	*5510*	*38*	*(53.2)*
Top five specialties by volume								
Physical Medicine and Rehabilitation	421	579	1.38	10	22	32	0.3	31.3
Internal Medicine/ Pediatrics	382	439	1.15	5	23	28	0.3	17.9
Orthopedic Surgery	742	987	1.33	3	17	20	0.3	15.0
Plastic Surgery	168	222	1.32	3	13	16	0.2	18.8
Vascular Surgery	60	77	1.28	4	11	15	0.2	26.7
Group total (average)	*1773*	*2304*	*(1.29)*	*25*	*86*	*111*	*1.3*	*22.5*

Count data are taken from (with permission) National Resident Matching Program. *National Resident Matching Program, Charting Outcomes in the Match: International Medical Graduates, 2018.* Washington, DC; 2018. Accessed March 2, 2020

represented 81.2% of all non-US IMG applications occurring that year. The combined match rate for these five specialties was 53.2% ranging from 35.4% for psychiatry to 62.9% for pediatrics. On the other hand, the volume of non-US IMG applicants to the bottom five specialties represented only 1.6% of the applications: vascular surgery had the fewest applicants (0.2%), followed by plastic surgery (2.4%), orthopedic surgery (2.9%), internal medicine/pediatrics (4.1%), and physical medicine and rehabilitation (4.7%). These specialties' combined match rate was much lower at 22.5%, ranging from as low as 15% for orthopedic surgery to 31.3%

for physical medicine and rehabilitation. The match rate for each specialty was positively and significantly correlated with how competitive these specialties were ($R^2 = 0.53$; $p = 0.02$), meaning that the higher the number of spots available, the higher the match rate for each specialty.

Match rates should not be used as the only measure by the IMG applicant to estimate their chance of matching into a specialty, particularly for the most competitive ones. For instance, one may think that almost one in every five IMGs that apply to plastic surgery ends up matching into that specialty according to match rates alone. However, from the authors' experience and given the low number of applicants seen in these competitive specialties, these match rates are not generalizable. Most IMGs applying to these specialties were probably known to at least one of the programs they were applying to through a clerkship rotation, observership, research-related activities, or via other networking avenues. For instance, the majority of non-US IMGs applying to dermatology and orthopedic, plastic, and neurological surgeries had five or more publications, and the mean number of publications for those who matched ranged from 12 for dermatology to 47 for neurological surgery. Since the availability of positions is a nonmodifiable factor, these data can be used by the IMG applicant to set realistic expectations and to plan accordingly (financially and time wise) should they still be interested in pursuing residency into one of these specialties.

Willingness to Consider IMGs

Despite data showing that there is no difference in patient outcomes when they are treated by IMGs relative to US medical graduates (USMGs) [7–9], discrimination in the selection process is one of the challenges IMGs face when attempting to get into a residency in the USA. Desbiens and Vidaillet [10] conducted a review of the literature and found that the bias against IMGs is manifested in three ways: one is the quota system, where programs set a proportion of IMGs that they will allow, which is enabled by the fact they can be accepted into a program outside of The Match®; another is the hierarchical system, where programs rank USMGs first before IMGs regardless of their qualifications; and lastly, the unfortunate categorical refusal to even consider IMGs. Part of this bias against IMGs may be due to the perceived inability to evaluate whether they are adequately prepared for a residency in the USA [11]. However, the Educational Commission for Foreign Medical Graduates (ECFMG) rigorous certification process should take this bias out of the equation as not only international medical schools and medical education credentials have to meet certain requirements but also the IMG must take the same examinations as USMGs [12]. Nonetheless, this bias still exists due to a variety of reasons [10] that IMGs cannot control and that are beyond the scope of this chapter.

In order to quantify and provide perspective of the degree to which programs are IMG-friendly, we reviewed and extracted recent data from a national survey of program directors conducted in 2018 [13] to evaluate the proportion of programs that would never, rarely, or often consider non-US IMGs for interview among the most competitive specialties. This survey evaluated responses from 1333 programs in 23 specialties. According to this study, 30% of programs do not even consider, 46% seldom do, and only 21% often considered non-US IMGs for interview nationwide. This phenomenon is more pronounced for competitive specialties such as orthopedic surgery where 79% or 21% of programs never or rarely consider non-US IMGs, 59% or 41% for dermatology, 57% or 36% for interventional radiology, 53% or 42% for plastic surgery, 44% or 53% for otolaryngology, 35% or 49% for diagnostic radiology, 22% or 65% for neurological surgery, 21% or 52% for general surgery, and 7% or 86% for vascular surgery, respectively. None of the dermatology and orthopedic surgery programs consider IMGs for interview on a regular basis. To contrast these figures, 18% of internal medicine programs would never, 42% rarely, and 39% often consider non-US IMGs for interview (Fig. 10.1). Furthermore, there are programs that often consider IMGs even at a higher proportion, such as neurology (47%) and pathology (74%), but the availability of positions for those specialties is over 10 times less than that for internal medicine. Therefore, it is not surprising that the majority (54%) of non-US IMGs apply to this specialty.

Unfortunately, the IMG applicant does not have control over the discrimination factor. Instead, the IMG may use this information when strategizing which program to apply to and there are ways to ascertain whether a specific program considers IMGs. The American Medical Association (AMA) Fellowship and Residency Electronic Interactive Database (FREIDA™) offers an online service, FREIDA

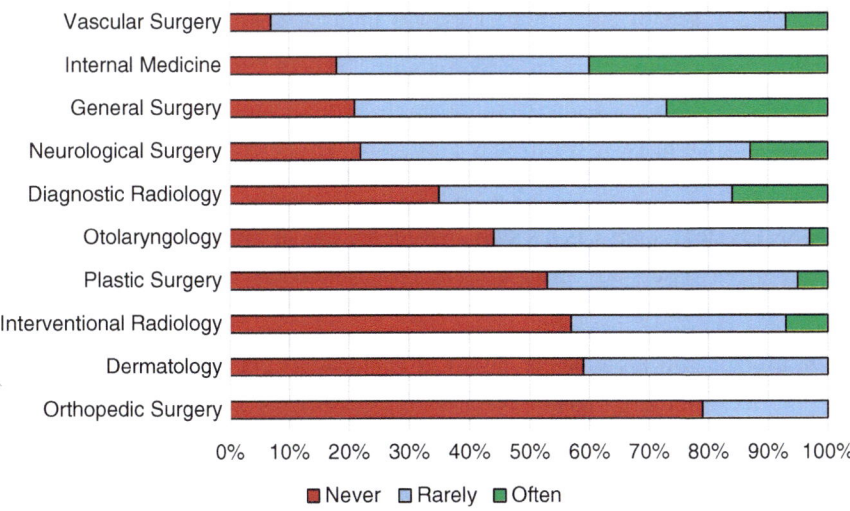

Fig. 10.1 Residency programs' IMG-friendliness defined by the frequency they consider IMG applicants for interview for the most competitive specialties. Note: Internal medicine included as reference as it is the most popular specialty among IMG. Data are taken from (with permission) National Resident Matching Program. National Resident Matching Program, Data Release and Research Committee: Results of the 2018 NRMP Program Director Survey. Washington, DC; 2018

online®, that allows to search for residency or fellowship of over 11,000 Accreditation Council for Graduate Medical Education (ACGME)-accredited programs [14]. The applicant can search programs by specialty and filter by geographical location, salary, types of visas offered, and even percentage of IMGs among others (for those programs who voluntarily provide that information). The latter can be used strategically by the IMG applicant to determine whether a specific program takes IMGs at all. However, further investigation is neceessary when programs provide demographic data in FREIDA(R) showing that there are a proportion of IMGs among their residents. Even when there is a proportion of IMGs in a particular program, this may not necessarily indicate that IMGs are typically considered during the application process. The IMG should further examine each program to determine whether it takes IMGs for postgraduate year-1 (PGY-1) categorical spots, whether the program takes IMGs only for preliminary spots such as general surgery or internal medicine, and/or whether IMGs have filled out spots in higher levels when a resident drops out of a program. To discern between the aforementioned scenarios, the authors recommend searching through the resident roster in programs' websites to determine if there are IMG categorical residents in postgraduate year-1 (PGY-1) positions. Some programs will provide residents' medical education background, which can be easily used to determine whether the PGY-1 is an IMG and whether IMGs in higher levels of training started with a preliminary year at another program. Another surrogate of IMG-friendliness that can be investigated online is the presence of IMG faculty on staff, or programs' IMG-dependency as defined by a high proportion of IMGs [15]. These strategies are not perfect; however, they may help the IMG applicant to rule out programs especially if there are financial limitations at the time of the application.

USMLE Steps

Scoring well on the USMLE exams (referred to as "Steps" thereafter) is an important accomplishment of every residency applicant regardless of specialty. Out of all the USMLE steps, Step 1 is not only considered one of the most difficult tests in medical education [16] but also the most important measure of success in the residency application process and, therefore, we will focus this discussion mainly around this exam.

On average, US programs receive 129 applications per position offered [13], which poses challenges for programs to provide a full review of all the applications received. According to NRMP data, less than half (47%) of applicants receive an in-depth review of their application [13], and this is likely due to the initial screening process that rules out applicants if they do not meet certain criteria. Step 1 is the first screening factor by many residency program directors and among the top 5 used to rank applicants after interview. This national trend holds true for competitive specialties such as plastic, orthopedic, neurological, and general surgeries, dermatology, interventional radiology, among others. This exam is so heavily emphasized by programs nationwide that 30% or 58% of programs would never or rarely consider for interview an applicant that has failed Step 1, respectively [13].

Passing is not the only important factor for Step 1, but also achieving an outstanding score. Indeed, two-thirds of programs only considered applicants who meet a certain target Step 1 score in 2018 [13]. Therefore, we aimed to provide approximate target scores for competitive specialties. For this purpose, we extracted Step 1 and Step 2 Clinical Knowledge (CK) scores data from the 2018 nationwide Program Director Survey conducted by the NRMP [13] for specialties in which non-US IMGs applied the same year [6] and grouped them into tertiles according to their median (or mean if median not available) Step 1 below which programs would not consider applicants for interview. The overall average cutoff values for Step 1 and Step 2 were 217 and 218, respectively (Table 10.2). Specialties with the highest

Table 10.2 Prevalence of use of Step 1 and Step 2 scores during the application screening process among programs where International Medical Graduates applied in 2018, by specialty

Specialty	Programs reporting use of target score (%)		Step 1 cutoff (median)	Step 2 cutoff (median)	Diff. between Step 1 and Step 2 cutoff	Tertile for Step 1
	Step 1	Step 2				
Internal Medicine	70	51	215	220	5	2
Family Medicine	38	36	205	210	5	1
Pediatrics	40	23	215	220	5	2
Psychiatry	36	21	210	210	0	1
Neurology	62	33	210	210	0	1
General Surgery	85	58	220	220	0	3
Pathology	54	38	210	210	0	1
Anesthesiology	86	47	215	220	5	2
Diagnostic Radiology	67	36	220	220	0	3
Obstetrics and Gynecology	76	51	215	220	5	2
Emergency Medicine	62	31	210	215	5	1
Child Neurology	55	31	210	210	0	1
Dermatology	82	18	230	N/P	N/A	3
Neurological Surgery	84	25	230	225	−5	3
PM&R	54	25	210	215	5	1
Internal Medicine/ Pediatrics	73	31	210	220	10	1
Orthopedic Surgery	98	45	230	230	0	3
Plastic Surgery	85	35	230	230	0	3
Vascular Surgery	86	71	210	215	5	1
Average	*68*	*37*	*216*	*218*	*3*	*N/A*

Abbreviations: Diff. difference, *N/P* data not provided, *N/A* not applicable, *PM&R* Physical Medicine and Rehabilitation

First four columns of data are taken from (with permission) National Resident Matching Program. National Resident Matching Program, Data Release and Research Committee: Results of the 2018 NRMP Program Director Survey. Washington, DC; 2018

cutoffs (upper tertile) included plastic surgery, neurological surgery, orthopedic surgery, dermatology, and neurology with a mean cutoff Step 1 score of 230. Among programs that used Step 2 during the screening process, the average score cutoff was equal or within 5 points of their Step 1 cutoff scores in most cases (18/19 specialties who provided both data points, [Table 10.2]). These data suggest that IMGs applying to competitive specialties should procure scoring above 230 for both Step 1 and Step 2 CK to at least make it through the initial screening process if the programs even consider IMGs at all. In our opinion, IMGs should aim even higher scores for both exams as there are programs that may give preference to USMGs over IMGs when comparing applicants with similar scores. This NRMP survey also offered scores above which programs almost always grant interviews [13]. Based on these data, applicants should target Step 1/2 CK scores above 250/250 for plastic surgery, 245/245 for orthopedic surgery, 245/240 for neurological surgery, 242 for dermatology (Step 2 data not provided), 230/235 for diagnostic radiology, and 230/230 for general surgery. Strategies for achieving such high scores are beyond the scope of this chapter.

Although a lot of emphasis is still given to Step 1 scores in the residency application process, this will soon change as the USMLE announced earlier this year the decision to change the Step 1 three-digit score to a pass/fail scoring system [17]. This change will likely have a positive impact on the educational experience of medical students in the USA; however, it may make the application process even more challenging for IMGs [16]. For example, doing away with Step 1 score would shift the IMG focus to reinforce their application through even higher Step 2 scores, additional research experiences, competitive clinical electives, letters of recommendation from recognized specialists in the field, and enhancing their networking. Before this change, an outstanding Step 1 score could have compensated for fewer publications or clinical experiences. Therefore, our recommendation for the IMG applicant is to prepare well for the USMLE steps and score as well not only in Step 1 but also in Step 2. There are available simulation USMLE exams that can be purchased and taken online to estimate the score the applicant would get at a given time. These should be used with caution as there is a margin of error; however, when used wisely they can let the applicant know where he stands compared to other test-takers. Also, this may allow the applicant to get an idea whether his current knowledge would allow him to get a score over the minimum score used during screening process in a particular specialty, or even better, over the score that typically warrants an interview in competitive specialties.

US Clinical Experience and Letters of Recommendations

Clinical experience in the USA is one of the critical key components of a successful IMG applicant [18]. Even though some IMGs have more years of clinical experience than the typical USMG, and some may even had completed a residency in their home country, they are still required to have additional clinical experience in the

USA [16]. As of now, there is no universal process or pathway for IMGs to secure clinical experience. Instead, this depends on the IMG ability to secure elective rotations if they are still in medical school or observerships if they have graduated already. The advantages and disadvantages of elective rotations and observerships are summarized in Table 10.3. In elective rotations, senior international medical students have the opportunity to have the same clinical experience, educational curriculum, and responsibilities as if they were US medical students. This guarantees IMGs hands-on experience within the US healthcare system, allows them to be evaluated during their rotation by faculty, and provides a basis for these faculty members to write them letters of recommendation. On the other hand, those IMGs who have already completed their medical studies cannot secure hands-on experience through elective rotations due to liability issues, leaving observerships as the only options for clinical experience and exposure to US programs/faculty in the majority of cases. An exception is the University of Washington Certificate Program for International Medical Graduates, a program offered for IMGs interested in applying to a one- or two-year preliminary position in general surgery. Observership rotations are less ideal as they provide limited clinical exposure to a component of

Table 10.3 Advantages and disadvantages of elective clinical rotations vs. clinical observerships

	Elective rotations	Observerships
Advantages	Allow exposure to the US healthcare system	Allow exposure to the US healthcare system
	Able to interact, interview and examine patients, able to scrub and assist in procedures and active member of the care team as any senior US medical student is allowed to	May be not as expensive if secured by own means
	Same educational experience (curriculum) as senior US medical students	Paid agencies available that help finding securing positions
	More likely to secure a stronger letter of recommendation if IMG performed well	May be offered on a case by case basis instead of through an application process
	Objective performance is assessed and scored in same way as US medical students (i.e., honors, high honors)	May be able to secure letter of recommendation
		May allow flexibility of starting and finishing dates
Disadvantages	Must be done during senior year of medical school	Not allowed to assist in patient care in any way (unable to scrub operative cases, unable to examine patients, etc.)
	Can be expensive. Often require prorated tuition fees	Letters of recommendation, if secured, will not be able to comment on clinical skills and clinical performance
	May require USMLE boards as part of application	

patient care (i.e., outpatient setting), which in turn limits faculty's ability to comment on their ability to perform well as residents.

It is not possible to ascertain the number of clinical experiences each applicant had at the time of their application along with their characteristics (i.e., observership vs. clerkship, whether performed in the USA or not, etc.) by specialty through The Match® report data. Therefore, we are unable to provide data-driven recommendations specifically for IMGs. Nonetheless, to the best of our knowledge, the IMGs that are successful in matching into competitive specialties have had US clinical/ healthcare exposure, through elective rotations, observerships, or at the very least through research experiences (e.g., research fellowship and research volunteer). We also recommend that future IMGs plan with enough time in advance to achieve this important requirement in the application process. We propose at least a year of anticipation to a clinical rotation to allow time for identification of rotations, processing once application is submitted, financial arrangements, and visa application and issuance (if applicable). This time can be significantly reduced if the IMG is already located in the USA. Elective rotations for international medical students such as the ones offered by Harvard Medical School [19] or Stanford Medical School [20] can be found online by searching for a combination of the appropriate keywords (e.g., international, visiting, student, program, exchange, and clerkship).

For those who elect to do observerships, these non-hands-on clinical experience opportunities can be found in different ways. Some IMGs may contact faculty and/ or programs directly inquiring about these opportunities as some programs/institutions may accept international observers without having a publicly advertised "observership program." Other IMGs may elect to use paid observership programs which provide assistance in securing these rotations [21]. These can be expensive for IMGs and are typically not at large academic or renowned institutions. Lastly, some programs may offer formal observerships.

In summary, if international medical students have made their decision to pursue residency in the USA and if their finances allow it, they should seek to apply and secure international visiting student elective rotations. During these rotations, the medical student should strive to excel, so a letter(s) of recommendation can be obtained. If for timing, traveling, financial, or any other reason(s) this is not possible, clinical observerships should be the alternative, and the observer should engage with faculty and residents as much as permitted in their rotation, so their chances of securing letters of recommendation increase.

Research Experience, Mentorship, and Dual Degrees

Undoubtedly, research experience including peer-reviewed publications, book chapters, and regional/national presentations can positively influence a program director's decision as to whether or not to interview an IMG applicant [13, 22]. This is especially true at institutions where faculty members highly value scholarly activity [22]. As with the aforementioned items that help an IMG standout relative to

USMG applicants, one can assume that research experience is almost a necessity for an IMG wishing to match into a residency program in the USA, particularly for competitive specialties such as surgical subspecialties, neurosurgery, and dermatology. Also, we have observed that in a given cycle for competitive plastic surgery positions, it is not unusual for an IMG applicant to have greater than 30 or more peer-reviewed publications, while USMG applicants may have less than 10 publications. We have also observed that IMGs are more willing to spend dedicated research time even if they do not get paid.

For IMG applicants interested in applying into a competitive US residency program, such as for integrated plastic surgery, an average of 1–3 years is devoted to research [23]. For independent plastic surgery applicants, meaning those applicants applying for a plastic surgery position following completion of general surgery, a range of 1–2 years is typical for dedicated research and this is often performed in the middle of their general surgery training [23]. In dermatology, research experience has become essential for non-US IMGs [24]. IMG applicants applying in neurosurgery and matching successfully in top ranked programs have higher H-indices, more publications, and are more likely to take research year(s) than USMGs [25]. For non-US IMGs wishing to apply in general surgery in the USA, the support for dedicated time-off for research is unclear. Recent unpublished data suggests that program directors advocate against IMGs taking time off after graduation to engage in research activity prior to general surgery residency. On the other hand, a study out of East Carolina University demonstrated that IMGs applying in general surgery had more scholarly works than USMGs [18]. Nonetheless, we strongly encourage partaking in research activities at least on a part-time basis alongside medical school curriculum even for those IMGs applying in general surgery. Similarly, it is important to note that time spent in research does not guarantee a successful match, rather it adds to the overall competitiveness of the application. One thing is for sure, research will not hurt an applicant unless there is minimal productivity during that time. In general, we agree with 1–2 years of dedicated research experience for IMG applicants wishing to pursue a competitive residency training in the USA such as dermatology, surgery, and plastic surgery. It is also universally recognized that research in the specialty of interest is more beneficial than unrelated scientific pursuit. For instance, an applicant interested in applying in dermatology should attempt to find research opportunities within the dermatology specialty and not, for instance, in general medicine or radiology. That being said, for competitive specialties such as plastic surgery and dermatology, any research is better than no research, and so if the only opportunity available is unrelated to the specialty of interest, then the applicant may choose to pursue that opportunity.

Perhaps as important as the academic productivity during the research time are the relationships established with mentors and the opportunity for letters of recommendation. It is expected that research mentors should in the least be able to serve as positive references during the application process. However, most program directors will expect a recommendation from a research mentor in support of the IMG applicant, particularly considering the full-time nature of the research work and related interactions. In the least, IMG applicants should request a letter of recommendation from a research mentor whom they worked with most closely and perhaps is most well known in the specialty of pursuit. Similarly, research experience provides an opportunity for networking with other academic clinicians (e.g., plastic surgeons and dermatologists) which can lead to additional clinical and/or research opportunities.

Pursuit of advanced degrees is another way that IMGs can strengthen their application, and some programs rank applicants higher if they have dual degrees (e.g., MD MBA) [22]. Schenarts and colleagues demonstrated that IMG applicants for general surgery training positions had more advanced degrees than USMGs [18]. Whereas a Master's in Business Administration (MBA) and in Public Health (MPH) may take 1–2 years to complete or may be offered on a part-time basis, a Doctor of Philosophy (PhD) may take 4–6 years. Therefore, it is rare that a non-US IMG would pursue a PhD only to strengthen his application. Having an MBA may show leadership and organizational capabilities in an applicant, while having an MPH may reflect a liking for scholarly pursuit. However, it is our personal opinion that an advanced degree is not necessary and should not replace the aforementioned items such as strong letters of recommendation, observerships, research experience, and academic excellence.

Overcoming Financial, Language, and Visa Status Challenges

Financial, language, and visa status challenges will be covered in detail in other chapters and a comprehensive review of those topics is out of the scope of this chapter. When considering all that non-US IMGs must do to position themselves competitively for a successful match in a desired specialty, there is no doubt that there will be considerable expenses along the way, in addition to what is necessary for required overseas traveling and interviews. Open communication with mentors may help identify scholarship and research grant opportunities. Some of these funding opportunities can also be identified on national organization/conference webpages, such as the American Academy of Dermatology and American Council of Academic Plastic Surgery for dermatology and plastic surgery, respectively. For applicants who wish to commit a year or more to research, there are paid positions that are available. For instance, for applicants considering plastic surgery, the University of Pennsylvania offers four full-time research fellowship positions that are funded and past fellows have included non-US IMGs. Additional paid research listings in plastic surgery can be found on the American Council of Academic Plastic Surgeons webpage [26]. Other paid clinical and research fellowships in other specialties, such as the International Dermatology Fellowship Program offered by Wake Forest School of Medicine, can be found by searching individual program webpages [27]. For those individuals wishing to obtain advanced degrees, unless scholarship, grant, or institutional funding is obtained, the applicant will bear the costs that can easily reach $50,000–100,000.

As long as a non-US IMG applicant is fluent in English in addition to their native language, we have observed that bi- or tri-lingual status is highly advantageous in a clinical setting and should be highlighted in the application/interview. Some non-US IMGs, such as those from Lebanon, are often fluent in English, Arabic, and French. It is recommended, however, that non-US IMGs are fluent enough in English such that they are able to communicate, interview, and write research papers similar to and nearly indistinguishable from USMGs.

Finally, applicants should be open and forthcoming about citizenship and VISA status when applying for observerships/clerkships, research experiences, and training positions in the USA. If the applicant has the time and financial support to apply for a green card, that would obviate any concerns that the program may have regarding VISA status and associated limitations.

IMGs Pathway Example for Successful Match into Competitive Specialties in the USA

Based on the above, there are several pathways that can be considered for a non-US IMGs applying for a residency position in the USA, although there are commonalities across pathways (Fig. 10.2). The IMG should consider a US clinical observership/clerkship at some point during medical school, which is useful for networking, obtaining letters/references of recommendation, and for additional research opportunities. If the decision to pursue categorical/definitive training in the USA is made too late, for instance toward the end of medical school, applying for 1–2 preliminary clinical years in the USA may be preferable [28, 29]. These preliminary spots are more commonly available in general medicine and general surgery and have been shown to help secure categorical spots for continuing graduate medical education [28, 29]. For instance, if a non-US IMG applicant decides late that they want to pursue a dermatology or radiology training in the USA, he may apply for a

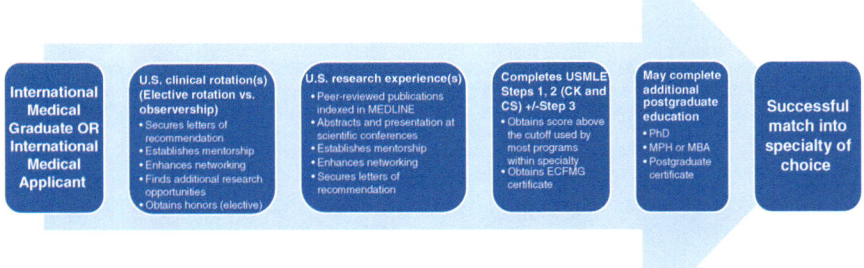

Fig. 10.2 IMG pathway example for successful match into competitive specialties in the USA

1–2-year general medicine preliminary position at a US institution. The preliminary year(s) offers the opportunity for the applicant to develop relationships with mentors and to prove their clinical capability/competency within the US health care system [24, 25, 28, 29]. After that time, the IMG can subsequently apply to a categorical/definitive training position in the USA. A study in neurosurgery showed that applicants with prior affiliation with US programs, by way of preliminary clinical time or research fellowship, were more likely to match at top-ranked neurosurgery programs [25].

As mentioned previously, research is essential for competitive specialties (e.g., dermatology, plastic surgery, neurosurgery, and interventional radiology) and there is no data to suggest that it is hurtful for other specialties such as general medicine and surgery [23–25, 30]. However, it is possible that non-US IMGs may obtain training positions in lesser competitive fields (e.g., psychiatry, family medicine, and even non-competitive general surgery) in the USA without dedicated time-off for research. For these latter specialties, we recommend reaching out to program directors at desired programs/specialties via e-mail or other communication 1–2 years ahead of the application cycle to discuss whether or not it is advisable to take time off for research.

The IMG applicant should complete USMLE Step 1 and Step 2 (CK and CS) prior to applying (Fig. 10.2). Even though Step 1 will be changing to pass/fail score reporting [16], a strong performance on Step 2, arguably the more clinically relevant of the step exams, will only strengthen one's application. This of course goes hand-in-hand with a strong academic performance in medical school. When additional postgraduate education such as advanced degree studies is desired by the applicant, it should be pursued in the USA and perhaps strategically in the desired geographic location/institution. Finally, when applying, data available on the dermatology and neurosurgery matches has shown that it may be advantageous to consider programs and institutions that have track records of taking prior IMGs [24, 30], particularly when the prior IMGs have been successful and well respected.

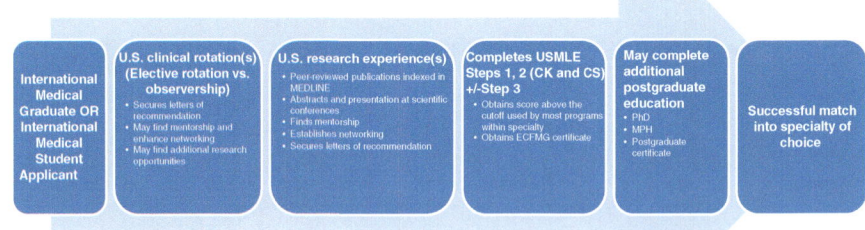

Summary of recommendations to overcome restrictions to specific fields
1. Organization and planning is key along the process.
2. Use publicly available data from program characteristics and The Match® to strategize and assess feasibility of specific specialties.
3. Consider programs/institutions that have a track record of successfully accepting IMGs.
4. Use data wisely to set expectations accordingly.
5. Scoring well, more emphasis on Step 2 now that Step 1 score report will change.
6. Prefer clerkships over observerships if given both options.
7. Secure good letters of recommendation through clinical and/or research experiences.
8. For competitive specialties (e.g., neurosurgery, dermatology, and plastic surgery), consider 1–2 years of research in the USA in said specialty and, preferably, in the desired geographic location/institution.
9. For lesser competitive specialties (e.g., family medicine and psychiatry), consider reaching out to program directors in desired institutions to discuss the need for dedicated research experience.
10. Networking and mentorship through clinical and research experiences can lead to additional opportunities and may help to secure interviews.
11. A good mentor can be the key to success not only in matching into your specialty but also through your academic career.

Conclusions

IMGs will continue to make up a considerable amount of our trainees and healthcare workforce in the future and this trend is projected to increase. Non-US IMGs can position themselves competitively compared to USMGs by scoring highly on Step exams, by exceling in medical school academics, and by pursuing research experience and observerships/clerkships in the USA. One or more clinical preliminary year(s) in general medicine or surgery is also an option for non-US IMGs as a way to demonstrate clinical competency in the USA and for networking and mentorship opportunities. Regardless, these driven and hardworking individuals benefit from support and mentorship along the way. From the IMG applicant perspective, the goal should remain to position yourself as competitively as possible in the shortest amount of additional time spent.

Acknowledgement The authors would like to thank Dr. Zhang and the National Resident Matching Program staff for their permission to use their data in this manuscript and for reviewing the integrity of it.

References

1. ECFMG. ECFMG statement on USMLE policy changes. ECFMG News. 2020.
2. Young A, Chaudhry HJ, Pei X, Arnhart K, Dugan M, Steingard SA. FSMB census of licensed physicians in the United States, 2018. J Med Regul. 2019;105(2):7–23.
3. Shiffer CD, Boulet JR, Cover LL, Pinsky WW. Advancing the quality of medical education worldwide: ECFMG's 2023 medical school accreditation requirement. J Med Regul. 2019;105(4):8–16.
4. National Resident Matching Program. National resident matching program, results and data: 2019 main residency match®. Washington, DC; 2019.
5. Chen JY. Residency match update and the most competitive specialty. J Am Coll Radiol. 2018;15:1335–6.
6. National Resident Matching Program. National resident matching program, charting outcomes in the match: international medical graduates. Washington, DC; 2018.
7. Zaheer S, Pimentel SD, Simmons KD, Kuo LE, Datta J, Williams N, et al. Comparing international and united states undergraduate medical education and surgical outcomes using a refined balance matching methodology. Ann Surg. 2017;265(5):916–22.
8. Tsugawa Y, Dimick JB, Jena AB, Maggard-Gibbons M, Blumenthal DM, Gross N, et al. Comparison of patient outcomes of surgeons who are US versus international medical graduates. Ann Surg. 2019; https://doi.org/10.1097/SLA.0000000000003736.
9. Norcini JJ, Boulet JR, Dauphinee WD, Opalek A, Krantz ID, Anderson ST. Evaluating the quality of care provided by graduates of international medical schools. Health Affairs. 2010;29(8):1461–8.
10. Desbiens NA, Vidaillet HJ. Discrimination against international medical graduates in the United States residency program selection process. BMC Med Educ. 2010;10:1–5.
11. Tinsley JA, McAlpine DE, Balon R, Mufti R, Williams M, Riba M. Another explanation for the apparent discrimination against international medical graduates by residency programs [6] (multiple letters). Am J Psychiatr. 1999;156(3):496a–7.
12. Educational Commission for Foreign Medical Graduates. ECFMG certification. 2019.
13. National Resident Matching Program. National resident matching program, data release and research committee: results of the 2018 NRMP program director survey. Washington, DC; 2018.
14. American Medical Association. FREIDA™. 2020.
15. Whitcomb ME, Miller RS. Comparison of IMG-dependent and non-IMG-dependent residencies in the National Resident Matching Program. J Am Med Assoc. 1996;276(9):700–3.
16. Desai A, Hegde A, Das D. Change in reporting of USMLE step 1 scores and potential implications for international medical graduates. JAMA. 2020;323(20):2015–6.
17. Federation of State Medical Boards (FSMB) and National Board of Medical Examiners® (NBME®). Change to pass/fail score reporting for Step 1. 2020.
18. Schenarts PJ, Love KM, Agle SC, Haisch CE. Comparison of surgical residency applicants from U.S. medical schools with U.S.-born and foreign-born international medical school graduates. J Surg Educ. 2008;65(6):406–12.
19. Harvard Medical School. Exchange clerkship program. 2020.
20. Stanford Medicine. International visiting student program. 2020.
21. American Medical Association. Observership program listings for international medical graduates. 2020.
22. Kaplan Inc. 5 ways to stand out to residency programs. 2019.
23. Kokosis G, Barone AAL, Grzelak MJ, Alfadil S, Davidson EH, Lifchez S, et al. International medical graduates in the us plastic surgery residency: characteristics of successful applicants. Eplasty. 2018;18:e33.
24. Ramos-Rodriguez AJ, Timerman D, Kyriacou MI, Martin RF. A strategic evidence-based framework for international medical graduates (IMGs) applying to dermatology residency in the United States: a literature review. Dermatol Online J. 2019;25(8):13030/qt0sh2s8h1.

25. Chandra A, Brandel MG, Wadhwa H, Almeida ND, Yue JK, Nuru MO, et al. The path to U.S. neurosurgical residency for foreign medical graduates: trends from a decade 2007–2017. World Neurosurg. 2020;137:e584–96.
26. American Council of Academic Plastic Surgeons. American Council of Academic Plastic Surgeons – Job Board.
27. Wake Forest School of Medicine. International Dermatology Fellowship Program.
28. Rajesh A, Asaad M, Chandra A, Rivera M, Stulak JM, Heller SF, et al. What do former residents say about their nondesignated preliminary year? A survey of prelims' experiences in a general surgery residency program. J Surg Educ. 2020;77(2):281–90.
29. Rajesh A, Asaad M, Chandra A, McKenzie TJ, Farley DR. Outcomes of non-designated preliminary general surgery interns: A 25-year Mayo Clinic experience. Surgery. 2020;167(2):314–20.
30. Scheitler KM, Lu VM, Carlstrom LP, Graffeo CS, Perry A, Daniels DJ, et al. Geographic distribution of international medical graduate residents in U.S. neurosurgery training programs. World Neurosurg. 2020;137:e383–8.

Chapter 11
Choosing a Specialty Just to Get a Job

Vinod E. Nambudiri and Kevin E. Salinas

How Do IMGs Even Start Looking for a Job?

The process of immigrating to the United States can bring an extensive set of challenges. These challenges are oftentimes related to navigating immigration policies, adapting to a new healthcare system, and learning a new language. For international medical graduates (IMGs) interested in practicing in the United States, this process includes applying to residency and becoming a practicing physician—"getting a job." In order to better understand how the job search begins for IMGs, it is important to start from the very beginning.

First and foremost, when considering applying to residency in the United States, the earlier one can start preparing the better. As a student at a medical school outside of the United States, preparation can start through clinical rotations in the United States while in medical school. For individuals beginning the process later in their training, this process might include looking for post-doctoral research or clinical opportunities at American institutions to bridge the gap in time between the completion of medical school and the beginning of residency. Regardless of the timing, some exposure to the scientific and clinical realms in the United States is likely to be extremely beneficial in the pre-application process.

After completing medical training abroad, individuals interested in applying to residency programs in the United States must register with the Association of American Medical Colleges (AAMC) in order to access the register with the Electronic Residency Application Service (ERAS®). Additionally, applicants must

V. E. Nambudiri (✉)
Department of Dermatology, Brigham and Women's Hospital and Harvard Medical School, Boston, MA, USA
e-mail: vnambudiri@bwh.harvard.edu

K. E. Salinas
Harvard Medical School, Boston, MA, USA
e-mail: kevin_salinas@hms.harvard.edu

© Springer Nature Switzerland AG 2021
H. Tohid, H. Maibach (eds.), *International Medical Graduates in the United States*, https://doi.org/10.1007/978-3-030-62249-7_11

register with the Educational Commission for Foreign Medical Graduates (ECFMG®) and obtain a residency token for the ERAS®. Importantly, the token is necessary to submit applications through the MyERAS website. In order to obtain a token, applicants must complete a set of standardized testing requirements.

These requirements consist of completing the United States Medical Licensing Examination (USMLE®) Step 1, Step 2 CS, and Step 2 CK components, all within 7 years of the date the first exam was taken. If not completed in time, the 7-year countdown resets based on the date the second exam was taken, if applicable. Exams taken prior to the date of the second exam must be retaken along with any other pending exams. For example, if an applicant had taken USMLE Step 1 in January 2013, USMLE Step 2 CS in February 2014, and then waited to take USMLE Step 2 CK until March 2020, their Step 1 score would no longer be valid, as the March 2020 test date would have been more than 7 years after the initial test date for Step 1. As a result, the candidate would have to retake Step 1 before February 2021, 7 years from their Step 2 CS test date. If not, they would risk voiding their Step 2 CS score as well.

Once applicants have (1) obtained some research or clinical exposure in the United States, either before, during, or after the completion of medical school; (2) decided to apply to US residency programs; (3) registered with the AAMC for ERAS® access; (4) completed standardized examination requirements; and (5) obtained a token for ERAS® through the ECFMG®, they can begin to select residency programs that interest them to apply to. Residency programs begin accepting applications in September, and interview season can generally range from late October to early February. Programs may discontinue reviewing applications at any time as they see fit, and as such, applying early in the application cycle may be of benefit. Additionally, the interview season may vary dramatically across programs, specialties, and institutions, with some completing all of their interviews during a narrow time period in the fall, with others more spread out or delayed over the application season.

Applicants must register with the National Residency Match Program (NRMP®) and submit their program preferences in order to be successfully matched to a residency program. The NRMP® uses rank order lists submitted by both residency program directors and applicants to determine the applicants' final placements.

On the Monday of the third week of March, applicants are told whether or not they have matched to a program, but not the program to which they were matched. The Friday of that week, medical school Match Day ceremonies take place across the country and final results become available.

What Happens When IMGs Do Not Get the Job on Their First Try?

While the prior section highlights the general process of obtaining a residency position, historically only about half of IMG applicants who have applied out successfully matched into a first-year position [1]. Those who do not match have a second chance at entering graduate medical education (GME) during the application cycle through the post-residency Supplemental Offer and Acceptance Program (SOAP®). Through this program, applicants can compete for the Main Residency Match's remaining unfilled positions, which are limited in number compared to the number of spots that are available in the Main Residency Match.

The process begins on the Friday of the week before Match Week, when the NRMP notifies applicants of their eligibility status for the Supplemental Offer and Acceptance Program. This eligibility status depends on three factors. First, applicants must be registered for the Main Residency Match for that year. Second, applicants must be eligible to enter graduate medical education on July 1st of the year of the Match, as determined by the ECFMG®. Lastly, applicants must be partially matched or unmatched on the Monday of Match Week in order to participate in the SOAP.

If SOAP-qualifying students receive an "unmatched" or "partially matched" notification on the Monday of Match Week, they can participate in SOAP. These unmatched or partially matched applicants can view the list of unfilled programs released to them by the NRMP®. They are able to view the list of unfilled programs across all specialties, regardless of what specialty or specialties they initially applied into. They can then submit applications through ERAS® starting the Monday of Match Week through that Thursday, the day before Match Day. Programs extend offers to applicants on the Registration, Ranking, and Results (R3®) system administered by the NRMP®, with deadlines detailed in the offer.

A post-SOAP list of unfilled programs is uploaded on the Thursday of Match Week. All unmatched and partially matched applicants have access to this list and can contact unfilled programs directly.

If still unsuccessful in obtaining a match position, applicants can prepare to re-apply in the following cycle. In the past, applicants had to begin new applications and re-upload many of their supporting documents. To address this issue, in 2017, an "import" feature was introduced to ERAS®. Currently, some materials can be transferred directly from one application cycle to the next on the MyERAS platform, including medical student performance evaluations, medical school transcripts, photographs, postgraduate training authorization letters, and letters of recommendation that were used in previous ERAS® seasons, thereby streamlining the re-application process.

Notably, re-application also involves an in-depth evaluation of a candidate's application as well as preparation for re-submission. The question "What could I have done differently to obtain my desired outcome?" must be asked in some form. Depending on an individual's particular situation, future steps might include searching for opportunities for more relevant clinical experience in fields they are interested applying to. Similarly, applicants may consider networking with individuals in programs they would like to attend. Revising personal statements and drafting separate statements for each specialty they rank might be more important for others. To tackle some of these aspects of the re-application process, identifying a mentor who can help in strengthening experiences and quality of the application can be key! Lastly, budgeting finances to avoid limiting the number of programs for which one can submit applications and attend interviews may be another factor to consider.

This point is particularly important for applicants who have found themselves limiting their number of applications or interviews during earlier cycles.

Where Do IMGs Go When the Job-Hunting Gets Tough?

With regard to choosing a specialty, the American Medical Assocation (AMA) recommends that medical students ask themselves the following four questions [2]:

1. "Procedures or patient interaction?"
2. "How do you want to interact with patients?"
3. "What kind of work-life balance do you want?"
4. "Who do you want to treat?"

Given the comparatively low match rates and associated challenges that IMGs face when applying to enter the workforce versus US-trained physicians, it would seem that these questions may not be first on their mind when considering specialties, and recent data seems to back this idea.

A recent study published in the *Journal of Graduate Medical Education* used data from 2015 to assess IMG representation among trainees and the active physician workforce in the 20 largest residency specialties. Among its findings, it was found that IMG trainees made up 25% of the total graduate medical education (GME) trainee pool in 2015, but showed significantly greater representation in 5 of the 20 largest GME specialties: pathology (39%), internal medicine (39%), neurology (36%), family medicine (32%), and psychiatry (31%). Notably, the proportion of IMGs was lowest for radiation oncology (2%) and otolaryngology (1%) [3]. This distribution may influence the choice of specialty by applicants as it may provide insights into field where historically international medical graduates have been more successful at obtaining residency positions.

Unsurprisingly, trends surrounding IMGs in the active physician workforce show similar results. IMGs made up 24% of the active physician workforce but showed significantly greater representation in internal medicine (39%), neurology (31%), psychiatry (30%), and pediatrics (25%). Among active physicians, IMG representation was lowest in orthopedic surgery (6%) and dermatology (5%) [3].

Systemic Barriers to Getting a Job

While the material presented in this chapter so far emphasizes the difficulty and length of the residency application process, it is important to additionally recognize the systemic barriers that both create and complicate the challenges faced by IMGs. Many systemic barriers play a role in this process, and here the focus will be placed on the influence and power of networks, time constraints, perceived residency program prestige, residency program selection by IMGs, implicit bias, and finances.

In terms of obtaining clinical or research experience, these opportunities are oftentimes dependent on personal and institutional connections. If a foreign medical school has ties to US-based hospitals or medical schools, it may make away rotations or research collaborations easier to arrange for a student who is interested in pursuing postgraduate medical education and training in the United States. Similarly, if an IMG has classmates, friends, or relatives who are already established researchers or physicians in the United States, securing opportunities for clinical or research experience may not be as difficult. Moreover, these experiences can be a significant financial burden or even cost-prohibitive for some people due in part to program fees and living expenses. Without access to these networks and opportunities, however, applicants may be more willing or likely to take a job in whatever specialty they can successfully match into.

With regard to the 7-year timeframe for completing examination requirements in order to receive the ECFMG® token, this requirement can pose problems for those with extenuating circumstances who have difficulty completing all the exams in the given timeframe. Possible challenges may include inability to travel, financial insecurity, or the logistics of balancing medical school requirements with scheduling of these exams. Even for those who do successfully obtain a token and apply to residency programs, the pressure and time-commitment may impact their performance and limit their specialty options in the future. Others may feel that after taking 7 years to prepare, the specific specialty they are able to practice does not matter so long as they can practice as a physician in the United States.

Another important factor to consider is that not all residency programs are equally representative of international medical graduates. Some residency programs consist primarily of IMGs, while others are what is termed "non-IMG-dependent" programs [4, 5]. This trend can be explained primarily by two major factors. Firstly, during the application process, competitiveness of programs can be perceived as the proportion of US-trained allopathic graduates (USMD)s on the house staff. In fact, a recent study assessing the factors influencing USMDs residency selection showed that the presence of IMG students plays a role in US-trained allopathic medical students' perception of residency programs [6]. Thus, in order to maintain the competitiveness and potential associated "prestige" of their programs, residency program directors may continue to preferentially select USMDs over IMGs during the application process.

Secondly, the general bias against IMGs in many programs has been recognized and sites such as Matcharesident.com have sprung up as a response. Such sites help applicants identify IMG-friendly programs based on their scores, geographic preferences, visa status, and nationality, among other factors. Still, while aiming to be helpful resources, these websites may also contribute to self-selection and promote current trends in specialty selection among IMGs.

Implicit bias during medical residency interviews is another factor which may contribute to the challenges faced by IMGs as they navigate the application processes. Broadly, implicit bias refers to the unconscious ways that attitudes or stereotypes toward certain people affect our actions and decisions. In the interview setting, these biases can surround language, such as accents or perceived language barriers.

There may also be concerns about cultural competence, especially for individuals from cultural backgrounds not commonly represented in the United States. Additionally, many IMGs come from schools that are unfamiliar to residency program directors and, as a consequence, may not be considered as seriously as someone from a school with close ties to the program. Implicit bias may partially explain why even though USMDs and IMGs who match into specialties such as internal medicine systematically match into different residency program types (e.g., community-based, university-affiliated, or university-based hospitals), even though they have virtually the same mean USMLE Step 1 scores [5].

Finances also serve as a limiting factor for some applicants. For IMGs the importance of finances may manifest itself in having to travel longer distances to interview sites, as well as having to apply to an increased number of programs because of the historically low match rates. Overall, the application process is expensive and time-consuming. This problem might be especially significant for those interested in competitive specialties who cannot afford to travel to a large number of interviews necessary to maximize chances of receiving an offer at the end of the application cycle. Beyond the cost of interviews, reduced income during time spent during research, residency training, and any subsequent fellowship training may result in decreased incentive to pursue more competitive specialties. Thus, the finances surrounding much of the application process and the medical training system in the United States may shift applicants' focus instead to obtaining any residency position in any specialty as quickly as possible to obtain some return on the time and money invested in the process.

Another point worth mentioning is that after overcoming many of these systemic challenges and applying to residency, there is still a chance at an unfilled residency slot through SOAP for those who do not initially match into the preferred specialty of their choice through the main match. This option may tempt IMGs who otherwise would re-apply and pursue a different specialty that is available through an unfilled residency slot in order to begin the residency training as soon as possible and ultimately pursue the path of clinical work in the United States.

Personal Challenges on the Way

Beyond the systemic challenges that exist surrounding the residency match process for IMGs, there are also important personal factors that play a role in IMGs' ability to successfully obtain a residency position. One main factor we consider in this chapter is family, but there are many others that could exist for different applicants, including the complexity and case-by-base nature of immigration and being far from home.

As far as family is concerned, IMGs are typically older than the average applicant to residency and may have family abroad or that immigrate with them [7]. These family members, whether abroad or with them in the United States, may depend on the IMGs financially. This additional pressure to care for and financially support others may push applicants to make their way through the application process as quickly as possible. In the process, they may reduce the number of research years or commitment to additional experiences that might make them more competitive for specialties of their choice. Consequently, they may shift their focus instead to obtaining any residency position in any specialty as quickly as possible.

Overall, personal challenges, when combined with systemic challenges in the residency application system, may further funnel IMGs into specialties that are not their first choice. The decision to apply to a particular specialty or combination of specialties is an extremely personal one. Weighing all the above factors must be taken into consideration when the choices are made. It is not uncommon for IMGs to apply to multiple specialties when entering the match, and this may provide them with multiple training pads to ultimately a similar career. For example, IMGs may apply for both internal medicine and family medicine residency programs and at the end of their training ultimately pursue a clinical path in primary care.

The Contributions of IMGs to US Healthcare

In thinking about what pushes IMGs to "choose a specialty just to get a job"—as is the title of this chapter—the topics so far discussed have focused on current trends as well as systemic and personal challenges on the path to obtaining a residency position. These challenges make it more difficult for IMGs to obtain a residency position overall and may also contribute to making them less likely to pursue more competitive specialties. Still, despite the challenges they face and the negative biases held by many residency programs toward IMGs in the United States, their contributions to the American healthcare system and American society in general must not go ignored. By understanding the positive impact of IMGs in the United States, changes can be made to facilitate their progress through the residency application system.

To provide context, IMGs that are pursuing GME training in the United States who do not hold US permanent resident status or US citizenship often arrive through the J-1 visa program. Notably, J-1 visa holders are required to return to their country of citizenship for 2 years following their training. If they would like to stay in the United States, they can commit to 3 years of work in a medically underserved community. As a result, not only are IMGs more likely to work in primary care (as shown previously during the discussion on IMG representation in different specialties), but they also contribute to closing gaps in healthcare in medically underserved communities [8]. Several international medical graduates often stay in these communities to provide care for the longer term following the completion of their required service, thus ameliorating physician shortages for underserved populations.

Moreover, while some individuals may have concerns surrounding IMGs regarding their clinical competency, several qualities of care studies on care delivered by IMGs versus US graduates indicate that quality of care should not be a concern.

Not only is the care provided by IMGs typically equivalent to that of USMDs, but some research indicates that it might even be better. A peer-reviewed study published in *The BMJ* assessing mortality rates among Medicare patients treated by general internists (both IMGs and USMDs) in US hospitals found that patients of IMGs had lower mortality rates compared to patients treated by their US-trained colleagues [9].

Additional benefits of a diverse workforce in medicine also include improved cultural competence and broader research agendas in academic settings [5]. Since the benefits to having a diverse workforce—in other words, a workforce that includes IMGs—are multiple, policy efforts to remove some of the barriers IMGs face in entering the US medical system are warranted.

How Can We Support IMGs on Their Job Search Moving Forward?

With the understanding that the IMGs contribute in many positive ways to the US healthcare and medical education systems, it may seem more convincing now that the system can and should change to accommodate IMGs. Fortunately, there are tangible changes in medical education that could be made to removing barriers and bias against foreign graduates.

One of these potential changes involves modifying requirements for foreign graduates to enter certain subspecialties. For example, a preference in the application process for IMGs committed to working long term in smaller, underserved communities with few specialists may level the playing field. After all, as mentioned previously, IMGs are already more likely to practice in underserved communities.

Keeping in mind that several of the challenges IMGs face—including finances and language barriers—will not disappear even with intentional modifications in how applications are considered, other forms of support are also necessary. One potential route to support IMGs is through assistance with funding for transport and accommodation. Easing financial burden through transport and accommodation assistance may be particularly helpful for those also caring for family members abroad or with them in the United States. More broadly, supporting IMGs financially may ease their burden outside of the medical training system and give them the opportunity to pursue increasing levels of specialization.

Professional language and cultural competence training during residency for those from non-English speaking countries may also play a role in overcoming some of the challenges currently faced by IMGs [10]. By providing training in these areas, programs effectively diminish language and cultural competence as a concern in selecting IMGs for residency positions. A change of this kind would be particularly beneficial for individuals from backgrounds with a largely different language and culture than those of the United States, or for those trainees whose language of instruction in medical school was not in English.

Overall, these changes could ultimately level the playing field for IMGs and permit increasing numbers of IMGs to practice in underserved communities, provide novel ideas in research, and fill various diversity roles as specialists and sub-specialists.

The Road Ahead

Despite the various topics covered in these chapters, the dynamics surrounding residency entry for IMGs will continue to evolve on various fronts over the coming months and years. The USMLE's announcement on February 12, 2020, regarding a transition in USMLE Step 1 grading from a numbered score to a "pass/fail" report is one prime example of such a change. The de-emphasis of what was once considered a key differentiating factor in the application process has created much uncertainty as to what the system will look like for future IMG and USMD applicants.

Recent and future changes in immigration policy may also continue to bring new changes to the challenges faced by IMGs. For example, since 2017, the US government issued Presidential Proclamations 9645 and 9983, which ban various visa categories for 13 countries. By restricting exchange with people and ideas from various corners of the world, these political changes will undoubtedly impact many IMGs' opportunities to participate in research and other clinical exposures necessary to begin training in the United States. Furthermore, these changes may affect their ability to begin training as residents or even remain in the country as attending physicians depending on their immigration status [8].

These developments are just the tip of the iceberg as changes in the political climate and medical education slowly begin to unfold. As the difficulty for IMGs interested in entering the American medical system continues to increase, it will be more important than ever to ask whether IMGs must "choose a specialty just to get a job" and to examine the factors associated with doing so.

References

1. Liang M, Curtin L, Signer M, Savoia M. Understanding the interview and ranking behaviors of unmatched international medical students and graduates in the 2013 main residency match. J Grad Med Educ. 2015;7(4):610–6.
2. Murphy B. Choosing a medical specialty: 4 questions to help get you started [Internet]. American Medical Association; 2020 [cited 28 February 2020]. Available from: https://www.ama-assn.org/residents-students/specialty-profiles/choosing-medical-specialty-4-questions-help-get-you-started
3. Ahmed A, Hwang W, Thomas C, Deville C. International medical graduates in the US physician workforce and graduate medical education: current and historical trends. J Grad Med Educ. 2018;10(2):214–8.
4. Whitcomb M. Comparison of IMG-dependent and non-IMG-dependent residencies in the National Resident Matching Program. JAMA. 1996;276(9):700–3.

5. Jenkins T, Franklyn G, Klugman J, Reddy S. Separate but equal? The sorting of USMDs and non-USMDs in internal medicine residency programs. J Gen Intern Med. 2019;35(5):1458–64.
6. Stillman M, Miller K, Ziegler C, Upadhyay A, Mitchell C. Program characteristics influencing allopathic students' residency selection. J Am Osteopath Assoc. 2016;116(4):214.
7. Jolly P, Boulet J, Garrison G, Signer M. Participation in U.S. graduate medical education by graduates of international medical schools. Acad Med. 2011;86(5):559–64.
8. Radabaugh C, Welcher C, Skochelak S. Long-term potential implications of immigration barriers for medical education. JAMA. 2019;321(8):741.
9. Tsugawa Y, Jena A, Orav E, Jha A. Quality of care delivered by general internists in US hospitals who graduated from foreign versus US medical schools: observational study. BMJ. 2017;356:j273.
10. Kehoe A, McLachlan J, Metcalf J, Forrest S, Carter M, Illing J. Supporting international medical graduates' transition to their host-country: realist synthesis. Med Educ. 2020;50(10):1015–32.

Chapter 12
An Insight into the Journey of USMLE (United States Medical Licensing Exam): Understanding the Process

Nitya Beriwal

Overview

The journey of the USMLE (United States Medical Licensing Exam) involves a sequence of four exams which holistically analyze knowledge and clinical skills of a medical student or physician.

The examinations required include:

1. Step 1
2. Step 2 CK (Clinical Knowledge)
3. Step 2 CS (Clinical Skills)
4. Step 3

The first three exams can be taken in any order and are required for ECFMG certification.

Once that is achieved, one can register to apply for the Step 3 exam. See Fig. 12.1.

The exams cover educational material from basic sciences to the clinical sciences. They test integration of disciplines/organ systems and application of clinical skills.

Deciding to take the USMLE exams

We all want to be doctors who contribute effectively to society and leave a positive imprint on the lives of patients and the people we take care of. Our passion and aspirations act like a compass and direct us in our life. Deciding to pursue higher education or medical residency training abroad is a huge decision and milestone which needs proper thought. It is important to ensure that your aspirations and goals align with the path you pursue. If one decides to venture abroad, it is always to learn something new so that they can make a fruitful contribution to the world [1].

N. Beriwal (✉)
Lady Hardinge Medical College, New Delhi, India

© Springer Nature Switzerland AG 2021   183
H. Tohid, H. Maibach (eds.), *International Medical Graduates in the United States*, https://doi.org/10.1007/978-3-030-62249-7_12

Fig. 12.1 Summary of the
USMLE journey [32]

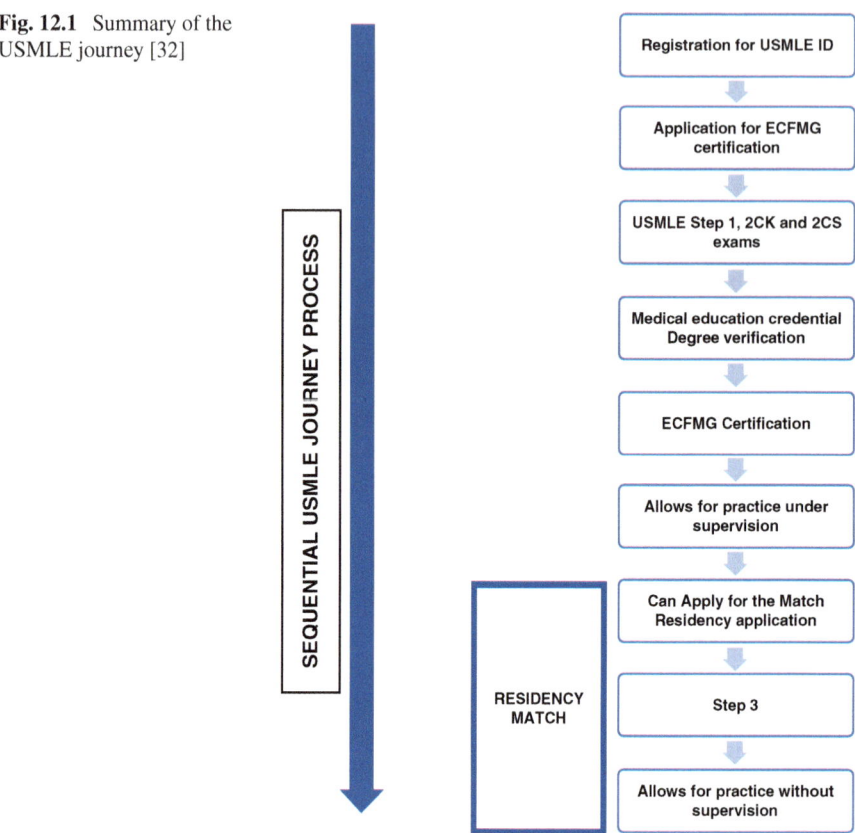

Important things to keep in mind before deciding to venture on this journey include the following:

1. *Establish your priorities and goals*

      It is best to make a roadmap for yourself. Take a sheet of paper and enlist how you want to see yourself in the next 5 years, 10 years, and so on. Ask yourself where your true passion lies, what do you think motivates you. Deciding the field you want to specialize in is the first step to realize where your passion truly lies.

Points to consider:

Decide your specialty of interest

It is important to determine where your interest truly lies. It helps if you understand your true calling early on as then you can align your energy and work toward your goal and dream branch.

Some questions to ask yourself:

Which discipline excites and motivates you?

What do you feel inclined toward?

What branch gives you a sense of reason?

Which discipline makes you feel content academically?

Do you like research?

Do you have an interest in public health or global health?

NOTE:

Some pointers that act as a basic guideline for helping you choose your branch:

(a) Medical or surgical
(b) Acute care or inpatient
(c) Pediatric or adult patients
(d) Interest in neuroscience
(e) Research or pure clinical practice

Future prospects

After you know your calling and have decided on your branch, it is crucial to consider the following pointers:

- Clinical exposure
- Research potential
- Fellowship prospects
- Work life balance

It is best to research on these pointers by using online forums and reaching out to friends, colleagues, and mentors.

2. ***Acceptability of current education***

The first step is to research regarding acceptability of your current medical qualification.

For USMLE, it is vital to check the status of your medical school and if your credentials are valid for ECFMG registration and certification in the world directory of medical schools (WDOMS). This is a widely accepted resource and enlists eligibility status of one's medical school for ECFMG certification [2].

3. ***Reach out to seniors***

Our friends, colleagues, and mentors are crucial for direction and guidance. Their experience not only directs us and shows us the way forward but also provides comfort during testing times. Please remember to always respect your seniors and value their time. Having fruitful discussion with seniors who have been on this journey provides valuable insight on the interplay of social, economic, and academic factors, which is very important to determine in this journey. They also act like pillars of moral support. It is vital to respect them for their journey and learn from them.

New guidelines being proposed from 2023 regarding accreditation of medical schools

The ECFMG is the main body that takes care of medical licensing for international medical students and graduates. However, this is carried out by the NBME for American medical students and graduates.

The ECFMG in 2010 established a new accreditation requirement for medical schools that will be effective from 2023 onward.

This was rolled out in an attempt to enhance medical education quality by establishing set standards to evaluate undergraduate medical education and ensure proper medical training standards in institutions across the world.

Based on these guidelines, medical graduates need to graduate from a medical school accredited by an accrediting agency that is recognized by WFME. WFME is the World Federation for Medical Education. This would be required for ECFMG certification starting 2023.

This process has been rolled out by the ECFMG in a sequential Four-Phase Implementation plan as follows:

Phase 1 (2018)
ECFMG released a new web resource to facilitate medical students to make informed decisions regarding deciding which medical school to enroll in.

Phase 2 (2020)
The WDOMS (World Directory of Medical Schools) now includes specific information regarding current accreditation status of medical schools across the globe.

Phase 3 (2021)
ECFMG has suggested that ECFMG physician reports will include information regarding current accreditation status of the medical school of the physician.

Phase 4 (2023)
ECFMG has suggested on their web portal that ECFMG certification will take into account accreditation status of medical school of the graduate.

Note: One should look out for recent accurate guidelines and further updates in this regard on the official website of ECFMG [3].

ECFMG Account Registration

It is important to register for a USMLE/ECFMG identification number and password, before one can apply for the various examinations.

Procedure/step-by-step guide:

1. Open the official website of the ECFMG.
2. From the Menu, select Online services.
3. Then select IWA (interactive web applications).
4. If you are a first-time user and have never applied for ECFMG ID before, click on the button indicated on the web portal.
5. Read the instructions page for the online authentication process carefully.
6. Ensure to fill complete and accurate information and to keep your current and active passport with you while filling the details.

7. Once you have an ECFMG ID and online password, you can begin applying for ECFMG certification.
8. The process of applying for ECFMG certification consists of two parts (both are available on IWA):

   1. An online application part on IWA platform

      The fee for applying for ECFMG certification is $145 as of February 27, 2020.

   2. Form 186: Certification of Identification Form (also on IWA platform)

      This form needs to be notarized online by NotaryCam service.

The online application needs to be completed. Post online application, ECFMG provides Form 186 which needs to be notarized using NotaryCam service [4].

Please remember to have your current and active passport with you during this process.

Application for USMLE examinations

Once you have been issued the USMLE/ECFMG ID and have completed applying for ECFMG certification, you can apply for USMLE exams Step 1, Step 2 CS, and Step 2 CK.

Please remember to read the latest official ECFMG information booklet and bulletin of information valid for your testing months. It is very helpful to ensure that you are aware of the updated testing policies and application process. The frequently asked questions page by the ECFMG is also very helpful.

The process of applying for USMLE exam consists of two phases:

1. Online application

   The online application can be completed within 14 days once you start filling it. It requires you to fill general information about yourself and your medical education.

2. Status verification by the medical school

This is a process by which ECFMG confirms your present status, that is, whether you are a student or graduate with one's medical school. It is a direct communication between one's medical school and ECFMG. It can be by two ways:

1. Electronic verification

   • This is done if your medical school has electronic access to EMSWP (ECFMG Medical School Web Portal)
   • Medical school completes status verification electronically.

2. Paper verification

   • This is done if your medical school does not have electronic access to EMSWP.
   • In this process, ECFMG provides candidate with Form 183 once application is submitted online.

- Form 183 has to be submitted to one's medical school.
- The medical school then fills this form and directly sends it to ECFMG.

3. ECFMG may also require additional documents; this is informed during the application regarding what credentials are required to be submitted.

The process is generally completed by ECFMG in 2 weeks, post receipt of all documents required [5].

USMLE Step 1, Step 2 CK, and Step 2 CS exams can be given in any order currently. However, there has been an update regarding rolling out of new guidelines in the near future prospectively, which can be found after the Step 2CS note in this chapter.

Once one has received their scheduling permit from the ECFMG, they can use their CIN (Candidate Identification Number) to book the desired date, center, and country of exam. All USMLE exams except the Step 2 CS and Step 3 are available in Prometric centers outside the USA. The official web portal for the Prometric can be used for searching available dates, booking a date, modifying the date, rescheduling exam, and all examination-related queries [6].

USMLE Step 1 Exam

The USMLE Step 1 exam has been one of the most important exams in the series of the USMLE exams. It is usually the first exam taken by most medical students and graduates in the series. It tests basic medical sciences by integrating it with applied clinical sciences.

The subject areas tested in the exam include:

1. Anatomy
2. Physiology
3. Biochemistry
4. Pathology
5. Microbiology
6. Immunology
7. Genetics
8. Nutrition
9. Pharmacology
10. Biostatistics
11. Behavioral sciences

Principal organ systems tested in the exam include:

1. Nervous system
2. Cardiovascular system
3. Hematology

4. Endocrine system
5. Gastrointestinal system
6. Musculoskeletal system
7. Skin
8. Renal system
9. Reproductive system
10. Respiratory system
11. Basic psychiatry

Important points about booking the Step 1 exam

1. It is recommended to book the exam 6 months prior to your desired eligibility period.
2. One has to decide and book a 3-month eligibility period for taking the exam.
3. A one-time 3-month extension is allowed for this eligibility period with some extension fee.
4. The exam date can be selected within one's eligibility period by visiting the Prometric website, once scheduling permit has been received.
5. The duration of the exam is *totally 8 hours*. It is a 1-day examination.

   – Tutorial: 15 minutes
   – Exam time: 7 hours
   – Break duration: 45 minutes

6. The exam consists of seven blocks of questions; the duration for each block is 1 hour.
7. After each block, candidate is allowed to take break. Duration of break between blocks is as per one's comfort. However, total break duration on the exam day cannot exceed 45 minutes + tutorial time saved if any.
8. Three-digit score is given after the exam. The passing score of Step 1 as of January 1, 2018, is 194.
9. The exam is a measure of proficiency in the basic sciences.
10. Results of the Step 1 are usually released within 3–4 weeks of the testing date. However, delays are possible during certain months, which are intimated from time to time on the ECFMG website [7].

InCUS guidelines
Invitational Conference on USMLE scoring

As of February 2020, InCUS has released that the USMLE program will change the way USMLE Step 1 score is reported from a numeric three-digit score to a pass/fail system, similar to USMLE Step 2 CS exam.

Numeric score system will be continued in score reporting for Step 2 CK and Step 3 exams.

This will be effective after January 1, 2022. Further details and updates regarding rolling out of this policy can be followed on the official web page of the USMLE [8].

USMLE Step 2 CK Exam

The Step 2 CK is the clinical knowledge exam. It tests the clinical proficiency and application of clinical knowledge by medical students and graduates.

It is usually taken by medical students after their final or fourth year.

The core areas tested in the exam include the following:

1. Internal medicine
2. Surgery
3. Obstetrics
4. Gynecology
5. Pediatrics
6. Preventative medicine
7. Psychiatry

Principal organ systems tested in the exam include the following:

1. Neurology
2. Cardiology
3. Hematology
4. Oncology
5. Endocrinology
6. Gastroenterology
7. Rheumatology
8. Dermatology
9. Nephrology
10. Reproductive system
11. Pulmonology
12. Clinical psychiatry
13. Ethics and patient safety

Important points about booking the Step 2 CK exam

1. It is recommended to book the exam 6 months prior to your desired eligibility period.
2. One has to decide and book a 3-month eligibility period for taking the exam, similar to Step 1 exam.
3. A one-time 3-month extension is allowed for this eligibility period with some extension fee, similar to Step 1 exam.
4. The exam date can be selected within one's eligibility period by visiting the Prometric website, once scheduling permit has been received, similar to Step 1 exam.
5. The duration of the exam is totally *9 hours*. It is a 1-day examination.

   – Tutorial: 15 minutes
   – Exam time: 8 hours
   – Break duration: 45 minutes

6. The exam consists of eight blocks of questions; the duration for each block is 1 hour. Each block has 40 questions.
7. After each block, candidate is allowed to take break. Duration of break between blocks is as per one's comfort. However, total break duration on the exam day cannot exceed 45 minutes + tutorial time saved if any. Maximum break if whole tutorial duration is saved is 60 minutes.
8. A three-digit score is given after the exam. The passing score of Step 2 CK as of January 1, 2018, is 209.
9. The exam is a measure of proficiency in the clinical sciences. It tests the application of core clinical concepts in patient-based clinical vignette-style questions.
10. The exam tests clinical concepts revolving around clinical diagnosis, prognosis, risk factors, management guidelines, treatment strategies, and ethical evidence-based patient care.
11. Results of the Step 2 CK are usually released within 3–4 weeks of the testing date. During certain specified months, potential delays are intimated from time to time on the ECFMG website. Candidates should plan their timeline after checking recent updates on the ECFMG website [9].

New Guidelines Addition of question stems
Exam content modification has been rolled out by the USMLE from mid-2020.

Thereon, the Step 1 and the Step 2 (CK) exams will have more number of questions on the following topics:

1. Communication skills
2. Evidence-based practice
3. Patient safety
4. Medical ethics

It has been rolled out that:

• Starting from May 2020, Step 1 will have questions testing communication skills.
• Starting from June 2020, Step 2 CK will have questions on evidence-based practice, patient safety, and medical ethics.

Recent updates should be followed by examinees on the official website of ECFMG [10].

USMLE Step 2 CS Exam

USMLE Step 2 CS (clinical skills) is a practical skills assessment exam. It is a 1-day exam which can be taken in centers only in the USA.

This exam tests clinical applied proficiency of a medical student or graduate. It tests clinical skills that are essential for provision of patient care and also health promotion strategies.

The exam consists of a series of clinical scenarios with standardized patients. Examinees have to take meticulous history, perform targeted examination, form differential diagnosis, counsel the patient adequately, and write patient note based on their clinical judgment.

The exam tests three areas:

1. Spoken English proficiency
2. Communication and interpersonal skills
3. Integrated clinical encounter

It is a pass/fail system based exam. There is no numeric scoring. Examinee has to pass all three components to pass the examination.

The exam can be taken in five test centers across the USA. The test centers include the following:

1. Houston, Texas
2. Los Angeles, California
3. Chicago, Illinois
4. Philadelphia, Pennsylvania
5. Atlanta, Georgia

The exam format consists of 12 sequential patient encounters. The duration of each patient encounter is 15 minutes followed by 10 minutes to type/write the patient note [11].

International medical graduates can register for this exam using the ECFMG IWA portal. A candidate is allowed to book a 1-year eligibility period during which they can apply for their desired date and location based on availability to take the exam. The Step 2 CS results are released based on a pre-planned reporting schedule which specifies the date of result for the set examination periods. Examinees should take this schedule into account while planning their timeline for the exam. The Step 2 CS reporting schedule can be found on the official webpage of USMLE [12].

New guidelines regarding eligibility for Step 2 CS exam
Based on recent guidelines proposed during the InCUS conference February 2020, there are speculations that application for Step 2 CS may require success in Step 1 before being eligible to book the exam. This guideline may come into force no earlier than March 2021 [13]. However, further confirmation and update must be looked out for on the official website of USMLE [14].

USMLE Step 3 Exam

Step 3 exam can be taken only if a candidate has successfully passed all three exams – Step 1, Step 2 CK, and Step 2 CS – and has become ECFMG certified.

The Step 3 exam is the final USMLE exam that leads to license to practice medicine in the USA without supervision. It assesses physician capability to assume independent responsibility and practice evidence-based medicine ethically.

The exam is a 2-day exam. Both exams can be taken on non-consecutive dates. The exam days test different domains of clinical knowledge and are as follows:

- Day 1: Foundations of Independent Practice (FIP)

  - Six blocks of 38–39 multiple choice questions
  - Hour allotted per block
  - 45 minutes break time and 5 minutes optional tutorial
  - Total exam duration: approximately 7 hours
  - This exam assesses clinical knowledge pertaining to diagnosis and management

- Day 2: Advanced Clinical Medicine (ACM)

  - Multiple choice part

    Six blocks of 30 multiple choice questions
    45 minutes per multiple choice block
    5-minute multiple choice tutorial

  - CCS part

    13 case simulations
    10–20 minute per case simulation variable
    7-minute CCS tutorial

  - 45 minutes break time
  - This exam assesses the ability to apply clinical knowledge in patient management.
  - This exam includes both multiple type questions and computer-based clinical case simulations (CCS).

Step 3 exam applications are done via the official FSMB (Federation of State Medical Boards) website [15].

The exam can only be booked by international medical graduates once they are ECFMG certified. This requires successfully passing Step 1, Step 2 CK, and Step 2CS USMLE examinations. It also requires verification of medical education credentials such as degree or diploma by the ECFMG [16].

The result of Step 3 examination is expressed as a numeric score. Based on a recent update on January 1, 2020, the minimum passing score for Step 3 is 198 [17].

Passing the Step 3 exam enables a physician to practice without supervision if required. This is the final USMLE exam for physicians. It can be completed before applying for residency training, but it can also be given in the intern year of residency training.

Commonly Used Resources

High-Yield Resources

- *UWORLD* question bank is the most widely used question bank. It is used to practice questions alongside studying textbooks and attending classes in your medical school. The information provided in the answer section of each question is gold and very important to enrich one's preparation. The educational objectives provided at the bottom of each question are of high yield [18].
- Students commonly use *First aid books for different Step examination* preparation. First Aid for USMLE Step 1 book is the most famous and widely used. It provides a summarized version of the most important topics one can prepare. One should read every word and annotate extra details and notes of classes in medical school and standard textbooks in it in a crisp manner, so you have a compiled resource to revise before your exam. The rapid review section at the end of the book serves as a good revision source [19].

Resources for USMLE Step 1 preparation

1. *First Aid for Step 1* [19]
2. *UWORLD* question bank for Step 1 [18]
3. Pathoma : Fundamentals of Pathology (Author Dr. Sattar)
   Review video series of Pathology [20]
4. NBME practice exams
   Practice test series by National Board of Medical Examiners [21]
5. Boards and Beyond video series
   Review video series covering all subjects and organ systems [22]
6. Sketchy medical
   Review series having picture mnemonics for Microbiology and Pharmacology [23].
7. USMLE Rx Q Bank
   Question bank curated by the authors of first aid books are available for all USMLE examinations [19]
8. BRS Behavioral Science by Barbara Fadem
   Textbook of Behavioural Science [24]
9. Physeo
   Review video course covering Physiology and integrating concepts [25]

Resources for USMLE Step 2 CK preparation

1. Uworld Q bank for Step 2 CK [18]
2. Uworld Q bank for Biostatistics [18]
3. Master the Boards for Step 2 CK: Conrad Fischer [26]

Resources for USMLE Step 3 preparation

1. Uworld Q bank for Step 3 [18]
2. Uworld CCS cases for Step 3 [18]
3. Master the boards for Step 3: Conrad Fischer [26]
4. Uworld Q bank for Biostatistics [18]

Resources for USMLE Step 2 CS preparation
1. First Aid for Step 2 CS [19]
2. Uworld Q bank for Step 2 CS [18]
3. Also a good study partner is must for practicing clinical cases

Practice Materials by the USMLE

- Practice materials for all Step examinations are available on the official USMLE website [14].
- These materials are very useful in understanding the pattern of the exam and provide an insight into the type of questions directly from the body responsible for the exam. It is recommended highly to go through them during your exam preparation as they provide an outline and foundation to guide one's preparation.
- The content one must go through is as follows:

  1. Content description and general information booklet

      It provides an overview of the outline of the exam.
      It specifies percentage of questions from different systems.
      It also specifies the crucial physician competency areas being tested in the exam and in what proportion.
      This information is vital for any exam candidate so that he/she can strengthen his/her weak areas to become a better physician and to also improve exam performance.

  2. Sample items

      Famously known as the "free 120" questions
      These questions are must-do for any candidate few days before the exam, as these questions are directly provided by the USMLE on their website.

  3. Tutorial and practice test items for multiple choice questions

      The tutorial is similar to the tutorial in the exam.
      It is a must-do the day before/a few days before the exam to become familiar with the exam software.
      Most candidates prefer to see the tutorial online 1 day before the tutorial and run through the 15 min tutorial in the exam to save time as it gets added to the total break time available for the candidate. If you prefer to rush through the tutorial in the exam it is highly recommended to do the audio headphone check. Please remember to do the audio check, as the headphone is crucial for the audio questions in the exam [14].

Fees Structure for USMLE Examinations

It is important to manage one's finances in the journey of USMLE. A major component of the finances is the examination fees. The fees for various USMLE examinations are enlisted in Table 12.1.

What is considered to be a good score?
The best resource to have an understanding regarding a good score to match can be obtained via the charting outcomes of the match data available on the NRMP web portal. One must remember that the USMLE scores are only one of the many parameters like research, medical school performance, and interviews that play a role in a successful match. The latest available data as of now is that of the NRMP Match 2018. The mean USMLE Step 1 score at which non-US IMGs matched is 234, and score at which US IMG's matched is 222. The mean USMLE Step 2 CK score at which Non-US IMGs matched is 240, and score at which US IMG's matched is 232 [31]. A pass is required on the USMLE Step 2 CS examination. Passing the Step 3 examination also confers an advantage. The average scores for a successful match vary based on the specialty of interest. Such details are easily available for the perusal of candidates in the "Charting Outcomes in the Match" summary provided on the official website of the NRMP (National Resident Matching Program) [31].

Table 12.1 Fee structure of USMLE examinations as of February 2020 [27, 28]

Exam	Fees
USMLE Step 1	$965 + ITDS[a] online using IWA
USMLE Step 2 CK	$965 + ITDS[a] online using IWA
Extension of eligibility period for Step 1 and Step 2 CK	$90 per exam using IWA
Testing region change for Step 1 and Step 2 CK	$85 per region change using Form 312
Rescheduling fee for Step 1 and Step 2 CK	Variable, $0–604 – contact regional Prometric center
USMLE Step 2 CS	$1600 online using IWA
Rescheduling for Step 2CS exam	Variable, $0–1300 online using Step 2 CS Calendar and scheduling (based on the date of cancellation before exam date)
USMLE Step 3	$895 for eligibility periods ending in 2020
USMLE Transcript	Paper transcript: $70 per request form up to 10 transcripts Electronic to ERAS: $80 per ERAS season

For latest details on fees structure, please refer to official websites of ECFMG and FSMB [27–29]
[a]*ITDS* International test delivery surcharge is additional fee if candidate chooses testing center outside USA and Canada for Step 1 and Step 2 CK examinations

Some Points to Remember

1. While preparing for USMLE, proper planning and formation of timeline are essential.
2. Read the latest information booklet on the official ECFMG website [29].
3. Regularly follow the WDOMS and the WFME websites for latest information on the accreditation status of your medical school [2, 30].
4. One should define one's study goals. Define the study resources you are going to use and allocate proper time to them.
5. Form a timeline to take different USMLE examinations based on when you plan to apply for the Match season.
6. Take advice from seniors regarding preparation strategy.
7. Solve practice tests such as Uworld self-assessment and NBME exams periodically during your preparation to analyze your weak areas to help strengthen them subsequently.
8. Read the exam guidelines on the USMLE website. Solve sample question items provided on the official USMLE website before the exam.
9. Take adequate rest before the exam. Remember to pack your admit card, scheduling permit, passport, and eatables the day before your exam.

References

1. https://www.usmlesarthi.com/is-usmle-right-for-you.html
2. http://www.wdoms.org/
3. http://www.ecfmg.org/accreditation/
4. https://iwa2.ecfmg.org/overview.asp
5. https://www.ecfmg.org/2019ib/apply-for-examination.html
6. https://www.prometric.com/test-takers/search/usmle.
7. https://www.usmle.org/step-1/
8. https://www.usmle.org/inCus/
9. https://www.usmle.org/step-2-ck/
10. https://www.ecfmg.org/news/2019/11/06/usmle-step-1-and-step-2-ck-content-changes-scheduled-for-mid-2020/
11. https://www.usmle.org/step-2-cs/
12. https://www.usmle.org/step-2-cs/#reporting
13. https://www.pastest.com/blog/usmle/incus-usmle-step-1-score-changes-to-passfail/
14. https://www.usmle.org/
15. https://www.fsmb.org/step-3/step-3-information/
16. https://www.usmle.org/step-3/
17. https://www.ecfmg.org/news/2019/12/10/change-in-minimum-passing-score-for-step-3/
18. https://www.uworld.com/

19. https://firstaidteam.com/
20. https://www.pathoma.com/
21. https://www.nbme.org/
22. https://www.boardsbeyond.com/
23. https://sketchymedical.com/
24. https://shop.lww.com/BRS-Behavioral-Science/p/9781496310477
25. https://physeo.com/
26. https://medquestreviews.com/
27. https://www.ecfmg.org/fees/
28. https://www.fsmb.org/step-3/step-3-faq/
29. https://www.ecfmg.org/
30. https://wfme.org/
31. http://www.nrmp.org/main-residency-match-data/
32. https://resident360.nejm.org/expert-consult/applying-for-residency-as-an-international-medical-graduate

Chapter 13
The Relationship Between Country of Origin and Performance on the USMLE

Haziq F. Siddiqi and Vinod E. Nambudiri

USMLE Performance by Country of Origin

As a critical series of exams that are necessary to complete prior to obtaining residency in the United States, thousands of medical students and early-career physicians around the world look to take the USMLE exams every year. Interestingly, USMLE performance varies by country of origin. This chapter reviews USMLE performance by a test-taker's country of origin, and examines several factors that may be associated with international medical graduates' performance on the exam.

One way to estimate USMLE performance by country of origin is through the number of certificates issued to each country by the Educational Commission for Foreign Medical Graduates (ECFMG). To receive an ECFMG certificate, a candidate must do all of the following:

- Pass USMLE Step 1 exam
- Pass USMLE Step 2 Clinical Knowledge exam
- Pass USMLE Step 2 Clinical Skills exam
- Verify successful graduation from their medical school

The distribution of ECFMG certificates is a proxy for USMLE performance by country of citizenship, reflecting the number of individual physicians from a given country who are able to successfully complete all components of the required certification. In 2017, 9839 ECFMG certificates were issued to IMGs (Table 13.1). Of

H. F. Siddiqi
Harvard Medical School, Boston, MA, USA
e-mail: haziq_siddiqi@hms.harvard.edu

V. E. Nambudiri (✉)
Department of Dermatology, Brigham and Women's Hospital and Harvard Medical School, Boston, MA, USA
e-mail: vnambudiri@bwh.harvard.edu

© Springer Nature Switzerland AG 2021
H. Tohid, H. Maibach (eds.), *International Medical Graduates in the United States*, https://doi.org/10.1007/978-3-030-62249-7_13

Table 13.1 Distribution of recipients of ECFMG certificates in 2017

Country	Country of medical school		Country of citizenship	
	No.	%	No.	%
Antigua and Barbuda	324	3.3	8	0.1
Australia	144	1.5	47	0.5
Bangladesh	63	0.6	51	0.5
Brazil	112	1.1	111	1.1
Canada	0	0.0	805	8.2
China	223	2.3	167	1.7
Colombia	102	1.0	99	1.0
Cuba	112	1.1	85	0.9
Dominica	680	6.9	4	<0.1
Dominican Republic	150	1.5	67	0.7
Ecuador	55	0.6	52	0.5
Egypt	255	2.8	241	2.4
Germany	58	0.6	55	0.6
Grenada	970	9.9	7	0.1
India	1017	10.3	1044	10.6
Iran	156	1.6	167	1.7
Iraq	104	1.1	122	1.2
Ireland	169	1.7	66	0.7
Israel	252	2.6	156	1.6
Japan	66	0.7	67	0.7
Jordan	150	1.5	154	1.6
Lebanon	138	1.4	115	1.2
Mexico	202	2.1	84	0.9
Nepal	91	0.9	108	1.1
Nigeria	183	1.9	254	2.6
Pakistan	673	6.8	624	6.3
Peru	61	0.6	63	0.6
Philippines	110	1.1	73	0.7
Poland	98	1.0	13	0.1
Russia	78	0.8	55	0.6
Saba	202	2.1	0	0.0
Saint Kitts and Nevia	310	3.2	1	<0.1
Saint Lucia	69	0.7	6	0.1
Saint Vincent and the Grenadines	84	0.9	3	<0.1
Saudi Arabia	134	1.4	118	1.2
Sint Maarten	370	3.8	0	0.0
South Korea	59	0.6	77	0.8
Sudan	76	0.8	64	−0.7
Syria	79	0.8	94	1.0
Turkey	93	0.9	87	0.9
United Kingdom	116	1.2	81	0.8

Table 13.1 (continued)

	Country of medical school		Country of citizenship	
Country	No.	%	No.	%
United States	0	0.0	3112	31.8
Venezuela	130	1.3	134	1.4
Countries with fewer than 50 recipients	1321	13.4	1098	11.2
Total	9839	100	9839	100

Adapted from ECFMG Data, Ref. [5]

these ECFMG certificates, over 30% – 3112 – went to internationally educated citizens of the United States (32%). This was followed by 1044 ECFMG certificates issued to citizens of India (11%) and 805 ECFMG certificates issued to citizens of Canada (8%).

The number of certificates reflects the influence of multiple factors. This includes the total number of physicians graduating from training in the specific country, as well as the number who aim to come to the United States to further their clinical training.

Factors That Influence Country Performance

Prior studies on the performance of Caribbean-educated IMGs on the USMLE have provided insights into some of the factors that determine country-level performance on the certification exams. In 2017, Caribbean-educated IMGs collectively received a total of 3009 ECFMG certificates, representing 31% of total certificates. While most other IMGs complete medical school in their country of citizenship, two-thirds of Caribbean-educated IMGs are US citizens [1]. Collectively, performance of these students on the USMLE has been increasing over time, possibly due to broader improvements in access to online medical education. From 2002 to 2009, the yearly first-attempt pass rate on USMLE Step 1 increased from 56% to 69% [1]. This likely reflects several factors, including the possibility of the strengthening of the caliber of trainees in these medical schools, innovations in medical school curricular content, more widespread availability of preparatory materials for the exam, or greater weight placed by applicants on Step 1 performance and thus increased time dedicated to improving scores.

Although performance overall has been increasing among graduates of medical schools in Caribbean countries, performance varies between the Caribbean countries. Collectively from 1993 to 2007, Step 1 pass rates of country ranged from 19% (Saint Lucia) to 84% (Grenada) [1]. The cause of this variance is likely multifactorial. For example, Van Zanten and Boulet described how differences in the language of instruction (Spanish, French, or English), accreditation process, and student backgrounds may account for some of this variation. Importantly, the exam is only administered in English, which may benefit students around the world who receive medical education in English compared to other languages. This may also benefit students for whom English is their first or native language relative to those for whom English is a second language.

Another useful study on country performance on the USMLE was conducted by Tekian and Boulet, who analyzed USMLE first-attempt pass rates for all Arab countries where English is the language of instruction during medical school [2]. The authors reviewed data from countries including Bahrain, Egypt, Iraq, Jordan, Kuwait, Lebanon, Libya, Palestinian Territory, Oman, Qatar, Saudi Arabia, Sudan, Syria, United Arab Emirates, and Yemen. The analysis included graduates of 150 medical schools across these nations. In total, the analysis included nearly 17,000 applicants from across these countries during the 15-year time period. Approximately 27% of the applicants studied were female.

The authors noted that the number of test takers from these countries increased dramatically from 1998 to 2012. They found that the USMLE Step 1 pass rate varied from 47% (Kuwait) to 95% (Palestinian Territories). The number of test takers varied widely across nations, with only 58 test takers from Yemen during the 15-year period, compared to 3408 from Egypt during the same time period.

The authors observed that variability in performance across the Arab world was also determined to be multifactorial. One of these factors was the desire to emigrate from their country of citizenship. This was influenced by income potential and desire for stability and security. Medical students from higher-income Arab countries, they argued, may be less incentivized to emigrate to the United States. Another factor was the average medical school selectivity and class size. Countries with higher physician density, which may correspond to lower admissions selectivity, were found to have worse performance on the USMLE.

Another factor which may account for discrepancies in performance based on country of origin is national support for USMLE studying. Having sufficient time to study and purchase study materials can be prohibitively expensive. Tekian and Boulet described that some countries such as Saudi Arabia provide national financial aid to help students pass their USMLE exams. While data on the presence of these programs was not available for other countries, it is likely that this influences performance. Similarly, trainees from across the world may experience variation in their performance on the USMLE exam based on how closely their medical school content and educational curriculum mirror the format and features of the USMLE Step 1 exam.

Finally, the role of national medical school accreditation programs has also been studied. Whether a country of origin has an accreditation system has been linked to the country's outcomes in USMLE scores. Van Zanten et al. specifically examined the impact of accreditation on USMLE outcomes [1]. They found that better performance on the Step 2 Clinical Skills exam was associated with female gender, testing within 3 years of graduation, native English-speaking status, and attending a school located in a country with a system of accreditation. This argues for a rigorous standard being applied to medical training in countries, which can encourage development of a better-prepared physician workforce that is able to outperform trainees from other countries on exams such as the USMLE.

In a different study by Tekian and Boulet, first-time past rates on Step 2 Clinical Skills and Step 2 Clinical Knowledge exams were examined. They found that the USMLE Step 2 Clinical Knowledge pass rate varied from 58.2% (Yemen) to 95.3% (Qatar). The number of test takers varied widely across nations, with only 67 test takers from Yemen during the 15-year period, compared to 3654 from Egypt during the same time period. The authors found that the USMLE Step 2 Clinical Skills pass rate varied from 62% (Oman) to 94.6% (Qatar). The number of test takers again was varied across nations, with only 24 test takers from Oman during the 15-year period, compared to 2795 from Egypt during the same time period. These data suggest several interesting findings. First, performance on individual USMLE exams by country of origin may vary, as some countries have higher rates of passage on Step 1 compared to parts of Step 2, and vice versa. For example, trainees from the Palestinian territory had very high pass rates on both the USMLE Step 1 and Step 2 Clinical Knowledge, but lower pass rates on Step 2 Clinical Skills. In contrast, trainees from the United Arab Emirates had low first-time past rates on Step 1, but high past rates on Step 2 Clinical Skills.

Taken together, these data suggest that international medical graduates are not a uniform population when it comes to thinking about pass rates on standardized USMLE exams. Understanding the implications of country of origin on USMLE performance may help applicants to understand where their predecessors have either excelled or struggled and thus prepare accordingly to overcome barriers to success in the residency application process. Given the importance placed on USMLE exam performance in the residency application process, this is an area where further exploration and understanding can be of significant mutual benefit for international medical graduates and the US graduate medical education system in general.

Clinical Implications of USMLE Performance

USMLE performance has also been linked to clinical outcomes during residency training in certain circumstances, including for IMGs. Different USMLE scores have been connected to differences in clinical performance. In a study of 1511 US medical students, Gauer and Jackson found that USMLE Step 1 and Step 2 CK scores "moderately correlate" with clinical clerkship performance [3].

Although this study only included American students, a different study by Norcini et al. showed that for IMGs, scores on the Step 2 CK are connected to patient outcomes [4]. In this publication, the authors retrospectively studied select hospitalizations where the attending physician was an IMG who had taken Step 2 CK. They then examined the relationship between in-hospital mortality and Step 2 CK scores. After adjustment for multiple factors including severity of illness, they found that performance on Step 2 CK had a statistically significant inverse relationship with mortality. Each additional point on Step 2 CK was associated with a 0.2% decrease in mortality [4]. While this study also had some limitations, it does suggest that there is some beneficial role for board examinations that test clinical knowledge.

This is an important area for further research for the international medical graduate community. In particular, given that these scores are often used to identify candidates for residency training, as well as provide medical licensing, understanding the true impact of scores on ultimately physician performance and patient outcome is vitally important. Additionally, understanding whether there are differences in the score impact for US physicians versus international medical graduates should also be an area of focus.

Upcoming Changes

There are two upcoming changes that will likely reshape the role of USMLE exams for IMGs. First, effective in 2023, individuals applying for ECFMG Certification will be required to graduate from a medical school that has been accredited by an accrediting agency that is formally recognized. This change will likely improve USMLE outcomes as well as improve the broader consistency of global medical education. As has been noted above, prior data indicates that score performance in countries with accreditation systems for their medical schools is generally higher on the USMLE exams than for trainees who attended medical schools from countries without such an accreditation system. Ultimately, this should hopefully have a positive impact on the physician workforce, as it will lead to more trainees in residency programs coming from institutions that have met the curricular criteria for accreditation.

In the short term, this may preclude students from non-accredited schools from receiving certification. In the long term, however, this may incentivize schools to pursue accreditation. It remains to be seen how this change will impact accessibility in the long term.

Additionally, whether or not this change will impact the performance on standardized exams that vary by country of origin remains to be seen. It is possible that variation will decrease, given the overall consistently high quality of education. Still, some country-specific variation may persist even following the implementation of such policies, due to the country-specific factors discussed previously.

A second major change was recently announced by the National Board of Medical Examiners (NBME) that the USMLE Step 1 exam will be transitioning to pass/fail grading. Accompanying this announcement, Dr. William Pinsky, President and CEO of ECFMG, stated: "The ECFMG supports the informed decision making of the NBME and FSMB Boards on these policy changes. We are looking forward to continually advocating for international graduates as well as participating in the important future conversations on residency selection and transition" [6].

It is likely that this change will lead to several modifications to the current residency selection process. First, there may be a greater emphasis on Step 2 CK as well as factors beyond USMLE scores such as letters of recommendation. Second, there may be a greater emphasis on holistic assessment of applications, which may provide as yet unforeseen opportunities for international medical graduates who previously may have struggled in the application process due to a low standardized test score. Because further details are not yet available, it remains to be seen how this will impact the ECFMG process, and whether or not applicants from particular schools or countries will be disproportionately positively or negatively affected by this change.

Conclusions

Many factors ultimately influence performance on any standardized examination, including the USMLE. In this chapter, we have reviewed the variation that exists between countries in their medical school graduate success in obtaining ECFMG certification, as well as data examining the performance of graduates from medical schools and specific countries. Several variables, including access to preparation for the exam, medical school curricula, language of instruction, and familiarity with testing format, may all influence candidate performance. Ultimately, more data is needed to understand this variation, as well as to better understand how performance on the USMLE exams may correlate with clinical outcomes.

References

1. Zanten MV. The association between medical education accreditation and the examination performance of internationally educated physicians seeking certification in the United States. Perspect Med Educ. 2015;4(3):142–5.
2. Tekian A, Boulet J. A longitudinal study of the characteristics and performances of medical students and graduates from the Arab countries. BMC Med Educ. 2015;15(1):200.
3. Gauer JL, Jackson JB. The association between United States Medical Licensing Examination scores and clinical performance in medical students. Adv Med Educ Pract. 2019;10:209–16.
4. Norcini JJ, Boulet JR, Opalek A, Dauphinee WD. The relationship between licensing examination performance and the outcomes of care by international medical school graduates. Acad Med. 2014;89(8):1157–62.
5. Educational Commission for Foreign Medical Graduates. Standard ECFMG certificates issued in 2017. Available from: https://ecfmg.org/resources/2017CertsbyMedSchoolCountryCitizenshipCountry.pdf
6. United States Medical Licensnsing Examination. Change to pass/fail score reporting for Step 1 [Internet]. InCUS. [cited 2020Mar12]. Available from: https://www.usmle.org/incus

Chapter 14
Unique Considerations of Certain Countries

Bilal Haider Malik, Ian H. Rutkofsky, and Dong Hyang Kwon

Introduction

In 2018 alone there were 46,344 applications received through Electronic Residency Application Service (ERAS) for residency match in the USA [1]. Out of which 18,427 applicants were regarded as international medical graduates (IMGs) [1]. It is important to note that even reaching the application submission stage through the ERAS, a candidate (both American medical graduate [AMG] and IMG) has gone through a lot of steps, but still the most crucial stage of interviews and matching remain. We aim to make this journey easy for our readers who are planning to embark on this long journey by providing them with the vital information they need to achieve their goals. There are a lot of hurdles a candidate has to pass through, which are of financial, cultural, lingual and legal (visas) nature. According to new information made available, there are definite considerations that US Medical Licensing Examination (USMLE) programme will change score reporting for Step 1 from a three-digit numeric score to reporting only a pass/fail outcome. A numeric score will continue to be reported for Step 2 clinical knowledge (CK) and Step 3.

B. H. Malik (✉)
CiBNP, Fairfield, CA, USA

Institute of Behavioral Neurosciences and Psychology, Fairfield, CA, USA

Internal Medicine, Research, California Institute of Behavioral Neurosciences & Psychology, Sacramento, CA, USA

I. H. Rutkofsky
Department of Psychiatry, HCA – Aventura Hospital and Medical Center, Aventura, FL, USA

Department of Research, CiBNP, Fairfield, CA, USA

D. H. Kwon
Georgetown University, Washington, DC, USA

Department of Pathology, MedStar Georgetown University Hospital, Washington, DC, USA

© Springer Nature Switzerland AG 2021
H. Tohid, H. Maibach (eds.), *International Medical Graduates in the United States*, https://doi.org/10.1007/978-3-030-62249-7_14

Step 2 clinical skills (CS) will continue to be reported as pass/fail. This policy is speculated to take effect no earlier than January 2022 with further details to follow later on from the concerned authorities. With this new information in mind and through our observations whilst dealing with US residency aspirants, we have identified that research from now on is going to make a lot of impact on candidate's CV, and being a published author in a PubMed indexed journal will add a very strong positive impact that might prove to be the difference. In this chapter, we have gone through a wide range of information available and tried to condense the most important points here so that we can make this journey somewhat more manageable for our readers. We have looked at the issues faced by the candidates from different parts of the globe and taken into consideration the unique circumstances these candidates face and tried to help them find the right information to make an informed decision.

USA (American Medical Graduates [AMGs])

The meaning of an international medical graduate is a medical professional who got a primary medical degree from a medical college situated outside the USA and Canada, which is not recognised by a US accrediting body, the Liaison Committee on Medical Education (LCME), or the American Osteopathic Association. The location/accreditation of the medical college, not the citizenship of the medical practitioner, establishes if the graduate is an IMG [2]. This implies that US citizens that have graduated from medical institutions outside of the USA and Canada are regarded as IMGs. Non-US citizens who graduated from medical institutions in the USA and Canada are not considered IMGs. American medical graduates after graduation also need to sit the USMLEs and score top marks to survive in the highly competitive market. They then apply for the match through ERAS and National Resident Matching Program (NRMP). It is believed that AMGs have better chances of obtaining strong letters of recommendation (LoRs) and getting a decent number of interview invites, leading to better residency acquisition rates. Reasons for better success rates for AMGs are better knowledge of the American healthcare system, attitudes, communication skills and networking opportunities with the local medical fraternity. After obtaining their matches, the candidates who are not US citizens or who do not have Green card have to apply for relevant visas to be able to join their matched programmes.

Canada

By and large, so long as a Canadian physician has a provincial licence, he/she is able to get a US licence in the state where he plans to work as a clinician. Under US immigration laws, foreign medical graduates (FMGs) cannot practise medicine in the USA without finishing a medical residency in the USA, and before doing so, they have to pass the US Medical Licensing Examination (USMLE), Steps I and II [3]. Graduates of Canadian medical schools are not regarded as foreign medical graduates, and their residency in Canada is seen as equivalent to residency in the USA. If the Canadian medical professional has passed USMLE – Steps I, II and III – and has an offer of work in the USA, he/she can practise medicine in the USA [3]. However, the majority of Canadian medical graduates sit the Licentiate of the Medical Council of Canada (LMCC) while a few sit the US examination.

Canadian Resident Matching Service (CaRMS) functions like the Dean's Office for Canadian medical students and graduates (i.e. pupils completing studies in or graduating from Canadian medical schools), using ERAS to apply in the USA. So it is essential to register through CaRMS for ERAS [4]. To be able to facilitate the procedure for applicants that desire to participate entirely in both the US and Canadian matches, CaRMS honours the agreement towards the US NRMP match [4]. One can register for both matches and apply to Canadian as well as US programmes. One is also able to submit a ranking order list to both the CaRMS and NRMP [4]. After getting the match, candidates need to apply for a relevant visa to be able to work in the USA.

Caribbean

Medical graduates who get their medical degree from a Caribbean medical school are called Caribbean international medical graduates (IMGs) and can be from different nationalities, including the USA. Being a Caribbean international medical graduate carries certain advantages, i.e. strong English proficiency, built-in US clinical rotations and experience, and curriculums are often close to the US system and US citizenship (Caribbean IMGs can be typically US citizens). St. George's University, Ross University and American University of Antigua (AUA) are the only three Caribbean medical schools that have approval by the Florida Department of Education, New York State Education Department, accreditation from Caribbean accreditation Authority for Education in Medicine and other Health Professions (CAAM-HP) and recognition from the Medical Board of California [5]. Medical University of the Americas (MUA) and St. Matthews University have New York approval [5]. Spartan Health Sciences University and Xavier University have provisional CAAM-HP accreditation [5]. The Liaison Committee on Medical Education (LCME) states that they do not accredit medical programmes outside the USA and Canada [5]. The Caribbean international medical graduates have to apply through the ERAS after completing USMLE.

UK

UK medical graduates (UK nationals or other nationalities) and General Medical Council (GMC)-registered doctors (UK nationals or different nationalities) are regarded as foreign medical graduates for the purposes of US residency match via ERAS and NRMP. They have to complete the USMLE Steps and then apply for the match via ERAS as an FMG. Even if someone has obtained their Certificate of completion of Training (CCT) or Certificate of Eligibility for specialist Registration

(CESR), they will still need to apply for the residency via ERAS after passing their USMLE. UK medical graduates and GMC-registered doctors practising in the UK might have an advantage and comparably more chances of getting a residency match because of proficient English language skills, NHS-based UK clinical training exposure, favourable research opportunities, strong LoRs and exposure to principles of medical education. GMC is also planning on introducing United Kingdom Medical Licensing Assessment (UKMLA) which will be a registration exam for both UK and international medical graduates (replacing Professional and Linguistic Assessments Board [PLAB] for IMGs) in the coming few years. It is believed to be based on similar principles from PLAB and USMLE keeping in mind the local curriculum, patient needs and NHS core principles of patient care provision. It is worth mentioning with Brexit insight that there might be an exodus of UK-trained European workforce, which might head towards the USA for future prospects. It is also worth mentioning that having membership of either of the Royal College (i.e. RCP [Royal College of Physicians], Royal College of Surgeons [RCS], Royal College of General Practitioners [RCGP], Royal College of Obstetricians and Gynaecologists [RCOG], Royal College of Anaesthetists [RCOA], etc.) can be seen as a positive by the interviewing panel for residency matches. The UK nationals can also have relatively easy access to the USA because of the US visa waiver policy, making it easy for UK nationals (financially and length of time-wise) to appear in the USMLEs [6]. Another advantage is financial as currency conversion rates from GBP to USD are also favourable.

European Union

European Union countries are Austria, Italy, Belgium, Latvia, Bulgaria, Lithuania, Croatia, Luxembourg, Cyprus, Malta, Czechia, the Netherlands, Denmark, Poland, Estonia, Portugal, Finland, Romania, France, Slovakia, Germany, Slovenia, Greece, Spain, Hungary, Sweden, Ireland and the UK. Graduates from European medical universities/schools or doctors (IMGs or EU nationals) are regarded as FMGs for residency applications and matches via ERAS and NRMP. Some graduates from universities where courses are taught with English as a medium of instruction, they can have the English language advantage. Another advantage can be financial, where Euro to USD conversion rates are quite favourable. Some EU nationals from certain EU countries can also take advantage of the US visa waiver policy, which can lead to a smooth experience of appearing in USMLEs in the USA [6].

India, Pakistan, Bangladesh, Nepal, Sri Lanka and Afghanistan

Medical graduates from these Asian countries are regarded as FMGs for residency applications through ERAS. Medical graduates from South Asian Association for Regional Cooperation (SAARC) countries, including India and Pakistan, make a very high proportion of FMGs applying for residency in the USA every year. Despite the increasing numbers of candidates, there are a lot of challenges faced by these candidates, which are as follows:

1. *Financial Issues.*

   Earnings for newly graduated and junior doctors that make up the highest proportion of aspirants are not enough to start the journey towards USMLEs and residency in the USA unless they have some form of strong financial support or savings. The journey can cost somewhere from $10,000 (USD) to $30,000 (USD), and with existing currency exchange rates to USD, it can become hard for the candidates and their financial supporters. This includes exam fees, travel expenses, boarding and lodging and application fees, to name a few.

2. *Visa Issues.*

   As most Asian countries do not have a visa waiver agreement with the USA, their nationals need to acquire visas to travel to the USA for exam and interview purposes. Visa process can be lengthy, expensive and demoralising for already stressed candidates. So such candidates must read information about the requisite visas and how/where to apply from the United States Citizenship and Immigration Services (USCIS) and their country's US embassy's website.

3. *English Language.*

   Asian countries are mostly non-English-speaking countries. So communication and English speaking skills may not be seen as a strength. So it is imperative that English writing, spoken and understanding skills are up to the mark.

4. *Cultural Differences.*

   There are a lot of cultural differences that are faced by candidates from Asian backgrounds. This includes social and work interactions, mindset, recreational activities and food choices, to name a few. Candidates can feel lonely under such circumstances and lose a bit of their morale, but keeping one's self focussed and socialising can help.

5. *Local Clinical Experience and Training.*

   Local clinical experience in the SAARC countries is not in line with clinical practices observed in the western world or the USA, so this might not be seen as an additional benefit during the interviews. So these candidates must attain some US-based clinical experience through externships or observerships which may or may not cost extra money.

6. *Research Facilities and Experience.*

   In most of these countries, the research facilities and experiences are minimal and the ones that even exist are not up to the standards regarded as sufficient by world's renowned organisations that regulate research. Research experience and publications have become important more than ever before during the residency applications and interviews. So candidates must take this aspect of their CV quite seriously.

China, Taiwan, Japan and Korea

Candidates from China, Taiwan, Japan and the Republic of Korea face somewhat similar issues as described above, but there are some positives:

1. Japan, Taiwan and the Republic of Korea have an advantage of visa waiver policy [6] with the USA.
2. The clinical experience can be of some value as their clinical training systems are somewhat aligned with the US curriculum.
3. These countries have some of the renowned research-active centres in the world, so applicants from these countries can benefit from the experiences gained through these research centres.

Israel, Qatar, UAE and Arab Countries (Middle East)

Candidates graduated and trained in the Middle East also face similar issues with some benefit of clinical training to those candidates that train in centres where the curriculum is aligned with the US clinical training curriculum for that field of medicine or surgery.

Israel and Palestine

Israeli citizens (Arab or Jewish) take Israeli board exams in Hebrew, Arabic or English, while Palestinians take Palestinian board exams. The Palestinian Authority has its own healthcare policies, laws, education, medical education and hospital systems. As per the information available, Palestine has been granted control over its own healthcare in the West Bank and East Jerusalem. There a couple of Palestinian medical schools and there are a few Israeli medical schools.

One of the Israeli medical schools caters to the Jewish population settled in the USA or Canada, with outstanding US residency match rates for its graduates. As per information available to us, Palestinians (non-Israeli citizens from the West Bank) can do a residency in Israel if they opt to take Israeli exams and get granted an Israeli ID card, which is not easy to obtain. They have to go through a strict process of applications and approvals.

With outstanding US–Israel relationships and good-quality (US curriculum aligned) training programmes in Israel, candidates from Israel stand a better chance of securing a US residency match. Also, Israel has residency programmes that accept USMLEs as well.

Qatar and UAE

Qatar and the UAE have residency programmes that accept USMLEs as well so they can be an alternative for candidates who are struggling to get US residency match and are ready to apply for these programmes in Qatar and the UAE.

Africa

Candidates from the African continent are also regarded as FMGs for the purposes of residency applications through ERAS and NRMP. The issues faced by the African countries' medical graduates are multifold. A few to mention are as follows:

1. *Visa Issues.*
   Visa issues can prove to be a significant hurdle in the journey of appearing for the USMLE Steps exams and can subsequently affect the timeframes and chances of the residency application through ERAS and acquiring interviews for the match.
2. *Financial Constraints.*
   Financial constraints faced by these candidates can prove to be a significant limiting factor during their USMLE and US residency journey. Exchange rates for most African currencies to USD are not favourable for the US residency aspirants from the majority of African nations.
3. *Clinical Experience.*
   Clinical experience from local hospitals might not be considered as an added plus point during the residency interviews as the clinical practices in these hospitals are not aligned with the US clinical guidelines and training not aligned with US training speciality curriculum. So a US-based clinical observership/externship must be seriously considered, which can mean added costs.
4. *Cultural Differences.*
   These candidates can face significant cultural differences concerning social interactions, mindset, work interactions, recreational activities and food choices. These differences can fill candidates with some negative thoughts, but this can be dealt with through focus and hard work.
5. *English Language Skills.*
   As members of the majority of non-English-speaking nations, this can be a drawback more so if the mode of instruction was not English and personal English proficiency of the candidate is below par. It can negatively impact one's progress through the process, so this requires a candidate's utmost attention.
6. *Research Facilities and Experience.*
   In most of these countries, the research facilities and experiences are minimal and the ones that even exist are not up to the standards regarded as sufficient by world's renowned organisations that regulate research. Research experience and publications have become important more than ever before during the residency

applications and interviews. So candidates must take this aspect of their CV quite seriously.

Australia and New Zealand

Medical graduates from Australia and New Zealand or doctors licensed to work in Australia and New Zealand are regarded as FMGs in the US system. They have to go through the same steps as any FMG. They have to apply through the ERAS as well. There are certain advantages that they enjoy, which can be relative but can prove to be vital. These are as follows:

1. Being majority English-speaking countries, graduates are regarded to be proficient in communication and English language skills, which can create a positive impact.
2. Clinical experience from these countries can also be regarded as beneficial during interviews as the healthcare system and medical training curriculum is mainly influenced by the UK healthcare and training system.
3. Having a membership of Royal Australian colleges through examinations also can be seen as an added benefit during the interviews.
4. Because of comparable exchange rates from AUD/NZD to USD, journey can be more manageable.
5. Journey for Australian and New Zealand nationals can also be easier as they can take advantage of visa waiver policy [6].

Countries with US Travel Restrictions

The US government has travel restrictions from Iran, Libya, Somalia, Syria, Yemen, Venezuela, North Korea, Myanmar, Eritrea, Kyrgyzstan, Nigeria, Sudan and Tanzania for various reasons. Candidates from these countries can find it much harder to apply and obtain a US residency match. So these candidates need to weigh their all options very carefully.

English Language

Proficient English language skills are considered to be an integral part of residency programmes. Candidates from majority English-speaking countries and from institutions where the English language is a medium of instruction certainly have an advantage. Residency programmes typically do not ask you for TOEFL/IELTS examinations to be cleared. Just a USMLE with highest possible scores is required.

If you are planning for US clinical experience (clinical externship/observership), then a few universities may ask you for it, otherwise not.

LoRs

Letters of recommendation (LoRs) are vital for your medical residency application. According to the NRMP Director Survey, letters of recommendation is ranked second among the top five most important factors [7].

Attributes of strong letters of recommendation are as follows [7]:

1. Recent – Within one year of applications.
2. Pertaining to US clinical experience – LoRs from observerships, externships or research experience done in the USA.
3. Specialty specific – specifically stating your strong points in one medical speciality.

Preparing for letters of recommendation is essential. Residency candidates are mostly categorised as follows [7]:

1. *Recent Graduates/First-Time Applicants*: Consider carefully about who you have worked with over the years. Make a list on the basis of how well they know you. They need not be your clinical supervisors but can be any clinician (preferably senior clinician) you worked with and who knows you.
2. *Older Candidates/Re-applicants*: Recent US clinical experience should be considered strongly if you are coming back after a break; it will also help you to have up-to-date references for the letter of recommendation. Observerships, subinternships and externships are preferred modes.

Once you are sure about who to put as your referees for the letter of recommendation, then ask them nicely and show your gratitude towards them for their help. Make sure to provide them with all the information they will need to write an excellent letter. Keep the following points in mind:

1. Arrange a meeting with your referees.
2. Make a strong CV.
3. Highlight your strong points during the meeting.

Bring the following documents to the meeting to provide to your referee for the letter of recommendation [7]:

- Your CV.
- Accreditation Council for Graduate Medical Education (ACGME) Core Competencies.
- Letter Request Form from ERAS application.
- Information about your chosen programme.
- Your personal statement.

Bring to their attention the following points [7]:

- The speciality you are applying for.
- ERAS deadline dates.
- Whether or not you want it waived.
- General directions about the content and pattern might be helpful.
- Examples of where you showed attributes like confidence, teamwork, dedication, knowledge and commitment could be provided to them.

Before submitting, your Letter Writer will need the following [7]:

- An Association of American Medical Colleges (AAMC) account.
- The Letter Request.
- Formatting is correct.
- Format is PDF.
- Letterhead paper is used.
- 500 KB or less.
- Letter Writer signs the letter.
- The Letter Writer or their designee can upload Letter of Recommendation (LoRs).

Once you have confirmed with your Letter Writer that LoR has been submitted, check your MyERAS account.

Visa (Electronic System for Travel Authorisation, ESTA)

1. *B1 Visa.*

Generally, B1 visitor for business visa might not be used to undertake clerkship in the USA. But this rule has two exceptions [8]:
- Engagement in a medical clerkship within certain parameters.
- Observation of business or other professional or vocational activities within certain parameters.

    – *Medical Clerkship* [8].
      9 Foreign Affairs Manual (FAM) 402.2–5(E)(3) defines the rules for utilising a B1 visa to undertake a medical clerkship:
    – The medical clerkship exception relates to an individual who is a student at a foreign medical school. Such an individual might enter the USA temporarily under B1 status to undertake medical elective clerkship at a hospital of US medical school. Such an individual may not receive any funds or wage from the hospital. The FAM defines "elective clerkship" as "afford[ing] practical experiences and instruction in the various disciplines of medicine under the supervision and direction of faculty physicians at a

U.S. medical school's hospital as an approved part of the alien's foreign medical school education".

- The FAM also clarifies medical clerkship as "medical students pursuing their normal third- or fourth-year internship in U.S. medical school as part of a foreign medical degree" [8].
- B1 visa cannot be used for any graduate medical training/residency. Graduate medical training/residency is restricted by sect. 212(e) of the Immigration and Nationality Act (INA) and requires a J1 visa generally [8].

J1 Visa

J1 visas are the most common visas that allow international medical graduates to participate in US graduate medical education (GME) programmes. The US State Department enables Educational Commission For Foreign Medical Graduates (ECFMG) to sponsor foreign national physicians for acquiring the J1 visa as described in Figure. Information is available from ECFMG's Exchange Visitor Sponsorship Program.

The following criteria must be met by an IMG to apply for a J1 visa [9]:

- USMLE® Step 1 and Step 2 CK (passed).
- ECFMG Certificate (valid).
- A contract or official offer letter for a position in a programme of training with a medical school or GME should be possessed.
- A statement of need is produced from the Health Ministry of the country of last legal permanent residence regardless of country of nationality.
- Home country physical presence, 2-year requirement.
- Coming back to their home country after completing their training in the USA for 2 years to distribute the knowledge they acquired in the USA.

Candidates can receive a waiver from 2-year home residence requirement of the J1 visa programme. Below are described the three circumstances to gain a waiver of the 2-year residency need [9]:

- The applicants show that they will suffer from persecution in their home country.
- Residency requirement will bring hardship to the applicant's children or/and spouse (who are US citizens or permanent residents in the USA).
- The applicant is sponsored by an IGA (Interested Governmental Agency) that has an interest in that physician's employment in the USA.

On receiving a J1 waiver and a state medical licence, they can obtain a work authorised status for US employment (immigrant visa or H1B visa) [9].

Figure describes the US residency pathway.

US residency pathway

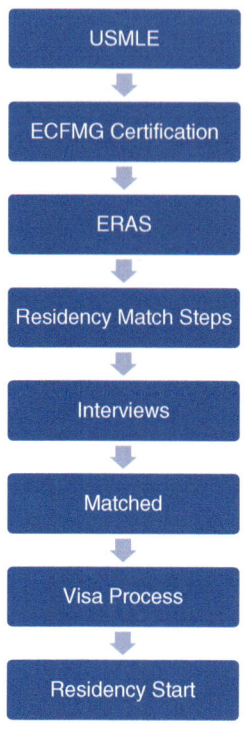

J1 visa pathway

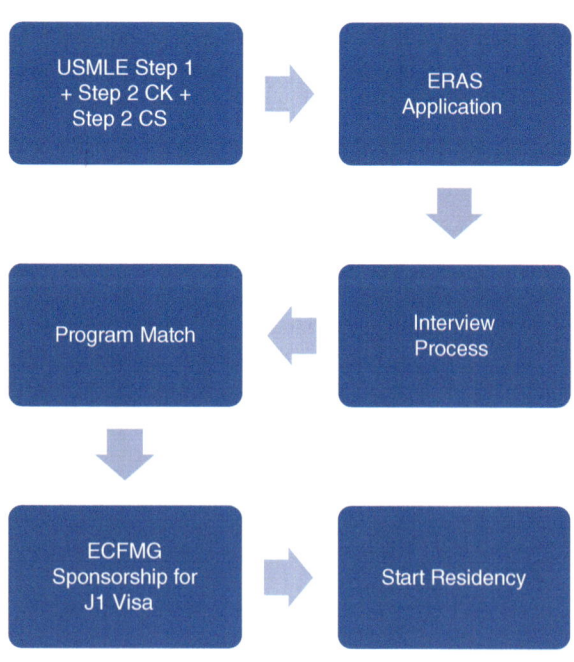

H1B Visa

Workers who have professional-level degrees in speciality occupations can get H1B visa. H1B visa carries no requirement of 2-year home residence [9]. Foreign nationals can enter the USA with H1B visa for up to 6 years for professional-level employment [9].

The H1B visa can be acquired by foreign medical graduates who have passed the necessary examinations, have a licence to practise required by the state, have obtained an unrestricted licence to practise medicine, or have graduated from the US or a foreign medical school [9]. However, to be eligible for this visa, the candidate must have passed USMLE Step 3 [9]. Figure 14.1 describes the H1B visa pathway.

Fig. 14.1   H1B visa pathway

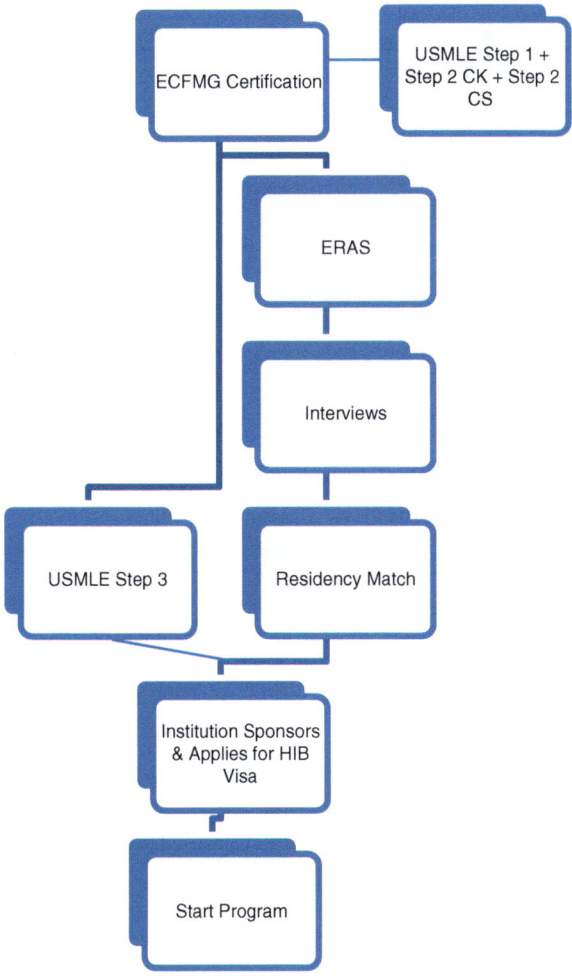

More information about visas and immigration can be found on the USCIS website.

Finances

There are many costs involved during the journey to residency in the USA. These include different fees (USMLE, ERAS and NRMP), USMLE preparation materials, interviews, travel, accommodation, food and clothes. Early knowledge can aid the applicants to plan for the future. Tables 14.1, 14.2, 14.3, 14.4, and 14.5 describe different costs involved [10].

These costs can be quite a lot for all the candidates, but more so for the candidates from Asia and Africa, so all decisions need to be taken with due care.

Ethnic Physician Organisations

Missions of ethnic physician organisations may vary. They range from promoting healthcare and focusing on raising awareness in their countries, connecting physicians of similar cultural background and striving to advance medicine in the USA. They have different fees and membership levels. ECFMG website has information about ECHO (ECFMG Certificate Holders Office), and these organisations are listed below [11]:

- Afghan Medical Professionals Association of America (AMPAA).
- American Association of Physicians of Indian Origin (AAPI).
- Albanian American Medical Society (AAMS).
- American Tamil Medical Association (ATMA).
- Argentine-American Medical Society (AAMS).
- Asian Pacific American Medical Student Association (APAMSA).
- American Lebanese Medical Association (ALMA).
- Armenian American Medical Society (AAMSC).
- Association of Haitian Physicians Abroad (AMHE).
- Association of Chinese American Physicians (ACAP).

Table 14.1 [10] – USMLE exams costs

USMLE costs[a]	
USMLE Step 1	$910 + International Test Delivery Surcharge, if testing outside the USA and Canada
USMLE Step 2 CK	$910 + International Test Delivery Surcharge, if testing outside the USA and Canada
USMLE Step 2 CS	$1565

[a]Subject to change, always consult the official website

Table 14.2 [10] – Additional USMLE costs

Additional USMLE costs[a]	
Extension of eligibility	$70 per exam
Step 1/Step 2 CK Testing Region Change	$65 per region change
Step 1/Step 2 CK Rescheduling Fee	$0–569 (depending on the exam, testing region and date of cancellation)
Step 2 CS Rescheduling Fee	$0–1285 (depending on the date of cancellation)
Score Recheck (Step 1/Step 2 CK/ Step 2 CS)	$80 per exam
USMLE Transcript (Paper Copy)	$70 per request (up to 10)
USMLE Transcript (Electronic)	$80 (once per ERAS season)

[a]Subject to change, always consult the official website

Table 14.3 [10] – ECFMG fees

ECFMG services[a]	
ERAS Token	$120
Application for ECFMG Certification	$75
Application for J1 Sponsorship	$325 + $180 to the Department of Homeland Security
Medical School Transcript Translation	$250 (if needed)
Certification Verification Service (CVS) Verification to State Medical Licensing Authority	$45

[a]Subject to change, always consult the official website

Table 14.4 [10] – ERAS fees

AAMC/ERAS – programmes per specialty[a]	
Up to 10	$99
11–20	$14 each
21–30	$18 each
31 or more	$26 each

[a]Subject to change, always consult the official website

Table 14.5 [10] – NRMP fees

NRMP[a]	
Registration Fee	$85 (first 20 programmes on the primary rank list)
Late Fee	$50
Couples	$25 additional per partner
Additional Programmes	$30 per programme

[a]Subject to change, always consult the official website

- Association of Philippine-American Physicians in Ohio (APPO).
- Association of Nigerian Physicians in the Americas (ANPA).
- Association of Physicians of Pakistani Descent of North America (APPNA).
- Burmese American Medical Association (BAMA).
- Bangladesh Medical Association of North America (BMANA).
- Burmese Medical Association of North America (BMA-NA).
- Chinese American Physician Society (CAPS).
- Chinese American Medical Society (CAMS).
- Dominican American Medical Association of New York (DMANY).
- Hungarian Medical Association of America (HMAA).
- Hellenic Medical Society of New York (HMSNY).
- Iraqi Medical Sciences Association (IMSA).
- Iranian American Medical Association (IAMA).
- Islamic Medical Association of North America (IMANA).
- Japanese Medical Society of America (JMSA).
- Kurdish American Medical Association (KAMA).
- Korean American Medical Association (KAMA).
- National Council of Asian Pacific Islander Physicians (NCAPIP).
- National Arab American Medical Association (NAAMA).
- North American Taiwanese Medical Association (NATMA).
- National Hispanic Medical Association (NHMA).
- Polish-American Medical Society (Medicus).
- Peruvian American Medical Society (PAMS).
- Polish-American Medical Society—Chicago (PAMS).
- Russian American Medical Association (RAMA).
- Romanian Medical Society of New York (RMSNY).
- Sudanese American Medical Association (SAMA).
- Syrian American Medical Society (SAMS).
- Serbian American Medical Association (SAMA).
- Thai Physicians Association of America (TPAA).
- United States Colombian Medical Association (USCMA).
- Ukrainian Medical Association of North America (UMANA).
- Vietnamese American Medical Association (VAMA).
- Venezuelan American Medical Association (VAMA).

Other Jobs

If unfortunately a match is not achieved in the first year, then there is no reason to lose heart and aim should be to make your CV strong for the next year. Candidates can do this by undertaking different related jobs (but remember to check information on their relevant forums and websites and acquire a suitable visa before starting these jobs [unless you are a US citizen]). Some are as follows [12]:

- *Research jobs.*

   To improve your application, doing research is an excellent option; some programmes are interested in developing future researchers. Some research opportunities are based in US hospitals, which can be doubly beneficial. Some research mentors may have personal terms with some programme directors and can advocate for you in addition to getting you other clinical opportunities. Also, if you have published your research work in a PubMed indexed journal, then that can be regarded as a very positive indicator on your CV and application.

- *Assistant physician.*

   Assistant physicians (AP), in contrast to Physician Associates (PAs), are a new type of healthcare providers introduced in the USA, who are primarily tasked to serve the patients in primary care settings in underprivileged rural areas. Qualifications wise, they have completed medical school and are ACGME/ ECFMG-certified clinicians [13]. Requirements for licensure include graduation from a recognised medical school, citizen or legal resident of the USA, passed USMLE Step 1 and Step 2, not accomplished completion of residency and proficiency in the English language. Requirements for practising include collaborative agreement with a sponsoring physician, 30-day internship with the sponsoring physician and work within 50–100 miles of the sponsoring physician, and this physician must undertake a review of 10% of the assistant physician's charts [13].

- *Medical interpreter.*
- *Medical secretary.*
- *Respiratory therapists.*
- *Certified surgical technologists (CSTs) and certified surgical first assistants work in the operating room on the surgical team.*
- *Emergency medical technicians.*
- *Genetics counsellors.*
- *Certified anaesthesiologist assistants are qualified to assist with anaesthesia patient care.*
- *Diagnostic medical sonography qualification can be obtained.*
- *Electrodiagnostic medicine technicians work in electrophysiology labs.*
- *Ultrasound technicians and lab directors.*
- *Massage therapy.*
- *Personal trainers work with people who need fitness counselling and coaching.*

Role of Observership/Externship/Electives

US-based clinical experiences are valued by the residency programmes in the USA. Through these experiences, candidates can request LoRs from senior faculty members who are already familiar with the needs and expectations of the residency programmes [14].

To students in medical school, most US medical schools offer clinical away elective. Some may be free, and some can have a fee. Many programmes run a dedicated site with most of the information for students. Candidates can often get interview invites from the hospital where they rotate, so always give it your best. Preparation is the key to start your rotation.

If candidates have graduated from medical school, then they are left with fewer options for clinical experiences in the USA. Fewer medical schools offer placements, so try and utilise your contacts and medical school alumni. American Medical Association (AMA) Observership Program is an option [14]. During observerships, use your skills to offer help to the residents include offering to help the interns by accompanying interns to the admissions and request to present these at the rounds, give presentations on problems and questions that arise during rounds and try to write up a review paper or a case report on any exciting case or observation [14].

IMG/FMG friendly specialities

International medical graduates (IMGs) seeking residency positions in the USA applied in smaller numbers but had more success finding postgraduate year 1 (PGY-1) positions in 2018, according to data from the National Resident Matching Program (NRMP) [15]. Tables 14.6 and 14.7 describe the IMG-friendly specialities and states respectively.

Table 14.6 [15] – IMG-friendly specialities

Speciality	Percentage of IMGs
Pathology	45.2
Internal medicine	43.2
Neurology	35
Family medicine	30.3

Table 14.7 [15] – IMG-friendly states

The IMG-friendly states
New York
Florida
Michigan
Pennsylvania
New Jersey

COVID-19 and Its Impact

At the time of writing this chapter, globally, we are facing a COVID-19 pandemic which has affected almost all the countries with varying degrees of severity. Different countries, including the USA, have taken many strict measures to safeguard their population from COVID-19, which means widening travel restrictions and changes in the schedule of planned activities like exams and interviews. So it is also crucial for IMGs to plan ahead of time about their finances, travel, applications and interviews.

Conclusion

This chapter provides an overview of the matters concerning the IMGs/FMGs en route to obtaining a residency match in the USA. We have looked at different aspects of the circumstances faced by the aspirant FMGs from different parts of the globe. We tried to focus on the financial, cultural, legal (visas) and lingual aspects. We also paid attention to the support and professional development side of the things, which in turn will help the FMGs to increase their productivity and chances of a successful residency match. The following are the highlights of this chapter:

- Plan early, preferably during your medical school years, about your USMLE journey.
- Plan to appear in your USMLE Steps 1 and 2 exams during the fourth or final year of your medical school.
- Plan to secure and undertake a clinical elective in the USA during your fourth or final year of medical school.
- Work on your CV and start as soon as possible.
- Plan to engage yourself in research activities and better so get yourself published in a PubMed indexed journal as it will increase your chances of a successful match.
- After USMLE Steps 1 and 2 apply for ECFMG certification.
- Know ERAS timelines and apply in an efficient and timely manner.
- Contact and meet your referees in time for letters of recommendation.
- Plan your finances well in advance and try to save wherever you can.
- Start the visa process well in advance since it can be time-consuming for most of the applicants.
- Network and use all your contacts optimally.

All the information has been gathered from different resources, so you guys must get in the habit of confirming the latest facts using appropriate resources and forums as information available is evolving at a rapid pace.

In the end, we recommend all our readers to obtain as much information as possible beforehand as it will help you better understand this chapter and the whole process of getting the residency. Good Luck!

References

1. No Title. [Internet]. [cited 2020 Jan 5]. Available from: https://www.aamc.org/system/files/reports/1/all.pdf.
2. Residency Application Requirements for International .... https://www.aafp.org/medical-school-residency/residency/apply/img.html.
3. Medical Employers - Healthcare Employment Network. [Internet]. [cited 2020 Jan 5]. Available from: http://medicalemployers.com/us-immigration-for-canadian-physicians.
4. Application to the US (ERAS) – CaRMS [Internet]. [cited 2020 Jan 5]. Available from: https://www.carms.ca/the-match/application-to-the-us-eras/.
5. U.S. Accredited Medical Schools in the Caribbean I SGU: Medical Blog I St. George's University I The SGU Pulse [Internet]. [cited 2020 Jan 5]. Available from: https://www.sgu.edu/blog/medical/find-the-best-medical-schools-in-the-caribbean/.
6. Frequently Asked Questions about the Visa Waiver Program (VWP) and the Electronic System for Travel Authorization (ESTA) I U.S. Customs and Border Protection [Internet]. [cited 2020 Jan 5]. Available from: https://www.cbp.gov/travel/international-visitors/frequently-asked-questions-about-visa-waiver-program-vwp-and-electronic-system-travel.
7. A Guide to Medical Residency Letters of Recommendation I Match A Resident [Internet]. [cited 2020 Jan 5]. Available from: https://blog.matcharesident.com/guide-medical-residency-letters-of-recommendation/.
8. B1 Visas for Medical Clerkships and Observing Business Activities [Internet]. [cited 2020 Jan 5]. Available from: http://myattorneyusa.com/b1-visas-for-medical-clerkships-and-observing-businessvocational-activities.
9. Immigration information for international medical graduates I American Medical Association [Internet]. [cited 2020 Jan 5]. Available from: https://www.ama-assn.org/education/international-medical-education/immigration-information-international-medical-graduates.
10. Fees for the 2018–19 US Medical Residency Application Cycle I Match A Resident [Internet]. [cited 2020 Jan 5]. Available from: https://blog.matcharesident.com/fees-2018-19-us-medical-residency-application-cycle/.
11. ECFMG Certificate Holders Office (ECHO) – ECFMG [Internet]. [cited 2020 Jan 5]. Available from: https://www.ecfmg.org/echo/.
12. Jobs for Physicians Without Residency – Non Clinical Doctors [Internet]. [cited 2020 Jan 5]. Available from: http://www.nonclinicaldoctors.com/careers-for-physicians-without-residency.html.
13. Malik BH, Krishnaswamy R, Khan S, Gupta D, Rutkofsky I. Are Physician Associates Less-defined Force Multipliers? Comparative Role Definition of Physician Associates within the Hierarchy of Medical Professionals. Cureus [Internet]. 2019 Dec 26 [cited 2020 Jan 5]; Available from: https://www.cureus.com/articles/25505-are-physician-associates-less-defined-force-multipliers-comparative-role-definition-of-physician-associates-within-the-hierarchy-of-medical-professionals.
14. Applying for Residency as an International Medical Graduate I NEJM Resident 360 <meta property="twitter:image" content="https://resident360files.nejm.org/image/upload/c_fit,f_auto,h_120,w_120/v1538599218/u8buf4o8mgdxgmfcczjk.png" /> <meta property="og:image" content="https://resident360files.nejm.org/image/upload/c_pad,f_auto,h_630,w_1200/v1538599218/u8buf4o8mgdxgmfcczjk.png" /> [Internet]. [cited 2020 Jan 5]. Available from: https://resident360.nejm.org/expert-consult/applying-for-residency-as-an-international-medical-graduate.
15. 4 medical specialties among the friendliest for IMG PGY-1 matches I American Medical Association [Internet]. [cited 2020 Jan 5]. Available from: https://www.ama-assn.org/residents-students/specialty-profiles/4-medical-specialties-among-friendliest-img-pgy-1-matches.

Chapter 15
The Role of International Medical Graduates (IMGs) in the US Healthcare System

Michael G. Fitzsimons and Bruna Maria Castro de Oliveira

Introduction

International medical graduates (IMGs) come to the United States for graduate medical education (GME) for many reasons including the quality of training and high-quality standards, predictability of career path after graduation, opportunity for board certification that is recognized worldwide, and the need to complete an American residency program in order to have the opportunity to practice in the United States and secure immigration status or citizenship [1]. Many IMGs remain in the United States after completion of residency and enter the medical workforce. Reasons include improved salaries, better lifestyle, personal and family safety, and professional satisfaction [2]. This movement is referred to as "medical migration" [3].

The US physician population is composed of approximately 25% IMGs [4, 5]. Such migration helps compensate for the physician shortage in the United States. Early policy was designed to enhance the pool of physicians, while more recent policy may discourage IMGs from entering residency or remaining after specialty training. This chapter will review the challenges faced by aspiring physicians during entry into the United States healthcare system, the role IMGs play in the United

M. G. Fitzsimons (✉)
Harvard Medical School, Boston, MA, USA

Division of Cardiac Anesthesia, Department of Anesthesia, Critical Care, and Pain Medicine, Massachusetts General Hospital, Boston, MA, USA
e-mail: mfitzsimons@mgh.harvard.edu

B. M. C. de Oliveira
Harvard Medical School, Boston, MA, USA

Department of Anesthesia, Critical Care, and Pain Medicine, Massachusetts General Hospital, Boston, MA, USA
e-mail: bcastrodeoliveira@mgh.harvard.edu

© Springer Nature Switzerland AG 2021
H. Tohid, H. Maibach (eds.), *International Medical Graduates in the United States*, https://doi.org/10.1007/978-3-030-62249-7_15

States, their distribution among different specialties, quality of care delivered to patients, contributions to academic research, role in medical leadership, and the experience that the IMG has practicing in the United States.

History of IMGs and Certification Policy in the United States

IMGs have no doubt contributed to the well-being of the citizens of the United States since the birth of our nation. The first efforts to address medical "internationalism" arose from the involvement of the United States in World War I. Esteemed physicians began to investigate how to establish reciprocal agreements on medical training among different European countries [6]. The National Board of Medical Examiners (NBME) was involved in these efforts. Graduates of foreign medical schools could apply to the NBME for certification. Europe produced more medical school graduates in the 1920s and 1930s than were needed, resulting in a surplus of physicians in the continent. This surplus also included Americans who were not accepted into training at home and journeyed overseas for their medical education. Questions of the quality of that training increased. Education at foreign medical schools was not scrutinized to the degree that American institutions were by the Flexner report [7]. The end of World War II (WWII) resulted in an increase in physician migration to the United States. The American Medical Association (AMA) Council on Medical Education and Hospitals created an advisory committee on foreign medical credentials in response to this migration [6]. Finally, in 1954 due to increasing numbers of IMGs, difficulty assessing the quality of medical education, and variable evaluation at the state level, temporary formal discontinuation of entry of all foreign medical graduates occurred.

The Educational Commission for Foreign Medical Graduates (ECFMG) was initially established in 1956 as the Evaluation Service for Foreign Medical Graduates (ESFMG) [8]. The ESFMG took on the role of evaluating IMG credentials, medical knowledge, and command of the English language. The ESFMG determined whether an IMG met the educational and examination requirements to enter training. The ECFMG asked that the NBME develop a testing system for IMGs. The NBME agreed to develop the examination despite concerns of foreign "brain drain," liability issues, and harm to its reputation. The first certificates were issues in 1958.

The ECFMG examination continued into the 1970s when concerns about the quality of medical training were raised again. A new and additional examination was added, the Visa Qualifying Examination (VQE). Content was identical to the NBME part I and II examination. The Foreign Medical Graduate Examination in the Medical Sciences (FMGEMS) replaced both the ECFMG and the VQE beginning in July 1984. IMGs were also required to complete the Federal Licensing Examination (FLEX).

The 1990s saw a desire to consolidate all testing and develop a single test for all individuals desiring to train and practice in the United States. The United States Medical Licensing Examination (USMLE) process was established in the 1990s.

The Higher Education Opportunity Act of 2008 established the National Committee on Foreign Medical Education and Accreditation (NCFMEA). This committee is authorized to evaluate standards applied to foreign medical schools and comparability of those standards to American medical schools [9].

The ECFMG established the 2023 Medical School Accreditation Requirement in 2019. This is an effort to enhance the quality and consistency of medical education worldwide. Individuals that wish to apply for ECFMG certification must graduate from a medical school that is accredited by an agency that is recognized by the World Federation for Medical Education (WFME) beginning in 2023 [10]. Legislation and cooperation among regulatory agencies have resulted in improved standards for medical schools throughout the world. Graduates today are more consistent than any time in the past.

Debate Regarding IMGs in the United States

Debate still exists concerning whether IMGs should be allowed to train and subsequently practice medicine in the United States. Those supporting IMGs note that sectors of the US workforce including higher education, technology, arts, and athletics already welcome and benefit from individuals from other countries [11]. IMGs already contribute significantly to healthcare in the United States and are a viable resource to fill the generalized physician shortage [11]. The physician shortage in the United States is only going to continue and IMGs answer this need. IMGs also work in specialties with the highest shortages of physicians and in geographic areas with less access to quality care. According to American Medical Association numbers, 62% of the IMGs in the United States practice in primary care specialties. That is double of the number of USMGs working as primary care physicians. Majority of IMGs (98%) are bilingual helping non-English-speaking patients to have access to medical care [12].

Arguments against support for IMGs in the United States are not based on the quality of the care. Even those that argue against IMGs acknowledge their tremendous historical contribution [13]. The arguments are based in the ethics of the role of the IMG and brain drain from other countries. The growth in graduate medical education after WWII was primarily driven by physicians seeking specialty training. IMGs were an easily obtained resource to fill the ranks, especially less competitive programs [14]. IMGs were an easily obtained resource to fill the needs of hospitals as available GME programs continued to expand [14]. Acceptance of IMGs into residency programs may contribute to the "brain drain" as the intellectual power of a country leaves for another. IMGs not only immigrate to the United States but to other developed countries including the United Kingdom, Canada, and Australia [15]. A largest percentage of these trainees come from lower-income countries. Additional arguments include the notion that IMGs may impose an extra educational burden on residency programs in the first 6 months to a year of residency. The learning curve is steep for these doctors that are not familiar with the US medical system and the epidemiology of endemic diseases in the United States. IMGs may have to learn characteristics of the American healthcare system that are not necessarily a part of that in their home country including patient-physician relationships, joint decision-making, the importance of accurate documentation, protection of patient information, and the use of evidence-based medicine. Language barriers can impair the rapport with other medical personnel and patients and result in inadequate documentation.

Current Status of IMGs in the United States

There are 11,490 residency and fellowship programs accredited by the ACGME in the United States according to the last National GME Census in 2018 [5]. There are a total of 136,028 residents and fellows with IMGs counting for 31,238 or 23% of the pool of trainees. Pathology (45.5%) accounted for the specialty with the largest *percentage* of IMGs followed by internal medicine (38.3%), neurology (31.5%), and family medicine (26.1%). IMGs were less well represented in surgical specialties. IMGs constituted 14.2% of trainees in general surgery, 3.4% in urology, 7.3% in neurological surgery, and only 1.5% of trainees in orthopedic surgery (Table 15.1).

Nearly a quarter of the trained physicians that practice in the United States are IMGs [16]. The largest *number* of IMGs are those in internal medicine where IMGs make up 39.2% of those actively practicing followed by family practice/general practice at 22.8% and pediatrics (24.9%) [16]. Specialties with the lowest IMG representation are dermatology (4.9%), orthopedic surgery (5.2%), otolaryngology (6.3%), and ophthalmology (7.1%). In general IMGs practice the most in primary care specialties with less representation in specialties than surgical (Table 15.2).

Table 15.1 Total number of resident physicians in ACGME-accredited residency programs, total number of international medical graduates (IMGs), and prevalence of IMGs by specialty

Distribution of international medical graduates (IMGs) in the US residency programs, 2018–2019	No (%)
Number of ACGME-accredited residency programs	11,490
Total number of residents	136,028
IMGs	31,238 (23.0%)
Pathology	1028 (45.5%)
Internal medicine	10,415 (38.3%)
Neurology	881 (31.5%)
Family medicine	3251 (26.1%)
General surgery	1318 (14.2%)
Neurosurgery	107 (7.3%)
Urology	46 (3.4%)
Orthopedic surgery	60 (1.5%)

Adapted from Brotherton and Etzel [5]

Table 15.2 Total number of practicing physicians in the United States, total number of IMG physicians practicing in the United States, and distribution of IMG physicians by specialty

Distribution of international medical graduates (IMGs) practicing in the United States, 2017	No (%)
Total number of physicians practicing in the United States	892,752
IMGs	218,540 (24.5%)
Internal medicine	45,274 (39.2%)
Family medicine	25,860 (22.8%)
Pediatrics	715 (24.9%)
Ophthalmology	1327 (7.1%)
Otolaryngology	603 (6.3%)
Orthopedic surgery	988 (5.2%)
Dermatology	591 (4.9%)

Adapted from Association of American Medical Colleges [16]

Most physicians practicing in the United States were born and trained in the United States. The most common origin of IMGs that immigrate to the United States are from India, the Philippines, Pakistan, China, Iran, Syria, Egypt, South Korea, and the former USSR [17]. The countries from which IMGs are most likely to have obtained their medical school education are India, the Philippines, Mexico, Pakistan, Dominican Republic, Grenada, Dominica, Egypt, China, and the Netherlands [17]. Physicians educated in India represent 27% of the IMGs practicing in the United States, more than any other country. Other nations that are heavily represented are the Philippines, Pakistan, Syria, Nigeria, China, Lebanon, the United Kingdom, and Germany [12]. Over the past 10 years, there has been a significant increase in the number of IMGs that possess US citizenship [18]. This number has surpassed IMGs in the United States from India [18].

Canadian Graduates Within the American Medical System

Canadians are *not* considered IMGs for GME. According to the GME census from 2018, graduates of Canadian medical schools represent less than 0.1% of the total medical trainees [5]. Their distribution among specialties is homogeneous with no one specialty highly represented [2]. According to the latest ECFMG report, the number of certificates issued to Canadian graduates has been rising since 2009 and now surpasses China and Pakistan [18].

Canada and the United States were already facing a physician shortage in 2006. Phillips et al. analyzed the migration pattern of Canadian-educated physicians to the United States and concluded that 67.8% (8162) of the 12,040 Canadian physicians living in the United States at the time were practicing in direct patient care, most as specialists (72.1%) and a smaller percentage in primary care (27.9%) [19]. Phillips et al. also found that Canada contributed with an average of 186 (37–268) physicians a year to the US healthcare system. American citizens that graduated from Canadian medical schools represented 14.2% of theses physicians [19]. Canadian physicians migrate to the United States for the opportunity to become highly specialized and consequently increase their earning potential, due to lower tax rates, and due to the rapidly increasing education debt in Canada [19]. Canadian graduates come to the United States to pursue postgraduate training in specialties that are not available in Canada. Canadian graduates who complete residency training in the United States are 9 times more likely to remain in the United States after finishing their training. This relationship is mutually beneficial, although the United States is clearly the major beneficiary. Such trade-offs are not typical for most physician-donor nations [19].

The decrease in Canadian workforce caused in part by migration to the United States is filled by IMGs that migrate to Canada from other countries. Saudi Arabia and other Middle Eastern countries are the primary origin [20]. The dependence on the Canadian healthcare system on those individuals became evident in 2018 when Saudi Arabia announced the discontinuation of their scholarship program after a diplomatic disagreement between the two nations [19]. The loss of the 800 medical trainees from the Canadian system was felt not only by those students and their families that had to abruptly interrupt their train and move but also by Canadian institutions and Canadian patients that rely on them [19].

Caribbean Medical School Graduates

The number of graduates from Caribbean medical schools certified by ECFMG has been rising over the past 10 years, with the United States being the number one country of citizenship of the candidates to receive the certification. Graduates of medical schools in the Caribbean islands are considered IMGs. According to the ECFMG database in 2009, 25.4% of the certified foreign graduates were from Caribbean medical schools [21]. This number is growing. Many of these IMGs return to the United States to complete residency training and subsequently join the physician workforce. In 2011, of the 2936 graduates from Caribbean medical schools that obtained ECFMG certification, 69% were American citizens. According to a survey by Jolly et al. in 2010, most US citizens that applied to international medical schools (majority of them in the Caribbean) have also applied to US MD-granting and/or DO-granting schools. These students are not eligible to obtain US federal loans and have to self-finance their education.

More than half of the IMGs who graduated from Caribbean medical schools are practicing in primary care specialties. Van Zanten analyzed the AMA Masterfile data from data from 2011 and determined that Carribeam medical schools contributed the highest percentage of their graduates to primary care specialties in the United States (56.7%) when compared with non-Caribbean IMGs (42.3%) and USMGs (32.9%)

[22]. With fewer medical graduates from the United States (USMGs) choosing primary care specialties, IMGs, especially those from Caribbean schools, will play an increasingly important role in US primary care. Most of these physicians are US citizens and more likely to stay in the country after they conclude their training.

Concerns have been raised about the quality of the training in those institutions with the increasing number of their graduates pursuing residency training and eventually practice in the United States. Studies have shown a lower performance of Caribbean medical students on standardized tests when compared to US medical graduates and other international medical graduates [22]. Studies are limited though.

International Nursing Graduates

Healthcare provider shortage in the United States is seen in other areas, including nursing. The shortage of nurses is expected to continue with a projection of 900,000 unfilled positions in 2030 [23]. Many hospitals attempt to overcome this shortage by relying upon foreign-educated nurses [23]. Data from 2005 indicates that 15,000 foreign-trained nurses passed the nursing licensure exam to practice in the United States. These nurses migrate primarily from the Philippines, India, and Canada [24]. Their presence in the US workforce is likely to be long-lasting since most of these nurses eventually became citizens or permanent residents.

The extensive presence of foreign-graduated nurses in the United States encouraged Mazurenko et al. to perform a cross-sectional study to evaluate the use of these healthcare providers as well as patient satisfaction. Despite the increased team diversity, like a broader range of knowledge, skill, abilities, and cultural identification, patient satisfaction was negatively impacted. Communication and cultural-related issues were the most predominant [24].

Geographic Distribution of IMGs

IMGs often work in areas especially hard hit by physician shortages and not filled by USMGs. The distribution of IMGs in the US territory is influenced by several elements including residency programs acceptance and immigration policies among others. Those states with the highest percentage of IMGs in GME programs are New York, Pennsylvania, Michigan, Illinois, and Texas [25]. Those states with the highest percentage of practicing IMGs are New Jersey, New York, Florida, Illinois, and Michigan [25].

The US government uses immigration laws to address the shortage of physicians in rural areas [26]. The Conrad 30 waiver program allows medical doctors with a J-1 VSA to apply for a waiver for the 2-year residence requirement upon completion of the J-1 exchange visitor program [27]. The healthcare facility must be in an area designated as a Health Professional Shortage Area (HPSA), Medically Underserved

Area (MUA), or a Medically Underserved Population (MUP) and receive a letter of "no objection" from the country from which they come [27]. The highest percentage of such recipients practice in internal medicine (43%) in private practice or clinic setting (45%) [28]. The National Interest Waiver (NIW) is offered by the US government to individuals with exceptional ability or advanced degrees, such as a physician. The NIW provides the opportunity to apply for a Green Card without a job offer and a labor certification if the physician agrees to work for a period of time in an underserved area [27].

Despite medical initiatives to train rural physicians, these areas continue to face shortage in healthcare providers. Challenges to attract USMGs to rural areas include lack of interest in the underserved areas from academically trained students and the appeal of higher-paying specialties given the increasing costs of medical education. Since 2011 the percentage of US-trained MD choosing primary care specialties has been on decline [29]. In 2019 the percentage of primary care positions filled by fourth-year medical students was the lowest ever registered [30].

Current Policy and Regulations

IMGs must go through a rigorous process to practice in the United States (Table 15.3). The current requirements for ECFMG certification are rigorous and include a primary source verification of educational credentials, passing the USMLE Steps 1, 2 Clinical Knowledge (CK) and Clinical Skills (CS). Once the certification is obtained, the IMGs are eligible to apply to an accredited residency program through the National Matching Residency Program (The MATCH). IMGs must complete residency in the United States to be eligible to apply for board certification.

Outcomes and Level of Care

There have been queries about the quality of care provided by IMGs despite the challenging process required to become a licensed physician in the United States. A study among residents in pediatrics noted that IMGs outperformed USMGs in clinical knowledge and skills but that communication, public health knowledge, and efficiency lacked behind, but their overall performance was viewed as positive [31]. Analysis has also demonstrated that IMGs perform well on national measures and on the board exams. There is a positive correlation between performance on the USMLE steps and clinical performance for IMGs. Curiously, IMGs performed better than American citizens that graduate from international medical schools on those metrics [32].

Tsugawa et al. compared the 30-day mortality in elderly Medicare patients cared by US graduates versus foreign graduates [33]. Despite the observation that the

Table 15.3 Residency timeline application for IMGs

Time period	Events
Preparation prior to ERAS application submission	Confirm Medical School ECFMG certified Consider observerships/clerkships in the United States Complete USMLE Steps 1, 2 CK and 2CS Obtain ECFMG certification Write personal statement Prepare your *curriculum vitae* Request MSPE
June	Obtain ERAS token Register with myERAS and upload your application
September	Apply to ACGME-accredited programs Residency programs start to review applications NRMP registration opens
November–February	Arrange and complete interviews
March	NRMP Match results available SOAP registration
May/June	ERAS 2021 season ends Obtain visa

Abbreviations: *USMLE* United States Medical Licensing Examination, *CK* Clinical Knowledge, *CS* Clinical Skills, *ECFMG* Educational Commission for Foreign Medical Graduates, *MSPE* Medical Student Performance Evaluation, *ERAS* Electronic Residency Application Services, *ACGME* Accreditation Council for Graduate Medical Education, *NRMP* National Residency Matching Program, *SOAP* Supplemental Offer and Acceptance Program

patients cared for IMGs had slightly more chronic conditions, mortality was lower on the group of patients treated by IMGs. Readmission rates were similar. Norcini et al. compared IMGs with USMGs and found no significant mortality difference [34]. Zhaeer et al. compared outcomes among surgeons who received undergraduate medical education in the United States versus IMGs [35]. Mortality, complications, and prolonged length of stay were equivalent.

Contribution to Biomedical Research

IMGs contribute not only as clinicians but also through biomedical research. They represent an important fraction of medical schools' full-time faculty and principal investigators (PIs) on NIH research grants.

The number of IMGs employed as full-time academic faculty more than doubled between 1984 (7866) and 2004 (17,085) [36]. The number of IMGs who were primary investigators (PIs) with National Institutes of Health (NIH) grants increased during the same period (from 16.5% to 21.3%), representing almost one fourth of the full-time faculty physicians who were PIs [36]. In 2017, IMGs represent 12.5% of NIH grant receivers and led 18.5% of the clinical trials. Almost half of these IMGs focus their research in basic sciences, unlike US and Canadian graduates' full-time faculties whose research focus on clinical medicine.

Among 82,737 US physicians in academic medicine in 2015, 15,075 (18.3%) were IMGs; from those, 2808 were full professors who had completed medical school in another country, representing 15.1% of all full professors. They were responsible for 18.0% of all publications, 18.5% of first-authored publications, and 16.5% of last-authored publications [37].

A research position in the United States can represent the first step toward becoming a fully trained, licensed physician. Some IMGs come to the United States as research assistants while preparing to apply for the residency match. That opportunity facilitates network development in their area of interest while adapting to the US culture and improving English skills. Many physician-scientists come to the United States as research fellows and, after consolidating a career in the biomedical research field, pursue the clinical training in the United States, ultimately combining both patient care and research into their practice.

Another possibly contributing factor is the fact that most IMGs do not have the financial burden of student loans that US graduates have, a factor that can sometimes discourage the later from pursuing a career in research medicine [36]. Physicians who chose to follow the research path encounter many adversities including lack of protected time for research, insufficient training, inadequate mentoring, and, lastly, financial attraction of full-time clinical practice.

The NIH has developed programs, such as the Loan Repayment Program (NIH-LRP), to encourage physicians, specially USMGs, to pursue the investigative path [38]. These programs are not available to foreign graduates and for IMGs, and to match in physician-scientist residency positions to pursue this path is extremely difficult. On the other hand, stimulating the migration of foreign medical graduates through research opportunities raises two major questions. One involves the ethics of removing talented physicians from underserved countries, and the other issue is the increasing the dependency of the US biomedical research on IMGs.

Immigration

The recent changes in immigration policies have had a profound impact in the US medical community and have raised ethical, moral, and geopolitical questions. The stricter visa policies, specially affecting the Muslin countries, is a threat to the future of the clinical and biomedical research in this country given the important contribution IMGs confer to this segment of the healthcare industry [39]. The visa delays and the uncertainty regarding long-term stay for IMGs created by new immigration rules also affect patient care directly given that 25% of the physician workforce in the United States is composed of foreign-educated doctors. The underserved areas are particularly affected given that the proportion of IMGs practicing is higher. Residency programs have been affected as well especially those that rely heavily on the H1-B visa program that was modified by President Donald Trump's administration. The government program that for years provided expedited H1-B visa processing for a special segment of highly specialized workers, including doctors, now has a processing time frame of at least 6 months with limited availability for premium processing [40]. That has caused distress among both groups. On one side, residency programs are not able to guarantee that residents will be able to start their training on time which affects the dynamic of the teams and the hospitals. On the other, trainees have to negotiate the tension of starting a new job in a foreign country added to the insecurity of their visa status, not to mention the disturbance caused by starting off track if there is a delay.

Diversity

It has been said that "American health is global health" [41]. Physicians from other countries have enriched the United States not only scientifically and clinically but also culturally. IMGs possess language skills and direct knowledge and experience with cultural differences and social experiences that those born, raised, educated, and trained in the United States may not [41]. These individuals can serve as cultural bridges between different countries and immigrant communities. They may not only serve to bring skills and knowledge from the United States to foreign countries but certainly also bring knowledge of distinctive care strategies to our system.

Chen et al. interviewed several IMGs to evaluate the unique skills and advantages this group of doctors brings to their workplace. IMGs have a singular professional asset from previous training in a different healthcare system that provides them a distinct knowledge background and set of skills. Some IMGs come to the United States for training having already completed residency training and practiced in their home country for many years. They have diagnosed and treated patients with conditions endemic to their home countries that are not prevalent in the United States [42]. Nowadays, with globalization and rapidly increasing medical tourism, endemic diseases as well as infections from other countries can be carried into the American healthcare system [43].

The disparities in health outcomes among minorities is a reality in the United States that is becoming gradually more evident [44]. Doctor-patient relationship is recognized as a central causative factor of this issue. Race, ethnicity, and language have a major influence on the patient-doctor relationship. Patients who are minorities and especially the ones who are non-English speakers tend to not establish a bond with the physician, receive less information, and participate less on their healthcare decision-making. Efforts to recruit a more diverse medical workforce have been seen over the years since minority patients are more likely to choose minority physicians [45]. Having a physician with similar ethnical/racial and language background increases medication adherence and therefore health outcomes. Measures to diversify medical workforce can have significant effect on public health in the United States [46]. Language concordance is associated with less confusion and less frustration and positively associates with patient's perception of quality of care. Patients who are non-proficient in English tend to rate the quality of their care higher when the provider speaks the same language [47].

Religion influences patient's interpretation of their illnesses, interactions with providers, adherence to recommendations, and seek for healthcare. That impacts specially populations that share a minority religious affiliation. Unfortunately, these patients experience discrimination in their interaction with the healthcare system because providers that are not from the same religious background may see their religious beliefs as ignorance and futility. Having a shared religious identity with the healthcare provider can have a big impact in health outcomes and patient satisfaction for these populations [48].

Role in Medical Leadership

The fact that IMGs make up a quarter of the physician healthcare workforce in the United States makes it logical that many would occupy positions of leadership. Meta et al. reviewed leadership of anesthesia departments in 2006 [49]. IMGs constituted 18% of chairperson positions comparable to the percentage of practicing IMG anesthesiologists. The American College of Cardiology has focused on diversity and inclusion as a priority [50]. IMGs make up nearly 30% of the cardiology workforce. IMGs make up 24% of ACC Member Sections' Leadership Councils (MSLC) and Task Force (TF) members. Even more (31%) occupied chairperson positions. Overall the impact of IMGs in leadership is poorly studied and much more work needs to be done.

Experience of IMGs

IMGs face many challenges along their path to become a licensed physician in the United States. Applying to residency without the support of a US medical school, mentorship guidance, or peers pursuing the same route makes the process more onerous. The process is also costly requiring multiple trips to the United States, test fees, and application fees, among other expenses. The chances of matching into the residency program choice or preferred specialty are limited when compared to USMGs.

Language and communication can be problematic for non-native speakers even those with command of the English language. Medical abbreviations, medical slang, cultural nonverbal communication, and regional dialects are among the challenges encountered every day by foreign doctors practicing in the United States [51]. IMGs may not be aware of differences in meanings of medical terminology and may not necessarily clarify when confusion arises [51].

Doctor-patient relationship and documentation can be compromised by the language difference.

It must also be recognized that IMGs may struggle with language issues outside of the medical care environment. Aspects of common acculturation such as popular conversation, variations in American culture, and survival skills, from obtaining driver's license to housing, impose another layer of adversity that can lead to isolation. Most IMGs end up turning to their own community, either with other IMGs from different nationality or immigrants of their home country that live in the area [26].

The United States is a diverse nation of immigrants. We have counted on individuals from foreign nations to make the country an economic and intellectual powerhouse. Many USMGs are likely the children or grandchildren of immigrants [52]. Yet, IMGs suffer discrimination from application to medical school or training and into clinical practice.

The challenges start early on, during the residency selection process. Woods et al. found four themes identified as barriers by IMGs [53]. These included difficulty obtaining externships to booster application strength, difficulty interview experiences, criticism of IMG heavy programs by USMGs, and difficulty finding employment after residency. Desbiens et al. investigated how IMG residency applications are processed compared to American graduates during the residency selection process for family medicine and psychiatry [54]. The results demonstrated that residency programs replied 80% more often to USMGs applicants even though applications quality was similar. They also performed a survey of surgical program directors regarding discrimination against IMGs applicants, and 70% of them recognized that there was inequity in the selection processes [54]. IMGs are often asked to meet requirements that go above those required by ECFMG or requirements for USMGs to match in a residency program [54]. Some residency programs have policies regarding IMGs, that they would rather have slots unfilled than matching a qualified IMG [54]. Balon et al. found that psychiatry programs responded more often to applicants of AMGs than IMGs [55]. The discussion of whether USMGs should have an advantage over equally or overqualified IMGs or whether the process should be based entirely on meritocracy should be investigated by medical education authorities.

Transparent policies should be developed for program directors to utilize to minimize nonacademic selection bias against IMGs. One possibility would be to include such policy in institutional diversity statements. Another approach could be changing the focus of the initial application screening, blinding the application reviewees to things like nationality and medical school of the applicants, and shift the focus to USMLE grades, research, and letters of recommendation, for example. One source of systematic selection bias against IMGs is difficulty associated with evaluation of medical training and qualification to enter US residency programs. The ECFMG has continued to innovate the process so that IMG eligibility is similar to the USMGs. IMGs now take the same USMLE exams as USMGs. IMGs are encouraged to arrange clinical experience at a US hospital to receive skills evaluation by US doctors and receive letters of recommendation for application. The interview process allows IMGs to demonstrate language and communication skills.

Additional factors that may have a negative impact on the residency selection process against IMGs include the financial and administrative burden created by the immigration process on residency programs and time delays that can now occur with the new immigration policies [56]. It is easier for residency programs to incorporate USMG into their system.

Despite what seems to be a standardized approach to the selection process, it is a well-known fact that IMGs are in disadvantage and several programs favor USMG during the process, specially the most prestigious programs affiliated with well-recognized academic institutions. Selection bias leads to a higher number of IMGs a higher number of IMGs who match into smaller programs in underserved areas [54].

The new US immigration policies have introduced another layer of difficulty for IMGs. The travel ban imposed to some countries in 2017 affected many physicians, researchers, and their families who abruptly lost their ability to work in the United States and created a collective sense of anxiety among many others with similar immigration status [39]. The new immigration rules affect not only these individuals and their loved ones but also the US health system that is already facing major shortage in healthcare workforce. According to the Immigrant Doctors Project, 7800 doctors working in the United States are citizens of Iran, Libya, North Korea, Somalia, Syria, Venezuela, and Yemen, countries included in the state department travel ban. Loss of these physicians may profoundly affect smaller hospitals in underserved areas [39].

Annual limitations of work visas may significantly affect healthcare. Khan et al. investigated the potential effect of this new policy surveying the number of physicians H1-B holders per state in the United States [40]. He discovered that 1.4% of all active physicians in this country are H1-B holders and certain states and institutions rely heavily on the program. The delays in processing and the specialized workers visa, like the H1-B, have affected the ability of residency programs to start matched applicants on time and also forced physicians already in training to take leaves of absence because they had temporally lost their right to work while the visa renewal is being processed.

Conclusions

Healthcare professionals migrate for many reasons at each state of their medical career from medical school through professional practice. Professional satisfaction, better training, long-term job stability, better salaries, improved lifestyle, and safety for self and family are the main motivations. The migration of skilled healthcare professionals raises concerns. Many of these highly educated workers have had their education subsidized by their home countries, many of which are developing countries with limited resources. Departure of this component of the academic elites contributes to "brain drain phenomenon" [57]. Yet, the human spirit to develop knowledge and skills to the highest level will continue.

Academic immigration will continue in all areas. Immigrants to healthcare experience challenges from application, through study and assimilation, and into clinical practice and beyond, yet healthcare cannot survive without their contribution at all levels including clinical area, research, and medical leadership. Medicine can lead society in the efforts to ehnace diversity and inclusion by recognition of the contribution of IMGs.

References

1. Hamnvik OPR. Applying for residency as an international medical graduate. *NEJM Resident 360* [internet]. 2019 [cited 2020 Mar 16]. Available from: https://resident360.nejm.org/expert-consult/applying-for-residency-as-an-international-medical-graduate.
2. Hallock JA, Seeling SS, Norcini JJ. The international medical graduate pipeline. Health Aff. 2003;22(4):94–6.
3. Parsi K. International medical graduates and global migration of physicians: fairness, equity, and justice. Medscape J Med. 2008;10(12):284.
4. Brotherton SE, Etzel SI. Graduate medical education, 2008-2009. JAMA. 2009;302(12):1357–72.
5. Brotherton SE, Etzel SI. Graduate medical education, 2018-2019. JAMA. 2019;322(10):996–1016.
6. Melnick DE. From defending the walls to improving global medical education: fifty years of collaboration between the ECFMG and the NBME. Acad Med. 2006;81(12):S30–5.
7. Flexner A. Medical education in the United States and Canada: a report to the Carnegie Foundation for the advancement of teaching. Carnegie Foundation for the Advancement of Teaching, Bulletin number four, 1910.
8. Education Commission for Foreign Medical Graduates. *About ECFMG: History.* Available from: https://www.ecfmg.org/about/history.html. Accessed 24 Nov 2019.
9. National Committee on Foreign Medical Education and Accreditation. U.S. Department of Education. *Accreditation and standards in foreign medical education.* Available from: https://sites.ed.gov/ncfmea/. Accessed 15 Jan 2020.
10. Education Commission for Foreign Medical Graduates. Medical school accreditation requirement for ECFMG certification. Available form: www.ecfmg.org/accreditation/. Accessed 24 Nov 2019.
11. Allman R, Perelas A, Eiger G. POINT: should the United States provide postgraduate training to international medical graduates? Yes. Chest. 2016;149(4):893–5. Available from: https://doi.org/10.1016/j.chest.2016.01.011.
12. O'Reilly KB. How IMGs have changed the face of American medicine. https://www.ama-assn.org/education/international-medical-education/how-imgs-have-changed-face-american-medicine. Accessed 15 Feb 2020.
13. Mandel J. COUNTERPOINT: Should the United States Provide Postgraduate training to international medical graduates? No. Chest. 2016;149(4):895–7. Available from: https://doi.org/10.1016/j.chest.2016.01.009.
14. Ludmerer LM. Let me heal: the opportunity to preserve excellence in American medicine. New York: Oxford University Press; 2014. p. 24.

15. Mullan F. The metrics of physician brain drain. N Engl J Med. 2005;353:1810–8.
16. Association of American Medical Colleges. 2019 State physician workforce data report. Available from: https://www.aamc.org/data-reports/workforce/report/state-physician-workforce-data-report. Accessed on 12 Nov 2019.
17. Foundation for Advancement of International Medical Education and Research. United States physician workforce issues. Available from: https://www.faimer.org/research/workforce.html. Accessed 28 Dec 2019.
18. Educational Commission for Foreign Medical Graduates. Top five countries of citizenship, certificants 1994–2018. Source: Available from: https://www.ecfmg.org/resources/data-certification.html. Accessed 28 Dec 2019.
19. Phillips RL, Petterson S, Fryer GE, Rosser W. The Canadian Contribution to the US physician workforce. CMAJ. 2007;176(8):1083–7.
20. Khan MH, Abdullah N, Stanbrook MB. Withdrawal of Saudi trainees exposes the vulnerability of Canadian healthcare. CMAJ. 2018;190(35):E1030–2. Available from: https://doi.org/10.1503/cmaj.181084. Accessed 1 Nov 2019.
21. Jolly P, Garrison G, Boulet JR, Levitan T, Cooper RA. Three pathways to a physician career: applicants to U.S. MD and DO schools and U.S. citizen applicants to international medical schools. Acad Med. 2008;83(12):1125–31. Available from: https://doi.org/10.1097/ACM.0b013e31818c6445. Accessed 13 Oct 2010.
22. Van Zanten M, Boulet JR. Medical Education in the Caribbean: quantifying the contribution of Caribbean-educated physicians to primary care in the United States. Acad Med. 2013;88(2):276–81.
23. Juraschek SP, Zhang X, Ranganathan VK, Lin V. United States registered nurse workforce report card and shortage forecast. Am J Med Qual. 2012;27(3):241–9. Available from: https://doi.org/10.1177/1062860611416634. Accessed 1 Nov 2019.
24. Mazurenko O, Menachemi N. Use of foreign-educated nurses and patient satisfaction in U.S. hospitals. Health Care Manag Rev. 2016;41(4):306–15. Available from: https://doi.org/10.1097/HMR.0000000000000077.
25. Ranasinghe PD. International medical graduates in the US physician workforce. J Am Osteopath Assoc. 2015;115(4):236–41. Available from: https://doi.org/10.7556/jaoa.2015.047.
26. Gastel B. Impact of international medical graduates on U.S. and global healthcare: summary of the ECFMG 50th anniversary invitational conference. Acad Med. 2006;81(12 Suppl):S3–6. Available from: https://doi.org/10.1097/01.ACM.0000243340.89496.43.
27. U.S. Citizenship and Immigration Services. Conrad 30 waiver program. https://www.uscis.gov. Accessed 1 Jan 2020.
28. Hagopian A, Thompson MJ, Kaltenbach E, Hart LG. Health departments use of international medical graduates in physician shortage areas. Health Aff. 2003;22(5):241–9. Available from: https://doi.org/10.1377/hlthaff.22.5.241.
29. Knight V. American medical students less likely to choose to become primary care doctors. https://khn.org/news/american-medical-students-less-likely-to-choose-to-become-primary-care-doctors/. Accessed 1 Feb 2020.
30. National Resident Matching Program. Results and data 2019 main residency match. https://mk0nrmp3oyqui6wqfm.kinstacdn.com/wp-content/uploads/2019/04/NRMP-Results-and-Data-2019_04112019_final.pdf. Accessed 1 Feb 2020.
31. Jimenez-Gomez A, FitzGerald MR, Leon-Astudillo C, Gonzalez-delRey J, Schubert CJ. Performance of international medical graduates in pediatric residency: a study of peer and faculty perceptions. Acad Pediatr. 2018;18(7):728–32. Available from: https://doi.org/10.1016/j.acap.2018.07.006.
32. Norcini JJ, Boulet JR, Opalek A, Dauphinee WD. The relationship between licensing examination performance and the outcomes of care by international medical school graduates. Acad Med. 2014;89(8):1157–62. Available from: https://doi.org/10.1097/ACM.0000000000000310.
33. Tsugawa Y, Jena AB, Orav EJ, Jha A. Quality of care delivered by general internists in US hospitals who graduated from foreign versus US medical schools: observational study. BMJ. 2017;356:j273. Available from: https://doi.org/10.1136/bmj.j273.

34. Norcini JJ, Boulet JR, Dauphinee WD, Opalek A, Krantz ID, Anderson ST. Evaluating the quality of care provided by graduates of international medical schools. Health Aff. 2010;29(8):1461–8. Available from: https://doi.org/10.1377/hlthaff.2009.0222.
35. Zaheer S, Pimentel SD, Simmons KD, Kuo LE, Datta J, Williams N, Fraker DL, Kelz RR. Comparing international and United States undergraduate medical education and surgical outcomes using a refined balance matching methodology. Ann Surg. 2017;265(5):916–22. Available from: https://doi.org/10.1097/SLA.0000000000001878.
36. Alexander H, Heinig SJ, Fang D, Dickler H, Korn D. Contributions of international medical graduates to US biomedical research: the experience of US medical schools. J Investig Med. 2007;55(8):410–4. Available from: https://doi.org/10.2310/6650.2007.00025.
37. Khullar D, Blumenthal DM, Olenski AR, Jena ABUS. Immigration policy and American medical research: the scientific contributions of foreign medical graduates. Ann Intern Med. 2017;167(8):584–6. Available from: https://doi.org/10.7326/M17-1304.
38. National Institute of Health. Loan repayment programs. https://www.lrp.nih.gov.
39. Johnson SR. What do U.S. immigration policies mean for the healthcare workforce? Available from: https://www.modernhealthcare.com/article/20180519/NEWS/180519929/what-do-u-s-immigration-policies-mean-for-the-healthcare-workforce.
40. Kahn PA, Gardin TM. Distribution of physicians with H-1B visas by state and sponsoring employer. JAMA. 2017;317(21):2235–7. https://doi.org/10.1001/jama.2017.4877.
41. Kidia KK. American health is global health. Ann Intern Med. 2017;166(8):589–91. Available from: https://doi.org/10.7326/M17-0323.
42. Chen PG, Nunez-Smith M, Bernheim SM, Berg D, Gozu A, Curry LA. Professional experiences of international medical graduates practicing primary care in the United States. J Gen Intern Med. 2010;25(9):947–53. Available from: https://doi.org/10.1007/s11606-010-1401-2.
43. Chen LH, Wilson ME. The globalization of healthcare: implications of medical tourism for the infectious disease clinician. Clin Infect Dis. 2013;57(12):1753–9. Available from: https://doi.org/10.1093/cid/cit540.
44. Mayberry RM, Mili F, Ofili E. Racial and ethnic differences in access to medical care. Med Care Res Rev. 2000;57(1):108–45. Available from: https://doi.org/10.1177/1077558700057001S06.
45. Ferguson WJ, Candib LM. Culture, language, and the doctor-patient relationship. Fam Med. 2002;34(5):353–61.
46. Traylor AH, Schmittdiel JA, Uratsu CS, Mangione CM, Subramanian U. Adherence to cardiovascular disease medications: does patient-provider race/ethnicity and language concordance matter? J Gen Intern Med. 2010;25(11):1172–7. Available from: https://doi.org/10.1007/s11606-010-1424-8.
47. González HM, Vega WA, Tarraf W. Health care quality perceptions among foreign-born Latinos and the importance of speaking the same language. J Am Board Fam Med. 2010;23(6):745–52. Available from: https://doi.org/10.3122/jabfm.2010.06.090264.
48. Padela AI, Curlin FA. Religion and disparities: considering the influence of Islam on the Health of American Muslims. J Relig Health. 2013;52(4):1333–45. Available from: https://doi.org/10.1007/s10943-012-9620-y.
49. Meta B, Galford J, Purichia H. Leadership of United States academic anesthesiology programs 2006; chairperson characteristics and accomplishments. Anesth Analg. 2007;105(5):1338–45. Available from: https://doi.org/10.1213/01.anee.0000284666.39224.05.
50. Asad ZUA, Sivaram CA. Diversity and inclusion in leadership positions of the American college of cardiology: how do the international medical graduates (IMGS) fare? JACC. 2019;73(9). Available from: https://doi.org/10.1016/S0735-1097(19)33635-6.
51. Dahm MR. Exploring perceptions and use of everyday language and medical terminology among international medical graduates in a medical ESP course in Australia. Engl Specif Purp. 2011;30(3):186–97. Available from: https://doi.org/10.1016/j.esp.2011.02.004.
52. Brown D. At med school, a new degree of diversity: classes reflect a foreign flavor. Available from: https://www.washingtonpost.com/wp-dyn/content/article/2007/05/31/AR2007053102433.html. Accessed 25 Feb 2020.

53. Woods SE, Harju A, Rao S, Koo J, Kini D. Perceived bias and prejudices experienced by international graduates in the US post-graduate medical education system. Med Edu Online. 2006;11(1):4595. Available from: https://doi.org/10.3402/meo.v11i.4595.
54. Desbiens NA, Vidaillet HJ. Discrimination against international medical graduates in the United States residency program selection process. BMC Med Educ. 2010;10:5. Available from: https://doi.org/10.1186/1472-6920-10-5.
55. Balon R, Mufti R, Williams M, Riba M. Possible discrimination in recruitment of psychiatry residents? Am J Psychiatry. 1997;154(11):1608–9. Available from: https://doi.org/10.1176/ajp.154.11.1608.
56. Horvath K, Coluccio G, Foy H, Pellegrini C. A program for successful integration of international medical graduates (IMGs) into U.S. surgical residency training. Curr Surg. 2004;61(5):492–8. Available from: https://doi.org/10.1016/j.cursur.2004.06.011.
57. Nwagwu EOC. Migration of international medical graduates: implications for the brain drain. Open Med J. 2015;2:17–24. Available from: https://doi.org/10.2174/1874220301401010017.

Chapter 16
The Role of Mentoring and Tutoring

Sarah Hayek and Mohsen Shabahang

Introduction

General Introduction

Mentoring and tutoring are vital components to the personal and professional development of any young physician. The privilege of becoming a physician, one who attempts to heal and positively influence the lives of others through recognizing and treating disease, requires years of dedication, training, and personal sacrifice. The guidance of mentors, role models, tutors, peers, and experienced physicians is imperative in order to produce highly effective and competent physicians, worthy of the trust of our patients. This chapter will give an overview of some of the specific challenges faced by international medical graduates (IMGs) and how mentoring and tutoring can provide support and guidance to this unique population. It is important to note that while similar, mentoring and tutor are two separate concepts.

Overview of Mentors and Mentorship

Mentorship is a concept that can mean many different things. In a professional setting, mentorship is most often defined as a deliberate and consistent relationship between two persons with the purpose of improving the professional and psychosocial condition of at least one of the partners [1]. This relationship often benefits both partners, but the intention is for one of the partners to look to the other as a guide to assist in their development and growth. It is worth noting that this definition of

S. Hayek (✉) · M. Shabahang
General Surgery, Geisinger Medical Center, Danville, PA, USA
e-mail: mmshabahang@geisinger.edu

© Springer Nature Switzerland AG 2021   245
H. Tohid, H. Maibach (eds.), *International Medical Graduates in the United States*, https://doi.org/10.1007/978-3-030-62249-7_16

mentorship is not universally agreed upon and that in many other cultures, mentorship is viewed differently. Many eastern cultures, for example, see elders as infallible authorities who are seldom questioned, and the relationships that develop are intended to be very unilateral and hierarchical [2].

Overview of Tutors and Tutoring

On the other hand, tutoring is a better-defined concept with a more tangible definition. Tutoring is a formalized and deliberate method for developing technical or knowledge-based skills. Typically, a tutor is one who has mastered a concept or skill, and this person is tasked with imparting their knowledge and wisdom to another who is attempting to improve in this area [3]. Tutors are not always a more seasoned person, they can be more senior or experienced professionals, or they can be peers who have mastered a certain topic or skill. The tutoring relationship tends to focus mainly on knowledge or skill development without focus on the psychosocial aspects of the student's development. Also, while mentorship tends to focus on large, wholistic concepts of professional and personal development, tutoring should be a focused development of an area identified as weak or needing growth within the student's professional skills.

Mentors and Tutors for IMGs

Mentorship and tutoring are two distinctly different concepts (Fig. 16.1); however, both are necessary for the development of young physicians. All physicians during the training portion of their career will require mentorship and tutoring. With the

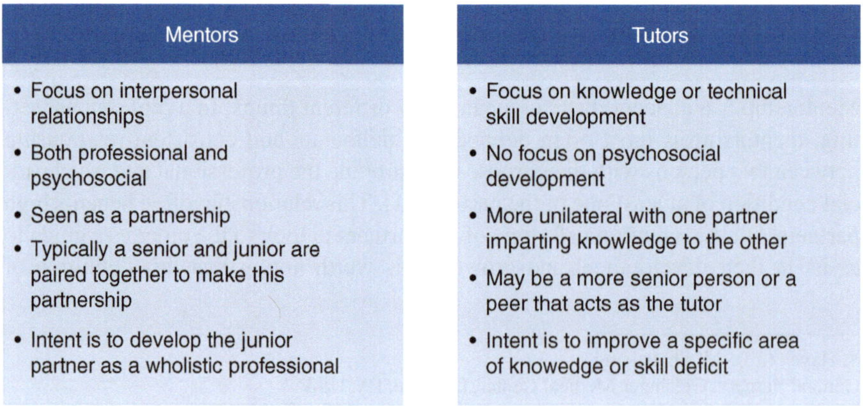

Mentors	Tutors
• Focus on interpersonal relationships	• Focus on knowledge or technical skill development
• Both professional and psychosocial	• No focus on psychosocial development
• Seen as a partnership	• More unilateral with one partner imparting knowledge to the other
• Typically a senior and junior are paired together to make this partnership	• May be a more senior person or a peer that acts as the tutor
• Intent is to develop the junior partner as a wholistic professional	• Intent is to improve a specific area of knowedge or skill deficit

Fig. 16.1 Similarities and differences between mentors and tutors

breadth of knowledge and skills required to become a competent and compassionate physician, it is unrealistic to believe that any student, even those that are the most gifted, will not require guidance and assistance in their development. For IMGs, the roles of mentorship and tutoring are even greater as they face more complex barriers and challenges when integrating into a new healthcare system and often a new culture.

Specific Challenges Faced by IMGS

Overview of IMGs as a Diverse Population

Although often described as a single group, IMGs are an extremely diverse group and face many different challenges. Some IMGs are United States (US) citizens who seek part or all of their medical training in another country, while others are non-US citizens who complete medical training outside of the USA and its territories. For those that are not US citizens, there may be significant challenges of acculturation or language barriers. Many IMGs face additional barriers involved with physically moving to the geographical region of their residency training including issues with obtaining visas for themselves and other family members, moving away from support networks, and having to leave behind belongings and relationships that are deeply meaningful to the individual [1–7]. Others may face discrimination from coworkers and patients alike based on religion, ethnicity, gender, and a constantly changing political environment [7, 8]. Some IMGs also face significant educational barriers entering the US medical education system as their prior medical education may have been vastly different from that which US physicians are accustomed to [9]. While many of these challenges are faced by US medical graduates as well, these challenges tend to be more pronounced and more complex in IMGs and result in specific mentoring and tutoring needs.

Culture and Language Issues Faced by IMGs

Acculturation is the process of personal integration into a culture. Typically, this means accepting cultural norms and standards of a new dominant culture in place of those of the prior culture. For IMGs who come from other cultures, this process can be challenging. In order to be considered a successful or competent physician within the USA and to have positive relationships with patients, a certain level of acculturation is required. Many IMGs struggle to recognize, understand, and embrace US cultural expectations. This is an area where specific mentorship from others who have gone through a similar process can be invaluable [10]. One of the biggest challenges of mentoring an IMG is that oftentimes the mentor does not understand all of the complex challenges being faced by the IMG. In order to provide supportive mentorship that can result in meaningful support through the acculturation process, assigning mentors who have experienced challenges of acculturation can be invaluable [11]. This is not always possible, and in that setting mentors should be willing and eager to learn about the complexities of immigration and the psychosocial ramification of such a life-altering event.

One of the most vexing challenges identified both by IMGs themselves and by those who have trained IMGs is the issue of language [12–14]. The level of language barrier faced by individual IMGs will undoubtedly be variable, but communication can be significantly impacted by lack of familiarity with the dominant language including local idioms, accents, and the complexity of medical terminology including the heavy reliance on acronyms in the US medical system. For many IMGs this can lead to frustration, breakdown in communication, and loss of confidence with resulting impact on patient care. It is important for any IMG who is struggling to overcome a language barrier to identify where his/her biggest challenges lie – comprehension, expression, written, verbal, or processing. Once the specific areas are identified, targeted tutoring such as working with standardized patients, taking online or in-person language classes, or other interventions such as avoiding speaking languages other than the dominant language can be put in place [12, 14].

For many IMGs who are facing these challenges, it is natural to seek out others who speak the same language or who practice the same cultural beliefs. This can result in improved sense of comfort for the IMG but can also lead to prolonged issues with language barriers and acculturation. Many have recommended that those facing cultural and language barriers practice complete immersion within the dominant culture or language. This includes adhering to certain cultural expectations or speaking the dominant language in all settings including at home [9]. These are some of the tutoring practices that have shown to provide rapid improvement in cultural and communication concerns resulting in improved professional development and confidence in the IMG. As a mentor, however, one needs to be aware of how this dramatic acculturation process can be disorienting and can cause a loss of sense of self [4].

A good mentor will recognize that while improved language skills and cultural assimilation into the dominant culture are likely to bring about improved professional growth, there can be psychosocial ramifications to this process. Certainly, improved communication and comfort within the culture can lead to improved daily satisfaction as the IMG develops stronger, more meaningful relationships with those that they work with and care for, but there is inherently a sense of loss that comes along with this process and this should not be overlooked.

In their 1984 study, Grinberg and Grinberg described four stages of acculturation. The first stage, they argue, is the stage of loss. Here is where the individual longs for their old comforting relationships and surroundings. Second comes the stage of confusion and anxiety, often accompanied by depression. In this stage the immigrant is typically faced with overwhelming demands to adjust to a new culture, to complete additional tasks associated with moving to a new country, and, in the case of an IMG, to perform well in a high-stress industry. Some will react by minimizing the significance of their cultural shifts, while others will magnify these changes and grasp onto their old norms as a lifeline to their former self. The third of acculturation is nostalgia and sorrow for the losses suffered through the process. During this time of sorrow and loss however, the immigrant begins to become more accustomed to the new cultural environment and less overwhelmed by sudden or unexpected discoveries. Finally, the stage of recovery is reached. Here the immigrant begins to think of themselves as part of the dominant culture, and the integration process is nearly complete [15]. These stages will occur over months to years. Mentors should be aware of the acculturation process and understand that it is not a static or linear process but ebbs and flows and even circles back to previous stages at times.

The Effect of Role Models in Mentoring IMGs

For IMGs who have done their medical training in another country, the entrance into the US healthcare system can be jarring. It is natural during times of great change to look for role models who have been through similar experiences. Role models serve a distinctly different purpose than do mentors and tutors. These are individuals who are visible in some way but a strong and meaningful relationship is not expected to develop. The purpose of a role model is to show that someone with a similar background to the IMG has navigated the barriers and challenges that the IMG is facing and has been successful. Depending upon the individual IMG's background, as well as the healthcare system that they are training in, these role models may be difficult to find.

As a mentor for an IMG, it is important to recognize the impact that role models can have. In their previous training, it is possible that the IMG saw successful professionals who looked like them, spoke like them, and shared a similar culture on a daily basis. When the IMG comes to a new country to complete their medical training however, people who share similar basic cultural and language backgrounds may be hard to find both within the healthcare system and within the community. Mentors can assist by identifying individuals who may act as role models to IMGs. Some healthcare systems have support networks built within them to help identify other physicians who are IMGs or who have specific cultural backgrounds [11]. There are also national societies and professional communities that have been developed such as multiple Ethnic Physician Organizations (more information can be found at www.ecfmg.org/echo/links-ethnic-physician.html). These communities of physicians who share common backgrounds can serve as role models, visible proof that the IMG is not alone and that other professionals with similar characteristics have successfully navigated the challenges of medical training in the USA. Role models not replace the need for mentors or tutors but rather are adjuncts that provide inspiration and proof that success is possible.

Support Structures for IMGs

The effects of isolation that occur from moving away from family and friends is a concern for many resident trainees. Medical training can be a demanding process with long working hours, exposure to illness and human suffering on a daily basis, and high levels of stress due to the responsibilities that come with being a physician who takes care of other people. A strong personal support system can be an invaluable resource for anyone facing such challenges and helps to foster important characteristics such as grit and resilience. For many IMGs, their personal support system will be drastically altered as they seek training in the USA. Family, friends, mentors, and role models that were previously relied upon may be difficult to contact, and daily interactions will be taken away [5, 8].

It is important for an IMG to be able to identify what gives them strength and support and increases their resilience. Our research lab conducted a study to understand how individuals applying to a general surgery residency program defined resilience. The study found that within a pool of combined applicants (US allopathic, US osteopathic, non-US IMGs, and US IMGs), the definition of resilience was multifactorial and not clearly defined. Multiple aspects of resilience were identified: support, learning from failure, adaptability, self-reflection, and perseverance. Mentors can help IMGs to identify which parts of resilience are most important to them and to develop skills and tools to help maximize these areas [16].

Issues with Belonging

For all persons, a sense of belonging is important to overall wellness and ultimately performance. Belonging makes us feel connected and deepens our satisfaction when interacting with others [17]. It is important to understand that belonging and being accepted are not the same. Acceptance shows tolerance while belonging shows a true sense of fitting in and having meaningful contributions and interactions which benefit both the individual and the group. Belonging can be challenging for anyone that is placed into a new situation such as entering a new healthcare system as a medical trainee. Once again, the challenge of finding belonging can be more difficult and more pronounced for an IMG as they struggle to overcome all of the other barriers associated with their status.

Many IMGs will face issues with discrimination and judgment. All people have biases. For some these biases are conscious and for others they are unconscious. For all sorts of reasons, we make assumptions about other people based on cues such as skin color, style of dress, gender, age, accent, and many other factors. For some IMGs, these cues may lead others to make assumptions about their ethnicity, education, or abilities as stereotypes and biases are projected onto the individual [7, 8].

Discrimination can be seen from microaggressions – small comments and actions that suggest a lack of respect – and with repeated exposure this can lead to burnout, fatigue, and poor wellness [18]. Discrimination can also be more overt, dehumanizing, and truly devastating to the individual [19].

While ideally discrimination would be dealt with by educating and intervening upon those who are the discriminators, this is an unrealistic expectation and does not help the individual who is being victimized in that moment. Mentors can help to work with the IMG to understand that discrimination shows a fault with the discriminator and not the victim. This can be especially challenging when these aggressions come from patients themselves, but there are methods for dealing with such interactions, and mentors should be aware of resources for victims of such discrimination [20]. They can also help to find support networks and to teach resilience practices so that the IMG may continue to move past ignorant comments and actions of others and to disconnect these from the IMG's sense of self-worth.

Special Issues Faced by Female IMGs

It is worth mentioning that female IMGs will face many of the same issues that other IMGs face as well as the issues that other female physicians face. This concept of facing multiple stereotypes at the same time has come to be known as intersectionality. According to work by Hall and colleagues (2019), intersectionality is when an individual is perceived to be from two or more minority groups and a mixture of stereotypes and assumptions are possible, some of which may conflict each other [21]. For example, women often face stereotypes about being more gentle or soft-spoken than men. Black people are sometimes assumed to be more aggressive than white people. A black woman presents as a mixture of these two minorities and may face varying degrees of discrimination or microaggression based on the perceiver's application of these biases. This type of discrimination can be challenging to predict and adapting to such discrimination is especially challenging.

For many other cultures, there are expectations and cultural norms that govern the actions of females. In some cultures, females are expected to dress in very specific ways or to avoid eye contact. These cultural norms which have been taught and modeled over the individuals lifetime are challenging to overcome for some women. Many women may see their actions as a sign of respect to males, elders, or more senior professionals, but these interactions may be mistaken when interpreted by those who have grown up in western culture. This is again an area where a mentor may be able to provide guidance on the cultural norms of the dominant culture and to help find other women who have been through a similar acculturation process in order to guide the IMG through the challenging process of learning the new culture and conforming while not giving up a sense of personal identity and heritage [8].

Practical Challenges Faced by IMGs and Becoming Certified to Train in the USA

For many IMGs there are practical barriers to becoming physicians in the USA. In the current political climate, there is much uncertainty and anxiety for many IMGs about the immigration process [22, 23]. Obtaining training visas is a large barrier for many IMGs. Depending upon the individual, this process can have a variety of challenges. Much of the burden of obtaining the proper documentation and required licensure falls onto the individual which adds financial, emotional, and time burdens. On top of these challenges are the issues of securing a training position in the USA that is willing to be a partner in overcoming these challenges. Mentors are not likely to be experts in the visa process but should familiarize themselves with the overall system and understand the basics of the J-1 and/or H-1 visa depending upon which is/are supported by their institution. It is also important to recognize the anxiety and frustration that this process can create. Empathy for the IMG as they attempt to complete their visa documentation or renew their visa can be very helpful.

The process of becoming eligible to apply to US residency programs requires foresight and advanced planning. In order to become a certified physician in the USA, one must attend a medical school that is appropriately certified, submit an application to the Educational Commission for Foreign Medical Graduates (ECFMG), pass the United States Medical Licensing Examinations (USMLE) Steps 1 and 2, be eligible to take the USMLE Step 3, and finally have official approval from the ECFMG. The IMG must also be eligible for a visa in the USA [24].

The USMLEs are examinations that US allopathic medical students take during their undergraduate medical education. These examinations are not traditionally included in the educational objectives of foreign medical education with the exception of some Caribbean and Philippine undergraduate medical schools. For those students who are training at an international medical school but intend to come to the USA for residency training, it is important to begin planning to study for and take these examinations early on in undergraduate medical training to prevent delays in the ability to apply to US residency programs. Virtually all US residency programs that participate in the National Resident Matching Program (NRMP) (the national system for assigning medical school graduates to accredited residency training positions) will require applicants to be certified by the ECFMG including having successfully passed USMLE Steps 1 and 2 [25]. Advisors and mentors to medical students who wish to apply to US residency programs should be aware of the requirements and help the IMG to plan for and arrange these examinations.

Important Changes to the USMLE Examinations

An important change to the USMLE system has recently been announced and may potentially have strong ramifications for IMGs. The National Board of Medical Examiners, the group that runs the USMLE, has just announced that the USMLE

Step 1 which has historically been a numerically graded examination will go to a pass/fail system in the near future (the current projection is 2022) [26]. This will have a large impact on IMG applicants. At this time, the USMLE Step 1 is one area of objective comparison between candidates of all backgrounds where an IMG can distinguish themselves by obtaining high scores. With a pass/fail system, the ability to show academic prowess and an objective, numeric accomplishment above other candidates will disappear. Mentors and advisors of IMGs seeking residency training in the USA should be aware of these pending changes.

Important Changes to the Certification Process of International Undergraduate Medical Schools

All IMGs who wish to obtain a residency training position in the USA must become accredited as an eligible applicant by the ECFMG. In 2023, the ECFMG will be implementing new regulations surrounding the accreditation process. Mentors and advisors need to be aware of these changes and make sure properly educate IMGs on these changes. Starting in 2023, all IMGs who wish to be certified as eligible applicants to US-accredited residency positions will need to graduate from a school that is certified by the World Federation for Medical Education (WFME) [27]. Any student who graduates from a medical school that does not have WFME recognition will be unable to apply as an eligible applicant to accredited US residency programs. This represents an important change and should be made clear to IMGs wishing to train in the USA – ideally prior to acceptance to undergraduate medical school but at least prior to completion.

Choosing a Specialty as an IMG

For IMGs, it is also important to understand the reality of the US residency training system. Prior research by our lab has shown that IMGs are not evenly distributed among medical and surgical specialties. There are specialties which have historically accepted a high number of IMGs into training positions and others which have historically accepted very few IMGs. It is important for IMGs to know the landscape and historic competitiveness of the individual specialties that they are considering for training. Ultimately the trends have shown that IMGs stand far greater chances of being accepted to a residency training program in fields of medicine and primary care such as neurology, internal medicine, family medicine, and psychiatry. On the other hand, surgical subspecialties and highly competitive medical specialties, such as orthopedic surgery, neurosurgery, and dermatology, very rarely accept IMGs into training positions [28]. It has also been shown that IMGs are expected to obtain higher standards on USMLE scores and other application metrics to be considered for a position for which there are US allopathic applicants also being considered. The rationale behind this seems to be that program directors feel that an

IMG brings inherent additional challenges to the training process that US allopathic graduates do not face. If there is a surplus of US allopathic graduates applying for training positions within a specific field, IMGs will find these fields exceptionally difficult to obtain training positions in. Mentors at the undergraduate medical level who work with students who wish to obtain a US training position as an IMG should be aware of these biases with the US system and help to guide the individual in their choice of specialty [29].

For some IMGs, the reality of the US training system and its biases against IMG applicants means that individuals choose specialties based on their likelihood of obtaining a position rather than the individuals desire to train within that field of medicine or surgery [30]. This can lead to a challenging dilemma for both the IMG and the mentor. While the IMG who matches into a residency program that is not their ultimately desired program undoubtedly has strong reasons for making this decision, the reality of what that means to the IMG on a daily basis may not be understood or anticipated. When discussing how program directors view IMGs in training programs with a variety of different specialties, our research lab discovered that this can be one of the most challenging aspects of training an IMG. If the field that the IMG has chosen does not bring them professional satisfaction, there can be serious concerns with physician burnout. It is estimated that 44% percent of physicians experienced serious burnout in 2019 [31]. This rate is even higher among trainees. In one large-scale study of general surgery residents in US residencies, 69% of trainees who responded to the survey met the definitions and standards for burnout [32]. Many things contribute to physician burnout including emotional stress, depersonalization, increased administrative requirements, and long working hours, but for those who do not find joy, intrigue, and fulfillment from their chosen medical or surgical specialty, these factors can be even more pronounced. Mentors and IMGs need to be honest about the individual's personal goals and recognize when a trainee does not find enjoyment and satisfaction in their daily practice.

For some IMGs who find themselves training in a field that they would not have chosen were it not for the challenges of gaining a training position in the USA, this challenge can be overcome by seeking additional training or fellowships in areas that are more intriguing and bring the individual higher job satisfaction. The concerns of a biased admissions process however are seen at the fellowship level of training as well, and thus, again, IMGs face more challenging odds when trying to secure positions within competitive fellowship training programs [33]. Mentors can help an IMG to identify the areas of the trainee's professional work that the trainees enjoy the most. Furthermore, mentors can strive to highlight the reasons that they themselves chose the field of medicine or surgery and how they find fulfillment in their practice. Unfortunately, some trainees will continue to be dissatisfied with their professional careers and progress toward burnout. In some cases, options for changing training programs or career paths are limited based on the individual's status and visa concerns.

Ways for IMGs to Strengthen Their Applications

Many IMGs struggle with ways to strengthen their application for residency training in the USA. To some extent this is specialty specific, but there are a few universal suggestions for IMGs to improve their chances of matching to a US residency position that all mentors of IMGs at the undergraduate medical training level should be aware of. The first suggestion is to do clinical rotations in the USA if at all possible. This shows that the IMG has previously been exposed to the US healthcare system and has been able to be successful. Evaluations and recommendations by US-trained physicians can be invaluable. Many program directors cite concerns about IMGs being successful within the US healthcare system. If a recommendation from a US-trained physician can be provided to show that the IMG is able to function at a high level within the US system, this can go a long way to alleviate those concerns from potential training programs [34].

Next, personal connections can make a huge difference. Even if rotations in the USA are not possible, attending national meetings and even presenting research at these meetings can result in networking opportunities that would otherwise be unavailable. Meeting physicians within the area of the IMG's interest can result in connections that may be beneficial in the future. Especially important can be networking events at national meetings where program directors and other influential physicians may be present. Other connections to well-known physicians can also be valuable as personal phone calls, emails, or other forms of contact with program directors can improve an IMG's chances of securing a training position in the USA. Many programs have automatic filters applied to the applications that they receive for training. For some programs one of the filters includes IMG status or non-US-citizen status. In these circumstances, no matter how strong the IMG's application may be in other areas, the program may never even see the application due to the filters that are present. A personal connection to another physician who can make phone calls on behalf of the IMG can make sure that the application is at least read [34].

Another concern is the ability of the potential programs to read the IMG's application. For those that come from training programs where English is not the dominant language, the ability to read the dean's letter or other materials including letters of recommendation may be affected. Within the USA there is no standardization of the scoring system of medical students, and even greater variation can be seen from foreign medical schools. Some of these scoring systems can be confusing and frustrating to understand for programs. Most training programs identify the review of applications as one of the most time-consuming and challenging annual tasks for their residency program. For these reasons many programs are unwilling or unable to spend additional time trying to read or understand applications which are confusing [34].

Many IMGs choose to engage in research opportunities. This is especially common as a gap between completing medical school and applying to residency positions. These research experiences can have both positive and negative impacts upon the application of an IMG. The opportunity to work in a research lab and to publish scientific papers and present at conferences increases exposure and strengthens the research and academic portions of an application. These opportunities can also lead to the development of relationships which can result in mentorship, friendship, and other connections that can lead to securing a residency training position. For some medical and surgical specialties, research can be very important and can increase the likelihood of gaining a training position [34].

For other specialties, however, research is not as valued. For these training programs, research can actually inhibit the chances of gaining a training position as it increases the number of years between completing undergraduate medical education and beginning clinical patient care and graduate training. Some training programs apply a filter for applications that automatically filters out those applicants who have graduated undergraduate medical school more than a set number of years ago. In these cases, research can sometimes increase the gap between medical school and residency [34].

It is important to also understand that for some IMGs, gap years between undergraduate medical school and residency training is not optional. Some countries require service commitments either as military personnel or physicians such as India's Compulsory Rotatory Residential Internship. For individuals who have these requirements and wish to complete residency training in the USA, it is especially important that they understand the climate of the US training system including making realistic and calculated decisions about chosen specialties and understanding the impact that additional gap years could have on their application. Mentors to these students should understand the realities of these challenges and advise student accordingly, setting up realistic expectations and maximizing all possible areas of their application to overcome the complications of these service commitments.

Another area which program directors cite as concerning when considering hiring an IMG is the use of the electronic medical record (EMR) in the USA and the diagnostic work-up of patients. Many other countries do not use EMRs and typing and basic computer skills are not universal in all countries. Some IMGs enter into training in the USA and struggle with how heavily many US healthcare systems rely upon technology. Typing notes and placing orders electronically, which is typically time-saving for most US physicians, can actually slow down the productivity of those who are unfamiliar with basic computer and typing skills. Adding this complexity on top of other communication challenges can lead to inefficiency and frustration. Tutors can be very helpful in teaching basic computer and typing skills and continued daily practice will often result in rapid increase in this skill set [34].

Similarly, the diagnostic work-up of patients in the USA tends to rely upon technology, imaging, and objective data more often than in other countries [8]. Some IMGs may enter the US system being confident in their diagnostic skills based solely or at least very heavily off of physical examination and history taking. In the

USA it is more common to order extensive laboratory tests, imaging, and other diagnostic tests that are often considered frivolous or cost prohibitive in other countries. While this certainly represents some excess within the US healthcare system and is being addressed by many healthcare systems, there are also medical/legal and insurance reasons that these tests are completed and are seen as required in some circumstances. Mentors can be helpful in assisting IMGs to understand the US healthcare system, but this is also an area where tutors can assist by helping to teach and guide IMGs in the typical diagnostic work-up undertaken for specific disease processes at their specific institution.

IMGs That Have Been Fully Certified Physicians in Other Countries

It is worth mentioning a specific subset of IMGs – those who have completed residency training or are fully certified physicians in their native countries. Under current state and national regulations, it is nearly impossible to become a fully accredited physician in the USA without completing a US residency training program. This is true even if the individual has completed a residency training program in another country or is a certified physician in another country [35]. For individuals who have completed training previously, this means returning to the beginning of training including the reduced salary, increased work hours, and lower position within the traditional hierarchy. Starting over can be frustrating for both the individual and those in charge of training an already trained physician. Old habits can be hard to break and conflicts can arise. Mentors should be aware of the possibility of increased tensions and complications while also respecting the prior education, training, and accomplishments of the individual. It is important to have open communication and to establish expectations and rules of engagement prior to the start of training this specific population of physicians in order to decrease frustration and concerns for both the IMG and those who take on the responsibility of training such unique individuals.

US Citizens Who Graduate from Foreign Medical Schools

Another subpopulation that deserves special mention are those individuals who are US citizens who sought medical training abroad and then wish to return to the USA for residency training. There are a variety of reasons that a US citizen would choose to train in another country. The most commonly cited reasons are the inability to secure an undergraduate medical school position and financial concerns [36]. These individuals often struggle and continue to face discrimination after completing medical school and are seen as different from US allopathic graduates. On the other hand, these individuals can notice advantages over non-US IMGs in that many programs view these applicants as having fewer challenges since the acculturation process and language barriers are not a concern [34].

Advising IMGs on Future Career Goals

For IMGs, career planning remains an important topic. For some, they have requirements attached to visa agreements that dedicate them to serve in rural or underserved populations following the completion of training [37]. This can at times require the IMG to delay or forego specialty training or fellowships. It is important to know this and have realistic expectations. For those IMGs who wish to obtain fellowship positions, there are some specific concerns to consider. If the IMG has successfully completed residency training in the USA, the concerns that existed of acculturation and language barriers tend to be less significant at this stage. Despite these decreased concerns of adjusting to the US healthcare system, there remain biases against IMGs at the fellowship level, especially for highly competitive specialties. Since not all fellowships are accredited or tracked in a centralized system, the exact data about the differences between US allopathic graduate acceptances and IMG acceptances to fellowship positions are not as reliable.

The individual specialty landscape is important to understand as IMGs prepare for future careers and make goals. Some specialties value research and will encourage or even require years of research training or a minimum level of academic publications and productivity. Other specialties focus on clinical experiences. Years since completing residency training can be viewed as positive or negative depending upon the specialty. For IMGs and mentors, it is important to investigate these factors early in the graduate training process. Even as early as the first year of residency training, IMGs should begin to identify their future career goals, and mentors should assist in this process. A plan should be formulated to enhance the application and CV for the IMG in order to increase their chances of obtaining the training positions or appointments that they desire. This is especially true for those seeking highly competitive fellowships, training programs, or academic appointments. Mentors should strive to help the IMG make important connections within the desired specialty and to understand the specific culture in order to properly advise the IMG in choosing and preparing for future ventures.

Specific Ways of Evaluating IMGs

It is important to be able to objectively evaluate IMGs in order to be able to track progress, identify areas of weakness, and provide feedback to individuals. For many IMGs, the process of evaluation and receiving feedback may be foreign to them as this is not a universal part of medical education across the globe [5]. This will also necessarily have an impact on how IMGs receive feedback and how their response is interpreted by senior faculty members. For some IMGs trained in other countries, the hierarchy of medicine is so absolute that they will interpret evaluation, assessment, and feedback from superiors as ultimate and absolute. Many IMGs may also actively avoid receiving feedback as they may see areas identified as needing improvement as failures and critical catastrophes. While it is still critically important to evaluate and provide feedback to IMGs, it is also important that those who are training IMGs are aware of this background and conscious of the cultural differences that may be at play.

Step 2 CS has a built-in Spoken English Proficiency (SEP) built into the examination. Harik et al. (2006) studied the correlation between English proficiency and the components of the SEP in Step 2 CS and found an overall correlation of 0.94 suggesting that the CS examination is a good surrogate for English proficiency [38]. An added benefit of this evaluation is that it is often already completed at the time of IMG application to a residency program and thus basic English proficiency should theoretically be established before training begins. This is one standardized examination, however, with fairly straightforward communication skills that are tested and does not necessarily evaluate for the subtleties of regional dialect and communication in complex situations.

Some specialties and programs have developed specialized assessment tools such as the Clinical Skills Verification (CSV) process, the Mini-Clinical Evaluation Exercises, and the Milestones. The CSV tool in particular has been studied and shown to be reliable across both US medical graduates and IMGs [39]. These systems of evaluation allow for formal evaluation and assessment which allows for structured, informed, and constructive feedback to be delivered to the IMG. It is helpful to repeat assessments and evaluations frequently so that progress can be seen, documented, and tracked. This is helpful both to mentors who are trying to promote progressive changes and to the IMG who may not recognize areas where improvements are occurring or may overestimate their progress in other areas.

Review of Currently In-Place Programming for Mentoring and Tutoring IMGs

There are a variety of different programs already in place to assist with the mentoring and tutoring of IMGs. Some countries or national healthcare systems have programming in place for IMGs (there is no national programming in the USA), and other programming is more regional or hospital/program specific. One study published out of Australia developed a pilot program for IMGs in transition [40]. This program involved gathering IMGs for routine conferences where informal discussions about daily challenges were held. IMGs were allowed to direct these conversations, identifying the challenges that they felt were most important to them. Fellow IMGs as well as native physicians were then able to discuss the issues and to formulate plans for how to handle future similar encounters. This program allows for IMGs to direct the conversations to the areas that they identify as most challenging or meaningful to their daily well-being and to also meet others who are going through similar situations so as to reduce the feelings of isolation.

Sockalingam et al. developed a 1-day orientation for IMG psychiatry residents in Canada. This program consisted of education on mental health, documentation practices, communication, feedback, and social considerations. Participants reported feeling more comfortable about beginning clinical practice after participating in this orientation [41]. Another study done in the UK by Bansal et al. implemented a 1-day course followed by a half-day course conducted 2 weeks after the first course. This course was designed to orient IMGs to patient-centered skills and was favorably received by participants [42]. Another valuable resource is the Society for Teachers of Family Medicine (STFM) which offers several online courses for IMGs and can be accessed through the STFM website, stfm.org.

Recognizing Signs of Mental Wellness and Burnout in IMGs

Mental health is a topic within residency training programs which has gained recognition as a significant issue within training programs in the USA. For IMGs, maintaining positive mental health can lead to improved acculturation and job satisfaction. On the other hand, a lack of mental health can have negative impacts of patients and outcomes and especially upon the individual suffering from burnout, depersonalization, or overall poor mental health [17]. Their study found that social support, increasing year of residency training, and immersion into the dominant culture were all correlated to the overall mental health scores of IMGs. Taylor-East et al. used the General Health Questionnaire and the Cultural Distance Questionnaire to identify that lack of leisure time was correlated to psychological stress in IMGs in Malta [43]. There are multiple validated mental health questionnaires which can be implemented, but those chosen by Taylor-East et al. are particularly suited to IMG populations.

A study by Kehoe in the UK suggests that preforming and individual needs assessment and setting clear job expectations at the start of training of an IMG leads to better outcomes and satisfaction in the training of IMGs [11]. These individualized assessments can help mentors to create targeted programming, interventions, and resource utilization to help promote positive mental health and to support individual IMGs with their unique needs rather than generalized interventions which are hard to apply to such a diverse population as IMGs.

It is also important to understand that burnout, while often triggered by different things for each individual, is a tangible and measurable concept. One of the most used ways of measuring burnout among trainees is the Maslach Burnout Inventory [44]. This is a standardized questionnaire which has been used for decades to conduct burnout research and is validated for use internationally. The Maslach Burnout Inventory is a good way to screen all trainees for burnout and to identify those who may need additional support. Mentors should be aware that not all persons display signs of burnout in the same way and thus screening is an important part of the process of recognizing individuals suffering from burnout. The cultural barriers of some IMGs may make it hard for mentors to recognize warning signs, and thus the use of a validated screening tool is highly encouraged.

Other Resources Available

It is important for mentors to be knowledgeable about the resources available to IMGs. Here is a brief, non-comprehensive list of some of the most useful resources for IMGs:

- Educational Commission for Foreign Medical Graduates (ECFMG): https://www.ecfmg.org/
- Electronic Portfolio of International Credentials (EPIC): https://www.ecfmgepic.org/index.html
- Global Educational Exchange in Medicine and the Health Professionals (GEMx): https://www.gemxelectives.org/
- Foundation for Advancement of International Medical Education and Research (FAIMER): https://www.faimer.org/
- World Federation for Medical Education (WFME): https://wfme.org/
- Doctors Speak Up: http://doctorsspeakup.com/

There are also several international medical and surgical organizations designed to support IMGs. These can be resources to find connections and advice from others who have been through similar situations. Some hospital systems may also have internal systems designed to provide support to IMGs.

Conclusion

Providing mentorship and tutoring for IMGs is a very complicated task. IMGs are spoken of as if they are a homogenous group with similar needs but this could not be farther from the truth. Individual IMGs come from an extremely diverse background and need individualized mentorship and tutoring strategies designed to fit their specific needs. Those who wish to mentor or tutor IMGs need to put effort into getting to know the IMG, understanding their background as well as their future goals. IMGs are a diverse, talented, and enriching population who make incredible contributions to the healthcare systems of their adoptive countries. Both the individual IMG and the institution that accepts an IMG must be prepared for challenges, but with the development of trusting and committed mentor relationships as well as targeted tutoring, IMGs can be an invaluable addition to healthcare.

References

1. Haggard D, et al. Who is a mentor? A review of evolving definitions and implications for research. J Manag. 2011;37(1):280–304.
2. Gawande S. Mentorship in India: changing scenario. J Educ Technol Health Sci. 2017;4(3):86–8.
3. Wood D, Wood H. Vygotsky, tutoring and learning. Oxf Rev Educ. 1996;22(1):5–12.
4. Chan M. International medical graduates: acculturation, repatriation and the third-culture kids of medicine. Edmonton, Alberta, Canada: John Wiles & Sons. Med Educ. 2015;49:850–8.
5. Gogineni R, et al. Identity development for international medical graduate physicians: a perspective. In: Rao NR, Roberts LW, editors. International medical graduate physicians. Switzerland: Springer International Publishing; 2016.
6. Huhn D, et al. International medical students - a survey of perceives challenges and established support services at medical faculties. GMS Z Med Ausbild. 2015;32(1).
7. Laird L, Abu-Ras W, Senzai F. Cultural citizenship and belonging: Muslim international medical graduated in the USA. J Muslim Minor Aff. 2013;33(3):356–70.
8. Aggarwal R, Anzia J. Identity issues specific to women and US citizens graduating from international medical schools: a perspective. In: Rao NR, Roberts LW, editors. International medical graduate physicians. Switzerland: Springer International Publishing; 2016.
9. Lineberry M, et al. Educational interventions for international medical graduates: a review and agenda. Med Educ. 2015;49:863–79.
10. Nair R. Mentoring: essential to an international medical graduate's education. B C Med J. 2014;55(9):429.
11. Kehoe A, et al. Supporting international graduates to success. Clin Teach. 2018;15:361–5.
12. Ramaswamy R, et al. Communication skills curriculum for foreign medical graduates in an internal medicine residency program. J Am Geriatr Soc. 2014;62:2153–8.
13. van Zanten M. Evaluating the spoken English proficiency of international medical graduates for certifications and licensure in the United States. In: Innovation and leadership in English language teaching. s.l.: Emerald Group Publishing Limited; 2011. p. 75–90.
14. Dahm M, Cartmill J. Talking their way to success: communicative competence for international medical graduates in transition. Med Educ. 2016;50:992–3.
15. Grinberg L, Grinberg R. A psychoanalytic study of migration: its normal and pathological aspects. J Am Psychoanal Assoc. 1984;32(1):0003–651.
16. Hayek S, et al. How applicants to general surgery define resilience. Chicago: Association for Surgical Education; 2019.
17. Atri A, Matorin A, Ruiz P. Integration of international medical graduates in U.S. psychiatry: the role of acculturation and social support. Acad Psychiatry. 2011;35(1):21–6.
18. Freeman L, Stewart H. Microaggressions in clinical medicine. Kennedy Inst Ethics J. 2018;28(4):1086–3249. s.l.: Johns Hopkins University Press.
19. Forrest-Bank S, Cueller M. The mediating effects of ethnic identity on the relationships between racial microaggression and psychological well-being. Soc Work Res. 2018;42(1):44–56.
20. Wheeler D. Twelve tips for responding to microaggressions and overt discrimination: when the patient offends the learner. Med Teach. 2019;41(10):1112–7.
21. Hall E, et al. MOSAIC: a model of stereotyping through associated and intersectional categories. Acad Manage Rev. 2019;44(3):643–72.
22. Liberia: US revises notification on cancellation of visa operation after meeting with Govt. deligation. s.l.: Frontapage Africa; 9 Dec 2019.
23. Rodriguez-Pose A, von Berlepsch V. Migration-prone and migration-averse places. Path dependence in long-term migration to the US. Appl Geogr. 2020;116:1–29.
24. Educational Commission for Foreign Medical Graduates. ECFMG Certification Fact Sheet. Educational *Commission for Foreign Medical Graduates*. [Online] 27 Aug 2019. [Cited: February 26, 2020.] www.ecfmg.org/forms/certfact.pdf.

25. National Residency Matching Program. Residency Applicant Eligibility. National Residency matching Program. [Online] 2020. [Cited: February 27, 2020.] www.nrmp.org/residency-applicant-eligibility/.
26. United States Medical Licensing Examination. USMLE Program Announces Upcoming Policy Change. United States medical licensing examination. [Online] 12 Feb 2020. [Cited: February 26, 2020.] www.usmle.org/announcements/?ContentId=264.
27. Educational Commission for Foreign Medical Graduates. 2023 Medical School Accreditation Requirement. Medical school accreditation requirement for ECFMG certification. [Online] 19 Feb 2020. [Cited: February 26, 2020.] www.ecfmg.org/accreditation/.
28. National Residency matching Program; Educational Commission for Foreign Medical Graduates. Charting outcomes in the match: international medical graduates. s.l.: National Residency matching Program and Educational Commission for Foreign Medical Graduates; 2014.
29. Clutts B, et al. Trends in United States residency match rates for international medical graduates. Abstract Presented at the Keystone Chapter of the American College of Surgeons Conference: s.n., 2018.
30. Pumariega A, Cagande C, Gogineni R. Chapter 13: Child and adolescent psychiatry. In: Rao N, Roberts L, editors. International medical graduate Physicians. Switzerland: Springer International Publishing; 2016.
31. Yates S. Physician stress and burnout. Am J Med. 2020;133(2):160–4.
32. Elmore L, et al. National survey of burnout among US general surgery residents. Journal of the American College of Surgeons. 2016;223(3):440–51.
33. Alsaied T, Baliga R, Madueme P. International medical graduates in cardiology fellowship: brain drain or brain gain? J Am Coll Cardiol. 2015;65(5):507–10.
34. Hayek S, et al. How do program directors view international medical graduate applicants when applying for residency training positions? Reading: s.n.; 2019. Keystone Chapter of the American College of Surgeons Annual Conference 2019.
35. American Medical Association. Residency program requirements for international medical graduates. American Medical Association. [Online] 2020. [Cited: February 28, 2020.] www.ama-assn.org/education/international-medical-education/residency-program-requirements-international-medical.
36. Gray S. Attending medical school on foreign ground. [Online] 1 September 2013. The Student Doctor Network.
37. The Ranchod Law Group. H-1B Visa options and requirements for doctors. [Online] 2020.
38. Harik P, et al. Relationships among subcomponents of the USMLE step 2 clinical skills examination. the step 1, and the step 2 clinical knowledge examinations. Acad Med. 2006;81(10):S21–4.
39. Dalack G, Jibson M. Clinical skills verification, formative feedback, and psychiatry residency trainees. Acad Psychiatry. 2014;36:122–5.
40. Harris A, Delany C. International medical graduates in transition. Clin Teach. 2013;10:328–32.
41. Sockalingam S, et al. A transition to residency curriculum for international medical graduate psychiatry trainees. Acad Psychiatry. 2016;40:353–5.
42. Bansal A, et al. Helping international medical graduates adapt to the UK general practice context: a values-based course for developing patient-centred skills. Education for Primary Care. 2015;26(2):105–8.
43. Taylor-East R, Grech A, Gatt C. The mental health of newly graduate doctors in Malta. Psychiatr Danub. 2013;25 Suppl 2:S250–5.
44. Maslach C, et al. Maslach burnout inventory. Mind Garden: Tools for Positive Transformation. [Online] [Cited: March 5, 2020.]. https://www.mindgarden.com/117-maslach-burnout-inventory.

Chapter 17
Medical Ethics and International Medical Graduates

Hassaan Tohid and Steven R. Daugherty

Background

According to Merriam Webster dictionary, ethics is defined as: "the discipline dealing with what is good and bad and with moral duty and obligation" [1]. Ethics is the act of doing the right thing, even if it goes against oneself. Spirituality and religion have highlighted this subject for thousands of years, yet the world faces difficulty in easily finding a person who is ethical in all areas of his life. Why is this discrepancy in human behavior? We may expect a shopkeeper to be hundred percent honest with us, but when we are in the same situation, we may not live up to that same ethical standard. We expect strict ethical behavior from everyone else but may be less critical of our own actions.

There are many reasons for this mismatch. We may think of ourselves as human beings, having no need for improvement or the tendency to give in to the temptation of inappropriate rewards or simply doing what is easiest. Knowing correct standards of conduct is one thing. Actually doing the right thing is altogether different. We tend to forget about ethical practices when we are really in a situation where our integrity is tested. Moreover, the most ethical conduct may not be clear in the confusion and fluidity of clinical practice.

So, no matter how well we have thought about these issues in the past, we must return to understand the subject of ethics again and again. The more we read and reflect on these issues, the more they will be embedded in our minds, and the more likely we will be able to do the right thing when hard choices present themselves.

The standards which make our actions ethical are different in different parts of the world. Local laws and customs set up different expectations as to what should

H. Tohid (✉)
California Institute of Behavioral Neurosciences and Psychology, Fairfield, CA, USA

S. R. Daugherty
Medical School Companion, Chicago, IL, USA

© Springer Nature Switzerland AG 2021
H. Tohid, H. Maibach (eds.), *International Medical Graduates in the United States*, https://doi.org/10.1007/978-3-030-62249-7_17

happen, indeed what needs to happen, between physicians and patients. To help physicians trained outside the United States adapt to medical practice in the United States, this chapter reviews the key ideas from which our ethical standards are derived and then explores how these standards might be applied differently in the United States compared to other places.

We are not arguing that the standards in the United States are somehow "better" but only that they are different and that adaptation to medical practice in a different setting requires an appreciation of those differences and the ability to change one's behavior accordingly. Our goal is to reduce confusion and foster an understanding of why these *differences exist, so that* physicians can be better prepared for the difficult choices that arise in daily medical practice.

Medical Ethics

Medical ethics is the moral compass that the doctors across the world use to ensure high moral standards for medical practice [2]. Good medical practice is not simply getting the right outcome but getting that outcome in the right way. We all want to "do the right thing."

For people raised outside the United States, their instincts as to what is right may be different from the expectations within the United States. The culture of many countries puts priority on a strong family system and assumes a standard of conduct that puts those family relationships first. Within the United States, it is the patient, not the family, who matters most. Patients, not family, are decision-makers. Patients, but not family, are entitled to information about their medical condition. Patients, not family, get to decide about the course of medical treatment or even if there will be any treatment at all. The family is valued and respected in the United States. But the family is not the patient, and in the end, the patient is at the cents of all that is decided and all that is done.

Values

Values are the foundational ideas that define our ethical universe. People with no values or ill-defined values behave in inconsistent manners and struggle to find the best ethical conduct. They can be merely reactive, without clarity about why they are doing what they do. Values are a filter that helps us make decisions in our lives. A person with high moral values will do the right thing, while the person with ill-defined values or wrong immoral values live with a constant uncertainty about what the right choice should be.

The textbook *Principles of Biomedical Ethics* by Tom Beauchamp and James Childress delineates four principles that should govern human values. These four principles are:

- Autonomy
- Beneficence
- Non-maleficence
- Justice

Autonomy

The word autonomy is a combination of two words, "autos" meaning self and nomos meaning rule, which means self-rule. This self-rule means that every individual has the right to self-determination. Now how does this autonomy fit into medical practice? What does that mean? It means that you cannot force anyone to do anything. You cannot enforce your decision upon anyone. It means that if you feel that the patient should take medication, but the patient does not want to take it, then you cannot force the patient to take the decision against his/her will [3].

IMGs need to know that in many countries the doctor-patient relationship is doctor-centered, where doctors behave like bosses and impose their decisions on the patients. In fact, some doctors yell at the patients and get upset if the patient refuses to take a medication and requested another medication. They sometimes say, "Am I the doctor or are you the doctor? Don't teach me what to do?" This kind of behavior comes when the doctors fail to learn the concept of autonomy. The patient has the right to say no or yes to the treatment advised.

The doctor can only advise and propose a treatment but cannot force the treatment. An easy way to remember this concept is to look at a waiter at a restaurant. The waiter greets you when you go to a restaurant, presents the menu of options, and asks for your choice and fulfills your order. How would you feel if a waiter says, "No, I will not serve you chicken; I will serve you beef because I feel it's best for you"? You would likely be upset and will probably not visit such a restaurant.

We clinicians are not too different from a waiter. We present options and answer the patient's questions so they have an understanding of what is possible, and then the patient decides based on that understanding. Every individual has the right to say "no" or "yes" to anything. No one, not even family, can force anyone about anything. Especially in the United States, since the United States is a free country, everyone understands freedom, and patients will not appreciate if you try to force a procedure or test without patient's consent. Do not be a boss or parent of your patient; be what you are, a doctor.

Case Example 1

A Jehovah's Witnesses follower is brought to the ER and is in critical condition. He is about to go into hemodynamic shock. If he does not receive blood, he will die. He states that I am a Jehovah's Witness and I do not want blood transfusion, and later he passed out. The doctors understand that since he has lost a lot of blood, his brain was not working to the fullest. Therefore, the doctor administers blood to save the life of the patient. Is this action of the doctor ethical?

A) *Yes*
B) *No*

Answer: The correct answer is B. The patient clearly said he does not want blood when was conscious. Therefore, the action by the doctor is wrong.

Can Patients Lose Autonomy?

Yes, if they are not mentally capable of understanding or making a decision. A patient who is unconscious cannot make a decision. That said, if the patient can be roused to consciousness, they regain their autonomy. We also cannot ignore a patient's prior decision if they lapse into an unconscious state. And, if the patient is unconscious and we turn to the family for guidance, we are asking the family to help us understand what the patient likely would want, not what decision the family wants to make.

If the patient is mentally incapable, they can also lose the autonomy to make decisions. But, and this is critical, we should start with the assumption that the patient remains the decision-maker and only stop listening to them when their lack of capacity is clear. The standard is whether we can get information from or give information to the patient. If we can, even if it is difficult, the patient remains the decision-maker.

Remember that patients with psychiatric diagnoses still have full autonomy to make medical decisions regarding their care. The same is true for mentally incapable patients. A patient with depression who refuses treatment for diagnosed cancer has the right to refuse treatment. It's the patient's ability, not the diagnosis, which matters here. We do not want to set up a process by which the physician can label a patient with a psychiatric diagnosis and then stop listening to the patient based on the asserted diagnosis. On the other hand, a patient who says, "I'm going to kill myself do not try and stop me" is assumed to lack capacity, and we do everything we can to stop the suicide and save their life.

The autonomy of the patient and the right to make decisions means that if the patient is dying and refuses medical treatment, you cannot save the patient. We respect that patient's autonomy even unto death.

Note that minor children (under age 18) have no autonomy and, therefore, do not make decisions regarding their own treatment. Decisions about a child's treatment are made by parents or legal guardians. Importantly, the parent's right to refuse treatment for the child has a strong limitation. Parents are not allowed to if they refuse life- or limb-saving treatment. This limitation on the parent's ability to refuse is true regardless of the parents' personal or religious beliefs.

A 13-year-old boy needs blood transfusion to survive. His parents and the boy himself refuse blood transfusion. The time is running, and the boy could die anytime. What should a doctor do?

Answer:

Proceed with blood transfusion. The boy is a minor and cannot refuse treatment, while the parents cannot refuse life-saving treatment.

Beneficence

The word beneficence means taking actions in the best interest of the patients. If the decision of the patient is not known, physicians should always take decisions in the best interest of his/her patient [4]. For example, if the patient is not able to communicate and there is no family member known or present, what does a doctor do? Should he treat the patient without signing the informed consent form? The simple answer to this question is, if medical attention is required, do what you think is best for the patient and you will be fine. The doctors should always take decision in the best interest of the patient, not the interests of the physician, the hospital, nor the family.

Good Samaritan Law

This law states that if a physician helps someone under a situation such as emergency in a nonmedical setting, he/she will not be held liable if there is an injury or death as a result of this action [5]. Note that the Good Samaritan laws do not protect nonphysicians or physicians without a license to practice medicine in the United States. Proper knowledge of Good Samaritan law is essential for the IMGs, so they understand that they can offer help to strangers in need.

Case Example 1

A doctor was driving to his hospital and saw a car accident. The passenger of
this car needed immediate CPR. The doctor saw this situation and continued
to drive because it was not his patient, and the doctor did not know about
insurance coverage and is afraid that he is opening himself up to legal risk if
the patient dies. Therefore, the doctor decided to continue driving and ignore
the accident. According to the medical ethics, the action of this doctor is?

A) Right, because the doctor could have lost his license and the patient is not
his patient
B) Wrong, because as a good human being, the doctor should have helped
the patient

Answer:
The correct answer is B; the decision of this doctor to continue driving and
not help this passenger was not the best approach because while helping the
patient if this patient had died, the Good Samaritan law protects the helper,
and the doctor would not have lost his license. When you have a choice, the
requirements of ethics override the minimum the law requires.

Non-maleficence

According to the Hippocratic Oath, it is more important to avoid harming the patient
than to do good [6]. If there is an equal chance of benefit or harm, then do not act.
We usually work this out by assessing the balance between benefit and harm.
Imagine that you have a patient who needs a medication A, and this medication A
has a side effect of headache, but if you do not prescribe this drug, then the patient
may die; then the benefits outweigh the risk. The harm is less with headache, and
not administering medication or prescribing is a bigger harm because the patient
can die without it. So, when you are weighing between two harms, choose the lesser
evil. On the other hand, if the drug has known side effects but only questionable
benefit, avoid prescribing the drug.

Non-maleficence also includes that being a physician it is the responsibility of a
doctor to ensure that the medication will not harm the patient. Not all drugs are good
for every patient; therefore, the doctor should study the side effects and take the
decision accordingly. The medication should not harm the patient; it should not
produce serious side effects, and if the side effect is inevitable, then choose the
lesser harm over the bigger harm of losing the life.

When maleficence is discussed, the principle of "double effect" is also brought
to discussion. The principle of double effect means that one action can lead to two
types of consequences. An example is a terminally ill patient, who has severe pain.
The doctor is now in a situation whether to administer high doses of morphine or
not. If the doctor administers high dose of morphine, it may have a negative impact

on patients' breathing and the patient may die. If the patient does not receive morphine, he will suffer more because of severe pain, and the patient is already dying and has no hope of survival. Under these circumstances, choosing the lesser evil is the best option. Since the chances of patients' survival are already dim, it is okay to try high-dose morphine to at least make his transition easier. This action of double effect is supported by the US Supreme Court.

Another example is pregnancy and abortion. A physician may consider abortion as unethical but probably must perform abortion if the mother's life is in danger. The fetus will be killed, but the mother will be saved. The intention is to save the mother, not to harm the baby. Not performing the abortion would lead to the death of mother and fetus both. Therefore, choosing an action with the least amount of negative effects is key criterion when assessing double effect.

I remember a case of my senior doctor who had to save a patient's life by offering a medication that could blind her fetus. The patient agreed, and eventually the patients' life was saved. The doctor showed non-maleficence by choosing the lesser evil. Happily, to our surprise, the baby turned out to be fine as well and had normal vision. Imagine protecting the baby's blindness had the doctor taken any other decision, the patient would have died and also the baby. But with this decision, the doctor saved the patient and the baby's life.

Justice

A just decision must always be taken. For example, if there is one ventilator available and there are many patients who need ventilator treatment, then the patient with the most need and the most hope of improvement should get the ventilator.

Conflicts

Autonomy Over Beneficence

If a treatment or decision is in the best interest of patient, but the patient refuses it, the clinician will listen to the patient.

A similar situation is euthanasia [7] where the patient is terminal but wants to help in speeding up time of death in order to avoid pain and suffering. Euthanasia is generally illegal in the United States but is now legal in 5 of the 50 states. Although euthanasia seems like it is the matter of patient's autonomy, it contradicts the concept of the doctor being a healer. A healer assisting in killing of his patient does not sound logical, which is why it is generally not legal.

In the United States, euthanasia is legal in California, Colorado, Oregon, Vermont, Washington, and Washington DC. Some other states do not consider it legal. Now for IMGs this knowledge is essential about the legal aspect as well as the ethical aspect. Always involve a senior or a supervisor if you are in a real-life scenario of euthanasia. Working as a team is the key, rather than taking such important decisions all alone. Proper considerations of all aspects are essential before making a decision.

The American Medical Association code of medical ethics suggests the following

Instead of engaging in euthanasia, physicians must aggressively respond to the needs of patients at the end of life. Physicians:

(a) Should not abandon a patient once it is determined that a cure is impossible.
(b) Must respect patient autonomy.
(c) Must provide good communication and emotional support.

Must provide appropriate comfort care and adequate pain control. *AMA Principles of Medical Ethics: I, IV* [8]

What Should IMGS Do?

Case Example 1
A first-year resident is alone with a patient in a remote residency program, and an end-stage cancer patient who has excruciating pain requests the resident to give him an injection that kills him so he can get rid of the pain. The patient's wife insists the resident help her husband to die with dignity because she also cannot see his pain. What should this resident do?

a) *If the state he is practicing legalizes it, then gives him the injection.*
b) *Refuse the injection because it is against ethics to kill the patient.*
c) *Inform the supervisor, and wait for the supervisor and other doctors to arrive and discuss the matter.*

Answer:
For a first-year resident, all important decisions must be okayed by senior physicians. This is not the resident's decision to make. Therefore, informing other staff members and waiting for the senior doctors and supervisors to arrive is the best approach.

Informed Consent

The patient must be informed about the treatment or procedure [9], ideally, both orally and in writing. Verbal presentation helps the patient to understand more easily, while the written document provides a legal record. IMGs need to remember this golden rule about practicing medicine in the United States that "Anything not written means not done." Therefore, it is essential to provide the informed consent form to the patient and have him/her sign it.

Note that for legal purposes, just having a signature is not enough. The patient must have a chance to read and consider the document. Paperwork which is signed quickly without being read may not stand up to legal scrutiny.

IMGs Must Remember

1. All informed consent documents *must* include the following five points:

   1. Nature of procedure
   2. Reason for the procedure
   3. Benefits of the procedure (the good being sought)
   4. Risks of the procedure (including the risk of doing nothing)
   5. Availability of alternatives (what other medical options are possible) [10]

2. The consent form should be provided in a written format and must be signed by the patient.
3. The patient must be an adult with an ability to understand the consent form.
4. The form should be in a language the patient understands.
5. A minor cannot give consent. Most people under age 18 (in a few states age 16) are considered minor. A parent or adult guardian must sign the form on the minor patient's behalf. However, under the rare situations of emancipated minor (minor not dependent on elders or married), the consent form can be signed by the minor.
6. The patient must be mentally stable to understand the form and give consent. A patient with mental disorder or with no orientation and ability to talk or communicate cannot provide informed consent.
7. Patients can choose someone else to make decisions on their behalf. This could be best seen in the situation where the patient is in a vegetative state and now the decision of ventilator being continued or discontinued must be taken. The patients can sign a form called "Advance Directive Form or DNR" as needed. If the patient signs DNR, then the ventilator will be discontinued. But if the patient chose someone else to be the decision-maker (health power of attorney), then that person will make the decision on the patient's behalf.

Confidentiality

It is rightly said that what happens in Vegas stays in Vegas. The same is true for the doctor-patient relationship. The conversation between a doctor and a patient should remain between the doctor and patient [11]. Many IMGs who come from a cultural background where community system is strong sometimes think that if someone is a family member of a patient, it is okay to tell him about the conversation or the patient's health-related information could be disclosed. This is not okay and acceptable under any circumstances, especially in the United States.

In 1996, President Bill Clinton signed the HIPAA law which protects patient's privacy [12]. According to the HIPAA law, any identifiable information of a patient cannot be shared with anyone without patient's consent, not even with a patient's family members. See below.

Can Confidentiality Be Breached Under Some Circumstances?

The confidentiality can be breached if there is a danger to life or health, for example, a husband diagnosed with HIV who wants to hide this from his wife or vice versa. The doctor must breach confidentiality to protect the life of the spouse. Most states also require a physician to report gunshot wound and impaired driver to DMV. Similarly, if a pediatrician feels that the child has been physically or sexually abused, he must report it to the Child Protective Services (CPS); the same is true for a non-pediatrician who sees bruises on a woman's body and suspects physical abuse; he may report it to the police if there is a clear evidence of abuse even though the wife denies any such abuse. Suicide attempt cases come under the confidentiality breaching scenarios.

Case Example 1

A 43-year-old patient during a conversation with a psychiatrist in an outpatient clinic says, "I have thought a lot and realized that I don't want to live anymore....I have decided to kill myself." The psychiatrist tried to convince him not to do it, but the patient refused. The psychiatrist asks him, "I understand, but do you have a plan?" The patient replies, "Yes I bought a gun and after I leave this appointment, I will go and kill myself." What should a psychiatrist do, considering that the conversation between a psychiatrist and a patient should remain strictly confidential?

a) *The psychiatrist should keep this information confidential and should not tell this to anyone. Otherwise, it will be a breach of confidentiality.*
b) *The psychiatrist should prescribe him with an antidepressant medication.*
c) *The psychiatrist should involve other staff members including the supervisor to handle this situation.*
d) *The psychiatrist should immediately call 911.*

Answer:
c) & d) Immediately involve other staff members and take appreciate decision. If it is an outpatient facility, then calling 911 will also help. (The physician should not allow the patient to leave, should involve any staff members necessary, and should call the police.)

Case Example 2

A 28-year-old woman told her doctor during a routine visit that "I have a gun and after I leave this office, I am going to kill my husband." The doctor tries to convince her not to do so. However, she refused to listen and rushes out of the doctor's office. What is the next course of action?

a) *Call 911 and inform them.*
b) *Call the husband and warn him.*
c) *Call the patient again and try to convince her one more time.*
d) *Don't do anything because it will be breach of confidentiality.*

Answer:
The correct answer is B because it is no more a confidentiality issue. The doctor needs to protect the husband. Calling 911 would be the next step after warning the husband. First warning the husband will provide the husband with some time to go to a safer place.

Case Example 3

A 31-year-old male patient is just diagnosed with gonorrhea. He requests the doctor, "Please keep it confidential. I acquired it because I had been seeing hookers lately, and my professional and personal reputation will be at stake. Also if my wife finds out, she will divorce me." What should the doctor do?

a) *Assure him that anything he told the doctor will remain strictly confidential.*
b) *Tell him that "of course I cannot tell this to your professional colleagues, but I have to inform your wife. I need to call her as soon as possible."*
c) *The doctor should just treat the patient and not worry about the wife or professional colleagues. Being a physician, a doctor has nothing to do with his patient's wife.*

Answer:
B) Informing the wife is necessary to protect her from an illness. This situation cannot remain confidential because the spouse is at risk of acquiring infection. The professional colleagues do not need to know this, but only the wife will be informed.

The Health Insurance Portability and Accountability Act (HIPAA)

When we talk about confidentiality, the chapter will remain incomplete until we discuss the Health Insurance Portability and Accountability Act (HIPAA). HIPAA law was signed in 1996 by President Bill Clinton. The law was signed mainly to improve the way we deal with healthcare information to create confidentiality systems within and beyond healthcare facilities and to keep protected health information (PHI) private [13].

The law has five titles:

- Title 1: Protects health insurance coverage for employees and their families in the event of switching or losing employment.
- Title 2: Prevents Health Care Fraud and Abuse; Medical Liability Reform; Administrative Simplification (AS) that emphasizes on the establishment of national standards for electronic healthcare transactions. The requirement national identifiers for healthcare providers, insurance providers, and employers are also included in Title 2.
- Title III establishes guidelines for pre-tax medical spending accounts.
- Title IV sets guidelines for group health plans.
- Title V controls company-owned life insurance policies [14].

Title 2 and HIPAA Privacy Rule

The Department of Health and Human Services (HHS) initiated five rules regarding Administrative Simplification:

1. The privacy rule
2. The transactions and code sets rule
3. The security rule
4. The unique identifiers rule
5. The enforcement rule

Privacy Rule

This is the most important rule IMGs should have knowledge about in regard to ethical concerns of confidentiality. For this reason, only this part is discussed in this chapter for the IMGs and other readers to understand. This rule regulates the use and disclosure of protected health information (PHI) by health insurers, employer-sponsored health plans, and medical provider (all of these are referred to as covered entities). Signed consent by patient is required to use or disclose PHI [15].

The Terminologies

Use of Information
Means how the information is used within a hospital or facility.

Disclosure of Information

How information is disclosed outside the hospital or facility.

Exceptions to the Privacy Rule

There is some exception to the privacy rule that IMGs need to know:

- A covered entity may disclose PHI to law enforcement if court orders, court-ordered warrants, subpoenas, and administrative requests are presented.
- To facilitate treatment, payment, or healthcare operations without a patient's written authorization
- Gunshot wound
- Stab wounds
- Injuries sustained in a crime
- Child or elderly abuse
- Infectious, communicable, or reportable diseases

The Type of Data Protected

Written, spoken, typed, printed on paper, or electronic (email).

How Can IMGs Easily Be Compliant to HIPAA Privacy Rule?

IMGs while working must:

- Never discuss any identifiable patient information in public. Ideally, the best approach is not to discuss your patients at a public location at all. These conversations could be done privately with the fellow doctors involved in the care of the same patient.
- Never leave their computers signed in and unattended.
- Never reveal patient information over the phone.
- Must never hide patient information from the patient himself. If the patient asks for his medical records, provide it.

Case Example 1

Two doctors are having lunch together in a hospital cafeteria. Doctor A asks doctor B: You are treating Mrs. Davidson these days. I see her coming often to your office. She is my mother's best friend. Is everything okay with her? Why is she coming? Doctor B should say:

A) *Poor woman is diagnosed with cancer and I am seeing her.*
B) *I cannot share any patient's information with anyone else who is not involved in the patient care.*

Answer:
The correct answer is B. Politely declining to answer such a question is the best approach. It will maintain the confidentiality, as well as protect the doctor from being HIPAA noncompliance.

Case Example 2

A team of parole and police officers arrives at a psychiatric facility with substance use patients and sex offenders. The parole officer asks the doctor on duty, "Is Mr. XYZ still admitted to this facility? Can we speak with him?" What should be the best course of action at this point?

A) *The doctor should comply with the law and provide the accurate information and take the officers to the patient.*
B) *The doctor should politely decline by saying, "I cannot confirm, nor deny the presence of this patient at our facility."*

Answer:
The correct answer is B; without a court order or information that the patient is an immediate threat to self or others, you cannot provide the information, even to the police or law enforcement team.

Cultural Ethics

IMGs come to the United States from almost all parts of the world. The biggest pool of IMGs comes from India, Pakistan, Bangladesh, and Middle East. Another large percentage of IMGs are from European countries. The Asian countries usually have a culture of community system where an extended family system is common. Although each culture has its own beauty and its own uniqueness, when students come to the United States, they must adapt to the US cultural expectations.

Many IMGs from some Asian countries find it difficult to always shake hands (pre-Covid-19) and say "thank you" and "please" to the patients. These social rituals are an essential part of doctor-patient relationship. Similarly, the eye contact is also important to make a human connection and establish a sense of trust. However, in certain cultures, due to religious or culture prohibition, people don't look into the eyes of the opposite gender. If this habit persists in the United States, patients may take it a sign that the physician is inattentive, doesn't care, or is even disrespectful. To be understood by patients, nonverbal and verbal communication should follow local, in this case US, custom. What you do in your personal life is your choice. But a communication style that establishes rapport is part of professional practice.

One of the authors of this chapter (HT) have seen in some people from the region he came from that they don't wait for the other person to finish their sentence, and it is absolutely okay in that culture. It is a sign of respect, and it means, "I am focusing on you and I am listening to you and engaging in a conversation with you. I have understood exactly what you mean." The other person feels heard, and listened to, and feels important. However, in the United States, if you cut off somebody who is still talking, you have crossed a boundary; you have disrespected him/her. Many IMGs struggle with this concept; they do not wait for the patient or the other person to be done talking completely. When the other person or specially a patient is interrupted, imagine what the patient will feel about the doctor. Again, whatever you do in your personal life is your business. But when interacting with patients, listening more and talking less is better professional practice.

Smiling is a particularly important part of the Western culture. In some countries, smiling while greeting is not a norm, and it could be mistaken for something else, especially if it is between opposite genders. But in the United States, if you greet your patient and do not smile, it will generally be seen as a sign of rudeness, arrogance, or disinterest.

To reiterate what we have said before, these comments should in no way be taken to imply that behaviors in cultures outside the United States are wrong but only that they are different and that the process of engaging patients, essential for medical practice, is best achieved by matching patient's cultural expectations. Nor do we mean to imply that everyone and all parts of the United States are the same. The United States is a large, diverse country comprised of many difference backgrounds. Rather, our recommendation is to develop a sensitivity to the expectations of each patient and approach them in a way that recognizes those expectations.

Religion and Medical Ethics

Different religions may differ in many aspects; however, on the following points, they all are in a unanimous agreement:

- Beneficence: All religions believe in doing good. It is referred to as altruism.
- Maleficence: Doing no harm is also an essential feature of all major religions of the world.
- Autonomy: This is also discussed in major religions. Every individual has the right to decide what is good or bad for himself.

These are some major similarities with modern medical ethics and major religions of the world. However, on the subject of euthanasia, religion and modern medical ethics could differ. For example, all major religions are against suicide. Yet in medical ethics there is a disagreement among the doctors. In some places it is illegal, while in some places it is legal.

Similarly, all religions support the act of random kindness, and offering and accepting a gift is okay; however, in medical ethics, the subject of gift giving and receiving is a topic of debate. See below.

Therefore, for IMGs it is important to study medical ethics and implement the principles in their professional and personal lives to understand what is considered ethical and what is not.

Conflict of Interest

Conflicts of interest are one of the most commonly discussed matters in regard to medical ethics [16]. A conflict of interest occurs when a physician is involved in multiple interests, where performing one action supporting one interest could work against other action which would be more favorable to the patient's interests. A "conflict of interest" occurs if a clinician will make more money if one treatment option is chosen. The interest of the patient, not the financial benefit to the physician, should be the sole focus.

All doctors take some form of payment for their services. This is okay because physicians are entitled to be compensated for their time and effort. However, when financial gain carries more weight or even becomes a priority, then it becomes a problem. Secondly, physician payment is not a hidden agenda; it's openly decided and documented. The problem lies with undisclosed interests such as sending patients to specific facilities in which the physician has a financial interest.

Examples of conflict of interest include situations in which business interests influence the actual results or publication of a clinical trial. This is the reason why it is important to disclose any possible conflict of interest in scientific manuscripts. Note that it is illegal for a physician to get commission from a pharmaceutical company for prescribing a particular drug. The IMGs should be aware of these common scenarios and should be careful about it when they start practicing medicine as a doctor in the United States. The risk here is not just ethical but legal. Any wrong decision and failure in judgment can be detrimental for their careers.

Common Examples of Conflict of Interest

Referral

It is considered unethical, and often illegal, for physicians to receive commission for sending a patient for lab tests to a specific lab, especially if he/she has a financial interest in that lab. Evidence suggests that doctors who refer patients to the lab with financial interest (it could be self-referral to one's own lab) tend to send more patients for lab tests [16]. Sending patients to get unnecessary test is clearly illegal. This is a clear conflict of interest, and it could lead to serious problems for the IMGs if they engage in such activities.

Receiving Gifts from Pharmaceutical Companies and Labs

The practice of receiving compensation from pharmaceutical companies in exchange of prescribing their medications is a common practice throughout the world.

Evidence suggests that doctors' decisions are influenced by gifts or compensation by a pharmaceutical company [17]. Some renowned universities, and all published ethics guidelines, have banned the practice of accepting gifts from pharmaceutical companies. Note that, by law, pharmaceutical companies must make public all payments they make to physicians for presentations or consulting. Therefore, IMGs need to be careful about this practice. This cannot just harm their reputation but can in fact put them in trouble with the authorities.

Receiving Gifts from Patients

A doctor should almost always say "no" to a gift presented to them by their patients. Many ethics experts believe that it is okay if the gift is of small amount (under 20 dollars). However, we suggest IMGs should be careful about this practice. It is always safer to say "no" to a gift and refuse politely by saying, "Thank you for your kind thought, but I just do not accept gifts from patients."

Accepting gift can lead to crossing the professional boundary. Gifts are symbolic. What is intended by the gift? Is the gift a statement for friendship or perhaps a suggestion for a romantic encounter? We also want to avoid creating the impression that gifts are necessary or may result in preferential treatment or better care. A doctor-patient relationship is just a doctor-patient relationship and nothing else. We want to avoid all confusion.

Intimate Relationship Between a Doctor and Patient

Intimate or sexual relationship between a physician and a patient is always a big NO. Under no circumstances a doctor should engage in sexual relationship with a patient [18]. In some states, you can wait 2 years to finish a clinician-patient relationship. However, we suggest IMGs should be extremely careful of this situation. Consider what might happen if a relationship begins but then ends badly and results in hostile feelings. The consequences could be severe from damage to reputation to being expelled from the job to losing the medical license. This conflict of interest especially is clear in a relationship such as psychiatrist-patient relationship but holds for all physician-patient relationships.

Futile Medical Care

Futile care is a medical treatment that does not benefit the patient anymore [19]. Sometimes IMGs will be in a situation where a treatment seems not to be effective anymore and they have to take a decision whether to continue or discontinue the treatment. If a doctor has reasonable cause to believe that this treatment will not help the patient, the treatment can be discontinued. This will not be considered as euthanasia, because in euthanasia the intention is to end the patient's life to avoid pain, while in futility the intention is not to end life but to end treatment, because there is no hope that the patient will survive. Continuing the treatment will deprive other patients from the same treatment who do have a hope of survival. For example, a patient on ventilator has no hope of survival, and there is another patient who does have a hope of survival; under these circumstances, a physician takes a "just" decision and ends the futile care.

However, if there is some slim possibility of recovery and the patient's family, representing the patient's wishes, wants the treatment to continue, then the treatment should be continued. Treatment continues even if the physician thinks it should stop.

Other General Ethics to Remember

Dress Code

Some doctors underestimate the importance of official dress code of a doctor. IMGs should be well dressed when practicing medicine and groomed and behave like a physician. The dress code helps in rapport building with a patient. It is quite natural to be impressed by a well-groomed and well-dressed doctor than a doctor who does not care about his dress code and look. The scrubs they wear should be cleaned, ironed, and organized.

Personal Hygiene

Personal hygiene is an important aspect of the life of a physician. Mature and smart doctors ensure that they are well groomed and cleaned. Daily showers are essential. Physicians should avoid the use of cologne or perfume because some patients have allergies. No patient would like a doctor who doesn't look after his/her personal hygiene. Patients judge the care they will receive based on the care the physician takes with him/her.

Boundaries

Maintaining a balance between professional and personal boundaries is essential for a successful career as a clinician. IMGs must learn some basic boundaries that are essence of the US culture. For example, you cannot force your fellow colleague to do certain things that you like. Everyone has the right to say "no," and a "no" means no.

Adding patients to your Facebook or Instagram is not okay. It is clearly crossing the professional boundary. The patients are not your friends. If a patient sends you a friend request, you can decline it. Many physicians find that they are best served by staying off of social media altogether. Similarly, you are not bound to share your personal phone number with the patients. Communication through a professional university or hospital email is ideal. Texting and emailing through personal phone or email address puts the IMGs at risk of being HIPAA noncompliant.

The same is true for accepting dinner or lunch requests by your patients. Thanking them for a nice gesture and declining the offer politely is the best approach.

Professional Manners

The USMLE Step 2 CS trains IMGs well for the professional manners such as knocking the door before entering the room and asking permission before examining. Due to Covid-19, Step 2 CS is suspended for a while; therefore, IMGs must practice these manners.

These manners also apply to professional relationship with the fellow doctors. It is not okay to enter a fellow colleague's room without knocking, and it is not okay to not smile and shake hands (once Covid-19 declines). Any manners taught in Step 2 CS are very much applicable while interacting with other doctors and staff members.

Interfering

In some cultures, it is okay to answering a friend's call on his cellphone. However, in the United States, it is not appreciated. The IMGs must learn the US customs and culture. It is disrespectful to read someone's mail or text message without their permission. It is probably okay under a life-threatening emergency, but under usual circumstances it is not okay.

If a fellow colleague is dating a staff member, it is none of anyone's business. Gossip creates ill feelings and makes relationships nonprofessional. What is someone's religious or political affiliation is also none of anyone else's business. Focusing on one's job and not worrying about fellow colleagues' or patient's religion, race, gender, and sexual orientation should be the professional conduct all IMGs should follow.

Discrimination

There is zero tolerance of discrimination of any kind at workplace. The United States is founded based on equality. Every individual must be respected regardless of their age, gender, caste, creed, culture, religion, or sexual orientation. Discrimination is not only wrong; it is against the law.

Research Publications and Ethics

Most IMGs are aware that they need research publications in order to be more competitive for US residency. Due to the lack of knowledge and experience, many IMGs have put themselves in trouble due to not properly conducting research. For example, three Indian-American doctors were arrested for scientific fraud in 2020 [20]. Any hint of fraud will likely end your career. In order to avoid such problems, IMGs need to be aware of the following practices that should be avoided:

1. Scientific fraud: Creating fraudulent and fake research findings in order to get publications.
2. Plagiarism: Plagiarizing is one of those mistakes, where intention doesn't matter. Many IMGs have been banned by various journals because of plagiarizing their research manuscript.
3. Buying publications: It is a common practice nowadays that some students like to pay someone to add their names in the publication without working hard. IMGs must be careful about any such activity. This is a career-ending offense if uncovered.

Ethical Issues That IMGs May Face While Working in the United States as a Physician

Here in this part of the chapter, we will discuss some issues that IMGs may face while practicing in the United States in the light of how things are in certain other countries versus how the things work in the United States. We will discuss the scenarios about how things are in some other countries initially, followed by how the things are in the United States. The point is not to criticize the way things are in other countries but compare and see how different the things work in the United States.

Scenario 1: Disclosing Patients' Location
How Things Are in Some Other Countries

A 43-year-old man visits a hospital during the patient visiting hours and asks a front desk personnel, "Hi could you please tell me where the patient John Doe is staying?" The front desk personnel replies, "Are you his family member?" The man replies, "Yes." The front desk personnel replies, "He is in room 204, second floor, the elevator is on the right."

Explanation

The front desk personnel guided a family member toward the patient's room number. The idea behind this behavior is that the patient and family members have already suffered a lot; therefore, depriving the patient from seeing his family and vice versa is not appropriate. We should help the family and the patient and remove any unnecessary barriers for them to see their family member who is admitted.

Some private hospitals in many urban areas will not allow this without asking for an identification card of the visitor. However, in many rural areas, the concept of asking for identification card is almost nonexistent. Several countries around the world don't have the laws like HIPAA; therefore, it is not a big deal if anyone knows about the patient's condition, and it is also assumed that usually the family members are already aware of the patient's condition. This may sound strange for a person accustomed to the US way of dealing with the same situation, but this is the normal way of many cultures.

How the Things Are in The United States?

Rules regarding patient confidentiality seek to balance the needs of family with a patient's right to privacy. In the past 20 years, these privacy rules have been codified in the Federal Health Insurance Portability and Accountability Act of 1996 (HIPAA). Remember that these general rules can be modified by customary practices and specific policies of individual medical institutions. Some hospitals are much stricter about confirming any patient information. Others are less so:

1. If a family member asks if a patient is in the hospital, the information is usually provided. Confirming the identity of the family member is good policy. Hospital security is increasingly strict, and visitors have to show identity and sign in when they enter the hospital premises.
2. Note that while confirming that a patient is in the hospital, no information about the patient's medical condition should be shared. The general rule is that information should flow from patient to family.
3. Even if hospital policy allows confirming that a patient is admitted, a patient must be given the chance to opt out of that policy. If you are a patient and do not want people, including family, to know that you are in the hospital, you have the right to say so, and the hospital is obligated to follow your personal wishes regarding confidentiality.
4. If the patient is unconscious, the physician may discuss the case with the family if they feel it is to the benefit of the patient. The discussions commonly involve gaining information about medical history, current medical conditions, and any current medications. Note that these discussions with family are the discretion of the physician and exclusively for the patient's benefit. The family does *not* have the right to know the medical details about the patient.

Scenario 2: Gunshot Wound Patients
How It Is in Some Other Countries?

A gunshot wound patient is brought to the hospital emergency department. The patient is bleeding profusely. The hospital staff and the doctors tell the family members of the patient, "This is a police case; please bring the police report; otherwise, we cannot treat him." The family insists on treating the patient because he is bleeding and can die without immediate treatment. The hospital staff says, "Sorry we cannot do anything to save his life without a police report."

Explanation

The hospital tries to stay away from legal issues and matters where police is involved, mainly to avoid unnecessary stress and protection against unwanted investigations by the law enforcement agencies.

How It Is in the United States?

Gunshot wounds are treated as medical emergencies. The principle is treat first, and then report. However, after treatment, by law, gunshot wounds must be reported to police or other relevant law enforcement agencies. Failure to make such a report can result in a physician's arrest:

1. Note that the wishes of patient or accompanying family are not relevant here. Even if they insist that the gunshot injury not be reported, the law must be followed, and a report must be made.
2. A report must be whether the gunshot injury was the result of an assault, accident, or suicide attempt.
3. Other issues requiring mandatory report are child abuse and sexual assault.

Scenario 3: Pay the Bill First
How It Is in Some Other Countries?

A patient with myocardial infarction is brought to the hospital and needs urgent help. The doctor sees the patient informed the family members that an urgent angioplasty is needed. The hospital staff says, "Please pay the bill first; then, we will start treatment." The family says, "We will arrange money; please start the treatment." The hospital refused to treat the patient.

Explanation

Many countries around the world don't have the health insurance system the way we have in the United States. Therefore, the only way the hospitals are paid is by the patients paying out of pocket, regardless of the expense. Therefore, under these circumstances, if the hospitals allow the treatment first because of humanity, many patients may never pay and will be difficult to trace and complete the payment after they are treated. The hospitals will not be able to pay their staff including the doctor's salaries and eventually will be closed permanently. The belief is it's better to have a hospital where you pay and get treated than no hospital.

How It Is in the United States?

In emergency situations, once the patient comes into the hospital, they are treated. Patients who come into the hospital are asked how they are going to pay, but even if they cannot pay, life- or limb-saving treatment must be provided:

1. If the patient has no means of payment (insurance, personal wealth) and they have a condition requiring emergency care, the needed care will be provided. However, once the patient is "stabilized," they may be transferred to a public

hospital where no payment is expected. The hospital must deal with the health crisis but is not obligated to take on longer-term care.
2. The number one reason for bankruptcy in the United States is inability to pay for medical treatment. Treatment occurs, but then the hospital usually tries to collect. Note that the hospital, or any physician, can choose to waive their fees, although as a rule they generally try to collect.
3. For hospitals to maintain their not-for-profit status (a considerable tax benefit), they must provide at least 20% of the care they give without compensation. For-profit hospitals do not have to follow this regulation.

Scenario 4: Patient Consent
How the Things Are in Some Other Countries?

A patient was informed by the doctor that he requires an invasive surgery. The patient denies the treatment and says, "Give me something noninvasive." The doctor gets upset and yells at the patient and says, "Are you a doctor? Do you know how you should be treated? Or am I the doctor?" The patient is forced to go through the surgery that he never wanted.

Explanation

The healthcare system in some countries is doctor-centered, which means that the doctor will decide the treatment and the doctor is the healer and has paternalistic attitude. The doctor behaved in such a way in the best interest of the patient because being a health expert the doctor knows the best treatment.

How the Things Are in the United States?

No medical procedure can occur without the patient's explicit informed consent. The physician informs, but the patient consents. Patients have an absolute right to refuse treatment. Patients are required to sign written documents demonstrating consent which contain all of the necessary information:

1. Informed consent means that the patient must "receive and understand" five pieces of information:

   - The procedure proposed
   - Reasons why the procedure is needed
   - The benefits of the procedure
   - The risks of the procedure (including the risks of doing nothing)
   - A review of *all* alternative treatments which are available

2. Note that a doctor who says, "If you will not follow my recommendations, then I cannot continue to be your physician" is guilty of "abandonment" and can be subject to civil and professional penalties.
3. If the patient is uneducated, then the physician must take the time to be sure they are fully informed.
4. Only patient's consent, not family consent, matters.
5. Yelling at a patient is never acceptable and will likely result in a complaint being lodged with the hospital and possible disciplinary action by whomever manages the medical staff.

Scenario 5: Patient Privacy
How Things Are in Some Other Countries?
Two doctors are walking in a hospital hallway and discussing the patient who was recently admitted. They are discussing the patient's condition so loud that another doctor hears it and gives them more ideas and suggestions on what should be the investigation they should order. The third doctor gets involved and gives more ideas on how to manage the patient.

Explanation
The idea behind this is that culturally it is not a problem if anyone overhears anyone's health issue in the hospital especially. Moreover, the more clinician's minds are involved, the better ideas and suggestions will be provided. It is in the best interest of the patient to involve more doctors, and it is okay if someone, even a nonphysician, overhears the conversation because doctors know what is in the best interest of their patients.

How Things Are in the United States?
As a rule, discussing a patient's case anywhere you might be overheard is a violation of the patient's right to privacy. Discussions should occur in situations where privacy can be reasonably assumed like in an office or a vacant room:

1. In practice, this rule is not strictly followed. Busy physicians may talk about a patient while walking together because that is the moment they have to communicate. But, understand, it is still a violation of the rules. Not every driver comes to a complete stop at a stop sign, but we all know that we are supposed to do.
2. Discussing patient with a colleague while out to lunch or dinner is also a breach of the rules.
3. Note that getting a consultation from another physician for the good of the patient is excellent medical practice and should be encouraged. But consultation should be sought and not come as the result of an overheard conversation.

Scenario 6: Patient Privacy with Other Patients
The pulmonology ward has over 25 patients admitted. The attending physician is on a round and talking to all the patients one by one. All the patients can hear the doctor talking while he is discussing the health-related issue with a patient.

Explanation
It is culturally okay if anyone hears anyone's private health-related information especially when all others are also patients with similar diseases.

How Things Are in the United States?
If many patients are on a large ward, or even if two patients are sharing a room, with similar diseases, the physician's discussion with one patient will certainly be heard by other patients. However, care should be taken to reduce what others might hear. Discussion with each patient should be at a volume which is loud enough to allow a caring conversation but not so loud as to broadcast details over the entire ward:

1. The physician should also set the expectation that patients will respect each other's privacy.

2. If topics of sensitivity must be discussed with a patient, such as difficult medical news or embarrassing diagnoses, the physician should try to find a more private spot for those conversations to occur.

Scenario 7: The Laboratory Tests
How Things Are in Some Other Countries?

A doctor orders lab test from a lab that is half an hour away, although the same test is available in the hospital lab. The patient asks the doctor why I should go 30 minutes away when I can have it done here. The doctor yells at the patient and forces him to obey his orders. Later on, it was discovered that the doctor gets commission from that lab that he recommended for each referral.

Explanation

Because of the paternalistic attitude and culture, doctors do normally yell at the patient in the best interest of the patient in order to motivate and help educate the patient. But under these circumstances, there is no explanation and excuse of this behavior. It is ethically wrong in almost majority of countries for a physician to get commission on referrals.

How Things Are in the United States?

Patients can elect to have their laboratory tests conducted at a facility of their choice. Most often, because it is more convenient, laboratory tests are simply sent to a facility affiliated with the hospital. This generally provides quicker and speedier access to results, as well as merging test results seamlessly into the medical record which is better for the patient. However, the patient can elect to have their laboratory tests done where they wish, just as they have the choice to decide where their prescriptions will be filled:

1. Commissions for referrals (laboratory tests, radiological scans, specialists) are illegal and can be grounds for suspension of medical licensure.
2. Yelling at a patient is considered unprofessional and may result in a complaint being filed or the patient deciding to find another physician. Given a choice, patients do not like to be yelled at.

Scenario 8: Baby Delivery
How Things Are in Some Other Countries?

A 28-year-old female patient just delivered a baby at a local hospital. The nurses on duty took the baby away from the mother to shower and clean the baby. The mother wanted to spend some time with the baby and requested the baby be given to her first and let her spend some time with her baby. The nurses replied, "No. According to the hospital policy, we cannot give the baby to you. Once you are a little better and ready to look after the baby, only then we will return the baby to you."

Explanation

There is mostly a good intention behind this action. The usual assumption is that the patient is weak and has just delivered the baby. It will be an added stress if we leave her to look after her baby. Let us take the baby away and let her rest and we will take care of the baby.

It is usually the hospital's policy that the nurses must follow.

How Things Are in the United States?

Although certain medical conditions may require the newborn to be isolated, allowing contact between mother and child is the usual procedure and highly recommended. The early connection facilitates bonding and attachment and lets the mother feel the physical reality of the new child. I know of a number of mothers with newborns who refused to let the child out of their sight for fear that the nurses would bring her back the wrong baby!

1. The mother is in charge and her wishes should be followed.
2. We also strongly encourage that the father (if available) be involved in all aspects of the birthing procedure and care for the infant.

Scenario 9: Another Baby Delivery Scenario
How Things Are in Some Other Countries?

A 38-year-old G1P1 woman is admitted to the hospital for baby delivery. The doctor suggests the patient should go for C-section. However, the patient refused the surgery and requested normal delivery and feels she can do it. The hospital is notorious of doing unnecessary C-sections to make money. When the patient refused, the doctor on duty got upset and yelled at the patient and forcefully conducted C-section.

Explanation

There is no explanation of any bad behavior. Performing unnecessary surgical procedures to make more money is wrong and cannot be justified.

How Things Are in the United States?

The patient, under the doctrine of informed consent, decides what procedure will be done. Court cases in the United States make it clear that the mother has the absolute right to refuse C-section, even if that physician thinks that the procedure would be best for the child. The pregnant woman is the patient and, therefore, the decision-maker:

1. Note that the father has no say in what procedure is selected. She is the patient, not him. It is her, and she gets to choose what is done with it.
2. Of course, the physician can recommend, even encourage, certain courses of action. But the ultimate decision rests with the patient, in this case the pregnant woman.
3. Yelling at a patient is unprofessional and never the right approach to gaining patient cooperation. As has been mentioned previously, physicians who yell at their patients tend to lose those patients and may be subject to negative evaluations by peers.

Scenario 10: Doctor Makes A Mistake
How Things Are in Some Countries?

During a surgery, the surgeon involved made a mistake by incising the left lower quadrant of the patient instead of the right lower quadrant. After realizing the mistake, the surgeon rectified the mistake by making the incision on the right side and performed the surgery. After the patient woke up, he was informed about the successful surgery and was discharged. Upon arriving home, he realized that there was an extra incision on the left side, about which he was not informed.

Explanation

Some doctors in some countries think they are the all-knowing experts. Therefore, admitting the mistake can hurt their ego, and they may lose the respect in the eyes of everyone else including the fellow colleagues. There is no explanation and excuse for the bad behavior. Almost all cultures and countries will agree that this doctor did the wrong thing by not telling the patient about his human error.

How Things Are in the United States?

Patients must be told everything, including about medical errors. Research and experience show that errors that are hidden and then uncovered are much more likely to result in angry patients and substantially more likely to result in the physician being sued for malpractice. Although admitting errors may seem hard or even damaging, when physicians are honest, patients are often very understanding, and the chance of a malpractice suit is markedly declined:

1. Liability insurance is required to practice medicine in the United States to provide the physician coverage if errors do result in malpractice litigation.
2. The surgeon in this case is a part of the problem in that the site for the surgery should have been marked by pen and signed off on by the patient before any incision was made. The surgical team also carries some blame in that they did not double-check to ensure the side was correct before the surgery began. The usual policy is for a "time-out" to occur during which the surgical team checks everything, including the site of the incision before the operation can begin. Everyone is responsible for checking everything, and any member of the surgical team can stop the procedure if something is not right. Smart surgeons welcome this process in that it reduces medical errors and corresponding legal issues.

Conclusion

Thousands of international medical graduates apply for the US residency each year. Despite studying ethics for USMLEs, the previous habit and lack of experience regarding ethical issues can impact IMGs' decision-making capability. Therefore, it is important that IMGs study the subject of ethics as much as they can, and when they are in any of the abovementioned situation, where they must take a decision, they should take a team decision initially by ideally involving a supervisor. They should ask their supervisor and senior doctors for suggestions until they are experienced enough to handle such situations all alone by themselves.

Acknowledgments The authors are grateful to Dr. Waqas Ahmed Burney from the University of California, Davis, for his valuable suggestions and ideas.

References

1. Ethic. Merriam Webster Dictionary. Available from https://www.merriam-webster.com/dictionary/ethics?src=search-dict-box
2. What is medical ethics, and why is it important? Medscape. Available from https://www.medscape.com/courses/section/898060
3. Arrieta Valero I. Autonomies in interaction: dimensions of patient autonomy and non-adherence to treatment. Front Psychol. 2019;10:1857. Published 2019 Aug 14. https://doi.org/10.3389/fpsyg.2019.01857.
4. Munyaradzi M. Critical reflections on the principle of beneficence in biomedicine. Pan Afr Med J. 2012;11:29.
5. Rozovsky LE. Doctors and the law of the Good Samaritan. Can Med Assoc J. 1971;105(4):387–9.
6. Tsai DF. Ancient Chinese medical ethics and the four principles of biomedical ethics. J Med Ethics. 1999;25(4):315–21. https://doi.org/10.1136/jme.25.4.315.
7. Gostin LO, Roberts AE. Physician-assisted dying: A turning point? JAMA. 2016;315(3):249–50. https://doi.org/10.1001/jama.2015.16586.
8. Euthanasia. AMA principles of medical ethics: I, IV. Chapter 5: Opinions on caring for patients at the end of life. Available from https://www.ama-assn.org/system/files/2019-06/code-of-medical-ethics-chapter-5.pdf
9. Faden RR, Beauchamp TL, NMP K. A history and theory of informed consent. New York: Oxford University Press; 1986.
10. Thewes J, FitzGerald D, Sulmasy DP. Informed consent in emergency medicine: ethics under fire. Emerg Med Clin North Am. 1996;14(1):245–54. https://doi.org/10.1016/s0733-8627(05)70249-2.
11. Shapiro R. Breaking the code: is a promise always a promise? In: Kushner TK, Thomasma DC, editors. Ward ethics: dilemmas for medical students and doctors in training. Cambridge: Cambridge University Press; 2001. p. 50–2.
12. Moskop JC, Marco CA, Larkin GL, Geiderman JM, Derse AR. From Hippocrates to HIPAA: privacy and confidentiality in emergency medicine – part I: conceptual, moral, and legal foundations. Ann Emerg Med. 2005;45(1):53–9. https://doi.org/10.1016/j.annemergmed.2004.08.008.
13. Health Insurance Portability and Accountability Act of 1996 (HIPAA). Center for Disease Control and Prevention. Available from https://www.cdc.gov/phlp/publications/topic/hipaa.html#:~:text=The%20Health%20Insurance%20Portability%20and,the%20patient's%20consent%20or%20knowledge.
14. HIPAA Title Information. DHCS. Available from https://www.dhcs.ca.gov/formsandpubs/laws/hipaa/Pages/1.10HIPAATitleInformation.aspx
15. The HIPAA Privacy Rule. Health Information Privacy. Available from https://www.hhs.gov/hipaa/for-professionals/privacy/index.html#:~:text=The%20HIPAA%20Privacy%20Rule%20establishes,certain%20health%20care%20transactions%20electronically.
16. Relman AS. Dealing with conflicts of interest. N Engl J Med. 1985;313:749–51.
17. Swedlow A, Johnson G, Smithline N, Milstein A. Increased costs and rates of use in the California workers' compensation system as a result of self-referral by physicians. N Engl J Med. 1992;327(21):1502–6. https://doi.org/10.1056/NEJM199211193272107.
18. Güldal D, Semin S. The influences of drug companies' advertising programs on physicians. Int J Health Serv. 2000;30(3):585–95. https://doi.org/10.2190/GYW9-XUMQ-M3K2-T31C. PMID 11109183.
19. Collier R. When the doctor-patient relationship turns sexual. CMAJ. 2016;188(4):247–8. https://doi.org/10.1503/cmaj.109-5230.
20. Indian origin doctors in the US fight charges of fake research based on fake data. National Herald. Available from https://www.nationalheraldindia.com/india/indian-origin-doctors-in-the-us-fight-charges-of-fake-research-based-on-fake-data

Chapter 18
The Alternative Career Pathways for International Medical Graduates in Health and Wellness Sector

Nashit Chowdhury, Mark Ekpekurede, Deidre Lake, and Turin Tanvir Chowdhury

Introduction

Who Are IMGs?

International medical graduates (IMGs) are the graduates from medical schools located outside of the country where the medical graduates intend to integrate professionally [1, 2]. They are also commonly mentioned as foreign medical graduates (FMGs) in academic literature, which is used as a Medical Subject Heading (MeSH) in the US National Library of Medicine as well [1]. Other terms that are interchangeably used include overseas trained graduates (OTGs), internationally trained physicians (ITPs), and internationally educated physicians (IEPs) [2]. These terms are commonly used in those countries where internationally trained medical graduates are important part of the physician workforce or migrate in larger numbers such

N. Chowdhury
Department of Family Medicine, Cumming School of Medicine, University of Calgary, Calgary, AB, Canada
e-mail: nashit.chowdhury@ucalgary.ca

M. Ekpekurede · D. Lake
Alberta International Medical Graduates Association (AIMGA), Calgary, AB, Canada
e-mail: deidre@aimga.ca

T. T. Chowdhury (✉)
Department of Family Medicine, Cumming School of Medicine, University of Calgary, Calgary, AB, Canada

Department of Community Health Sciences, Cumming School of Medicine, University of Calgary, Calgary, AB, Canada
e-mail: turin.chowdhury@ucalgary.ca

© Springer Nature Switzerland AG 2021
H. Tohid, H. Maibach (eds.), *International Medical Graduates in the United States*, https://doi.org/10.1007/978-3-030-62249-7_18

as the United Kingdom, Australia, New Zealand, Ireland, Sweden, Norway, and other immigrant-receiving countries.

In the United States and Canada, IMGs are considered those medical graduates who obtained their medical degree from anywhere outside the United states and Canada [3]. The IMGs in the United States and Canada are often divided into two categories: (1) *US-citizen IMGs* or *Canada-citizen IMGs,* who are the US or Canadian citizens but obtained their medical degrees outside the United States and Canada; and (2) *immigrant IMGs,* who are immigrant physicians and obtained their medical degree before moving to the United States or Canada [4, 5]. *Canada-citizen IMGs* are also termed in literature as Canadian Studying Abroad or CSA [4].

IMGs Across Different Countries

About one-quarter (24%) of the physicians currently practicing in the United States are IMGs [6]. IMGs come to the United States from over one hundred countries around the world. The top countries among them include India, the Philippines, Mexico, Pakistan, and the Dominican Republic [7]. However, not all states of the United States have similar proportions of IMGs. Some states have been known to be more IMG friendly and house a higher percentage of IMGs than other states in the United States. For example, New Jersey (45%), New York (41.9%), Florida (36%), Michigan (33.9%), and Illinois (34%) are the top five states where most IMGs work as physicians [8]. These states are also known to be more culturally diverse. Canada also has a similar proportion (25.9%) of IMGs constituting their physician workforce [9]. In some of the Canadian provinces, the percentage is notably high, such as Saskatchewan (52.5%), Newfoundland (36.6%), and Alberta (34.2%) [9]. IMGs are a crucial part of the US and Canadian healthcare system and especially for providing primary healthcare to remote, underserved areas in the United States and Canada [6].

The United States and Canada are not the only countries that depend on physicians who graduated from foreign medical schools [10]. According to data from the Organization for Economic Cooperation and Development, almost 58% of practicing doctors in Israel are IMGs. In Ireland and New Zealand, physicians trained outside those countries constitute nearly 40% of the total number of registered medical practitioners [11, 12]. The percentages of IMGs may be higher in some countries; however, the total number is the highest in the United States [10]. According to a study in 2017, the total number of IMGs practicing medicine in the United States was 218,059 [13]. In 2015, there were about 48,000 practicing IMGs in Britain and 35,000 in Germany, whereas the number for Australia, France, and Canada were reported between 22,000 and 27,000 [10].

Unlicensed IMGs in the United States and Canada

Nevertheless, the numbers of IMGs mentioned above include only the IMGs who succeeded to obtain their license and practice as a physician. There are a large number of IMGs who aspire to achieve the license to join the practicing physician workforce in those countries. Any systematically collected information on this group is non-existent. Academic literature on unlicensed IMGs is surprisingly scarce [14]. There are many blog posts, news reports, and online articles on their struggles and failures to integrate professionally, but there is no notable systematic research on them including their demography in the host countries and what alternative career choices are available for them when they cannot practice as physicians [14]. Only a few studies indicated rough speculation of their total number in the United States. For example, according to an online article in 2018, Massachusetts Immigrant and Refugee Advocacy (MIRA) Coalition reported an estimate of 65,000 unlicensed foreign-trained doctors across the country [15]. Very few reports are available on the number of unlicensed IMGs in Canada, but one study suggests there are several thousands of them in Ontario only [16]. Another study estimated that in 2006 there were 14,500 IMGs across Canada who could not obtain the license to practice by then [17]. But these numbers in Canada are probably an underestimation of the real scenario.

The statistics of the residency match from the National Residency Matching Program (NRMP) provides some approximation of unlicensed IMGs in the United States. In 2019, about 59% of IMGs got matched into residency positions. This was the highest match rate in more than 25 years [5]. Previous years had shown a matching rate of 50% or below [5]. This indicates that about half of the IMG candidates do not enter into a residency position and wind up doing survival jobs or switch to non-physician careers. By contrast, about 94% of US medical graduates (US-MGs) matched in 2019, and historically the match-rate for US-MGs is between 92% and 94% [5, 18, 19]. Studies indicate that some of the unmatched IMGs turn to nursing, some take jobs as physicians' assistants, some opt for a career in research, and many are forced to do survival jobs for the rest of their life [18, 19].

The situation is much rougher in Canada. The rates of successful completion of licensing examinations and obtaining residency spots have started to gradually decline for IMGs in Canada [20]. The Canadian Resident Matching Service (CaRMS) reported that only 103 out of 2984 Canadian medical graduates remained unmatched in 2019; whereas, 1334 out of 1725 IMGs went unmatched, which is a drastic comparison [20, 21].

Comparison of US-Citizen IMGs *or* Canada-Citizen IMGs *with* Immigrant IMGs

There are instances when US- or Canadian-born youth travel to other countries to study medicine. After completing their graduation, they come back to their home country and attempt to get into the practicing physician job market. As they are also treated as IMGs, they have to go through all the process of exam and licensure similar to *immigrant IMGs*. There has been quite an interesting observation across two reports regarding the performances of these two groups. It has been shown that

US-citizen IMGs have lower pass rates on the Step 1 and Step 2 clinical knowledge parts of the United States Medical Licensing Exams (USMLE) compared to other *immigrant IMGs* [22, 23]. However, despite a lower score in the licensing exams, *US-citizen IMGs* generally have a higher success rate in obtaining residency spots, perhaps due the consideration of other factors in the selection process [24, 25].

According to a report, during the residency match in 2011, *Canada-citizen IMGs* made up a quarter of the total IMG applicants; however, they secured approximately half of the residency positions allocated to IMGs [26]. On the other hand, *immigrant IMGs* showed a much lower success for residency matching than *Canada-citizen IMG* applicants (i.e., 6% and 20.9%, respectively) [26]. *Canada-citizen IMGs* definitely surpass *immigrant IMGs* in the residency match, which is an area that needs further exploration. While *immigrant IMGs* represented about two-third (65.9%) of the total number of IMGs in residency training in 2005, their proportions reduced to about half (48.7%) by 2011 [27]. But it needs to be noted that this change was most likely due to supply and demand as in 2005 Canada was facing a shortage of physicians and was actively trying to fill the shortage. Whereas, around 2011, the number of residency seats decreased to accommodate the need of that time, which would in return have a negative impact on the number of seats allocated for IMGs.

Challenges of Licensure

The relatively low success rate of IMGs to integrate into the labor market as physicians could be explained by the myriad of barriers they face. Studies found discrimination between identical applications of US-MGs and IMGs [28, 29]. IMGs do not receive positive response from various residency programs when they request information or apply to the programs including family medicine, psychiatry, surgery, and anesthesiology [30–35]. They also felt being singled out during the interview process where many interviewers clearly implied that they look for US graduates [31]. In Canada, most of the residency programs allow for only a set number of IMG candidates that ranges from 10% to 15% [4]. This so-called residency bottleneck is likely to be more challenging in the future as the number of graduates of the medical schools in the United States and Canada are climbing disproportionately compared to the number of residency positions [36–42].

Many IMGs fail to match to a residency program due to lack of recency of practice and/or graduation [36, 43]. Moreover, inability to get local clinical experience such as externship or clerkship complicates the pathway of integration as a physician in North America [31, 44, 45]. A lack of research experience also hinders IMGs to secure a residency spot particularly in any field of specialization such as dermatology and neurosurgery [46, 47]. Faulty strategies for attending interviews and ranking programs such as not selecting all the programs and passing over some interview invitations further narrow down the chances of getting matched [48].

Coming from diverse, ethno-cultural backgrounds, IMGs face the common financial, socio-cultural, and language challenges like any other newcomer population, which further complicates their efforts to integration into the medical profession. IMGs have been reported in the news as doing various survival jobs such as security guard, Uber/taxi driver, and pizza deliverer that would take away the time and energy needed to prepare and perform well on licensing examinations [49]. In addition, studies indicate IMGs may not communicate effectively with native patients, colleagues, and program supervisors [50, 51]. These factors may influence many program directors to show reluctance and be more careful while recruiting IMGs [52–56]. However, even after overcoming all these barriers when IMGs complete residency training successfully, they undergo the same discriminating procedures and barriers to find employment as independent physicians [45].

Alternative Career Pathways for IMGs

Definition of Alternative Career Pathways

There is no formal definition of alternative career pathways (ACP) for international medical graduates in the literature. However, a study that worked on alternative careers for the internationally educated health professionals including IMGs developed a working definition for alternative careers: "Alternative careers are those career options that immigrants pursue other than but related to the regulatory profession in which they were originally trained, that make use of and relate to an immigrant's skills and experience" [57].

Alternative careers may include some occupations that do not exist in the IMGs' home country but utilize their relevant knowledge and skills such as pathologist assistant. Moreover, career options for alternative careers may be in health-related fields such as physician assistants or completely unrelated to health such as engineering or business [57].

Importance of Alternative Career Pathways

Most IMGs come to the United States, Canada, or any other country with the goal of being a practicing physician and spend a significant amount of their time, money, and energy to pursue licensure. For many of the IMGs, this pursuit ends in failure resulting in feelings of frustration and hopelessness [20]. They are left with no professional identity and in a confused state where they have no idea of what else they can do and lose any hope of professional reintegration [20]. This unfortunate reality was captured by a study conducted in Canada by World Education Services (WES) in 2019 [58]. While most of the participants of that study (91.4%) hoped to be employed in the same area of their education and training, only less than half (47.2%) were successful to secure one. About a third changed to alternative sectors and almost a quarter of them remain unemployed [20, 58].

Failure to obtain licensure following successful completion of a long series of licensing examinations, limited residency spots, and an unwillingness to start from the beginning or after hitting a stumbling block in the pathway to licensure may direct many IMGs to seek employment in alternative fields, preferably health-related [59]. In recent years, the issue of "brain waste" problem has gained quite an attention for the increased report of underemployment of highly skilled immigrants including physicians who are working in jobs that require no skills or limited skills due to inability to secure a job in the area of their expertise [60, 61]. Physicians being featured on the news and media as taxi/Uber/delivery drivers became a silent wail of underemployment of immigrant professionals due to lack of professional license despite a rising demand for their profession [59, 61].

Underutilization and underemployment of skilled immigrants and refugees create a huge financial burden and economic loss on the individuals and the economy of the country [20]. According to the analysis of Migration Policy Institute in the United States and Royal Bank of Canada, underemployment of the skilled newcomers causes loss of tens of millions of dollars to the US and Canadian economy each year that could be in unearned wages by the immigrant professionals and which could have been pumped back to the economy of these countries [20, 37, 62, 63]. Taking an alternative career pathway, instead of repeated failed attempts to original career or doing low-skill jobs, boosts the prospect of better integration to the labor market by increasing opportunities for IMGs to utilize their skills and experience [57].

For most of the IMGs, usually alternative careers are chosen by them to earn a decent living and support their family while pursuing licensure. For others who decided not to go for medical licensure and who gave up the target of obtaining the license for practicing as physicians, the alternative career becomes their new career goal. The integration into a reasonable alternative career where their skills and knowledge are utilized and that act as a dependable source of earning a living as well as contribute to the host countries' economy [20, 57]. However, various factors including the requirement of upgrading the skills of IMGs related to the alternative job, obtaining a professional license, certification, or membership, and job opportunity for them in the market are strongly associated with this pathway [20, 57].

Generally, it takes a long time and strenuous efforts to get the license to practice medicine for international medical graduates in the United States and Canada. Nonetheless, working in an alternative job related to the experience and qualification of the person is a better option than doing a low-skilled survival job. Some of these alternative jobs such as research assistant or medical laboratory assistant may not pay high wages; however, they could be stepping-stones to high-paying jobs in the related field. For instance, experience as a research assistant will open the ways of being a research associate and research coordinator. Similarly, being a medical laboratory assistant can lay the foundation of being a lab manager down the road with further training and experience. Suitable alternative jobs for the IMGs can be a good way to identify and utilize their transferrable skills and get Canadian health-related job market experience.

Types of ACP in Health and Wellness Sector

The choice of alternative career depends on the individual IMG and the availability of the jobs. The IMGs are mainly driven with the aspiration of landing into their choice of main career pathway: the physician stream. In our discussion, the ACP is defined as the non-physician health and wellness–related career stream. The jobs or career choices within this ACP stream in health and wellness can be categorized based on the regulations around doing the jobs, the requirements for further training to getting the job, or need of certification and degrees to pursue this career. Categorization taxonomy of ACP jobs for IMGs in the health and wellness sector is illustrated in Fig. 18.1.

Regulated ACP in Health and Wellness Sector

Some non-physician health and wellness–related jobs are regulated in the United States and Canada. In other words, to be employable for these jobs one needs to obtain respective licensure and/or certification from a regulatory body. These regulated jobs can further be classified into two sectors: clinical and non-clinical. A selective list is provided in Table 18.1.

Regulated ACP: Clinical Jobs

A number of ACP jobs are clinical in nature such as chiropractor, registered massage therapist, and respiratory therapist. These require patient engagement at the bedside, and treatment of patients directly.

Regulated ACP: Non-clinical Jobs

These types of ACP jobs are non-clinical that may contribute to patient care, but these do not require a direct contact with the patient for the diagnosis, treatment or care of the patient such as nutritionists/dietitian, medical laboratory technologist,

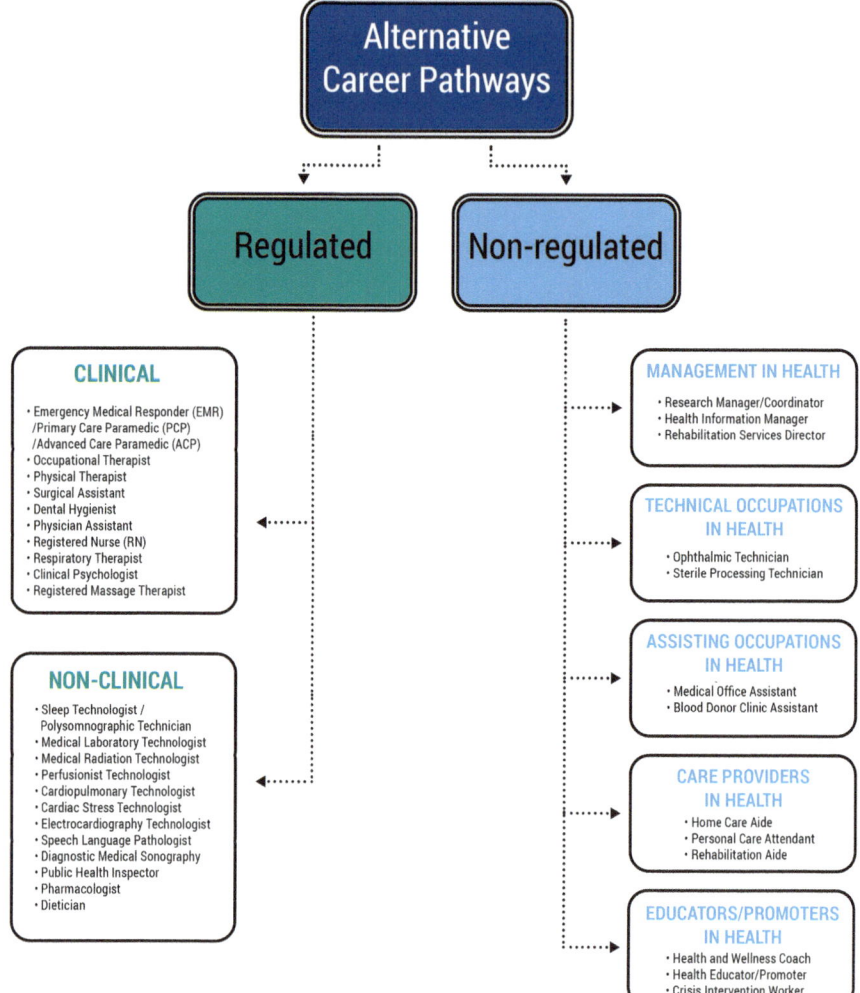

Fig. 18.1 Categorization taxonomy of ACP jobs for IMGs in health and wellness sector

and pathology assistant. Nevertheless, the requirements and standards of regulation may depend on the state or province. For example, while most states of the United States allow diagnostic medical sonographers to practice with relevant degree and training, four states: New Hampshire, New Mexico, North Dakota, and Oregon mandated American Registry of Diagnostic Medical Sonographers (ARDMS) certification to be eligible for practice as a sonographer.

Table 18.1 Selective list of ACP jobs for IMGs in health and wellness sector

Regulated	Clinical jobs	Examples include
Registration with the regulatory body required Registration and certification requirements may vary by state or province	Relating to providing bedside care, treatment, or performing other diagnostic and therapeutic procedures to the patients directly	• Chiropractor • Dental hygienist • Registered massage therapist • Occupational therapist • Physical therapist • Physician assistant • Registered nurse (RN) • Respiratory therapist • Surgical assistant • Clinical psychologist • Addictions counsellor • Board-certified behavioral analyst (BCBA) • Mental health counsellor • Family therapist • Emergency medical responder (EMR)/primary care paramedic (PCP)/ advanced care paramedic (ACP)
	Non-clinical job May support patient care, but does not provide direct diagnosis, treatment, or care for the patient	**Examples include:** • Dietitian • Medical laboratory technologist • Medical radiation technologist • Perfusionist technologist • Pharmacologist • Cardiopulmonary technologist • Cardiac stress technologist • Electrocardiography technologist • Sleep technologist/ polysomnographic technician • Speech language pathologist • Diagnostic medical sonography • Public health inspector

(continued)

Table 18.1 (continued)

Unregulated	Management in health	Examples include
License with regulatory or governing body not required to practice	Managers in healthcare plan, organize, direct, supervise, and evaluate the delivery of healthcare services. They may work in hospitals, medical clinics, nursing homes, government, community, and non-profit organizations. They may work in public and private organizations or be self-employed	• Research manager • Research coordinator • Mental health residential care manager • Health information manager • Rehabilitation services director • Health program manager
	Technical occupations in health Technical occupations require specific skills, abilities, and often knowledge of specific equipment needed to perform tasks. They are employed in medical laboratories, hospitals, clinics, and universities	**Examples include** • Ophthalmic technician • Renal dialysis technician • Sterile processing technician • Pharmacy technician
	Assisting occupations in health Those in assisting occupations support health services by providing services and assistance to healthcare professionals and other healthcare staff. These include administrative positions. They are employed in hospitals, clinics, assisted care facilities, community health centers, and other laboratories	**Examples include** • Blood donor clinic assistant • Medical office assistant • Autopsy assistant • Healthcare aide • Laboratory assistant
	Care providers in health Care providers provide personal care and companionship for seniors, persons with disabilities, and clients. Care is provided within the client's residence, in which the home support worker may reside. They are employed by home care and support agencies, private households, or they may be self-employed	**Examples include** • Home care aide • Live-in caregiver • Personal aide • Personal care attendant • Respite worker • Rehabilitation aide
	Educators/promoters in health Educators include those who may teach in social assistance programs, government agencies, organizations, school boards, and other educational institutions. This also can include jobs as faculty members or teachers in universities, technical colleges, and professional institutes. They may work within communities, for private, public, government organizations, and universities or colleges, or be self-employed	**Examples include** • Health and wellness coach • Health educator/promoter • Patient advocate • Indigenous outreach worker • Crisis intervention worker • Community health worker • University or college teachers and faculties

Non-regulated ACP in Health and Wellness Sector

The rest of the non-physician alternative career options could be labeled as unregulated health-related jobs that do not require a licensing or professional certification. A selective list is provided in Table 18.1. These jobs can be clustered into five groups depending on the nature of these jobs. These are described as follows:

Management in Health

These jobs require management skills of IMGs in planning, organizing, supervising, and evaluating delivery of healthcare services. IMGs may need to earn further institutional degrees to be employed in these jobs such as obtaining a Master's degree or PhD in the relevant field. Examples of these jobs include research coordinator, health information manager, etc.

Technical Occupations in Health

IMGs are usually required to undergo some training to master relevant technical skills for these jobs; however, their prior knowledge can be utilized to some extent. For example, as an ophthalmic technician, IMGs' extensive knowledge about ophthalmology is in good use, but they are usually required to complete a 6-month to 1-year long course to get this position.

Assisting Occupations in Health

These jobs can potentially utilize many of IMGs' technical/clinical skills obtained during their medical training and clinical experience. For example, the knowledge about human body and surgical skills of IMGs will be largely employed in the job of autopsy assistant. These types of jobs generally require institutional education and/or extensive training.

Care Providers in Health

IMGs can work as non-clinical care providers to seniors, persons with disabilities, and clients. Examples of these jobs include home care aide, personal care attendant, and rehabilitation aide. On-the-job training is usually sufficient for these kinds of jobs.

Educators/Promoters in Health

Another excellent opportunity to employ IMGs' vast health-related knowledge is to work in health education and promotion. They can act as health and wellness coach, patient advocate, community health worker, and in similar roles and contribute to community health and wellness. On-the-job training or bridging programs developing knowledge about local healthcare systems and interpersonal skills can help IMGs ace such careers. IMGs also can pursue teaching and faculty positions in educational institutions such as universities, technical colleges, and professional institutes. But these types of careers need Master's and/or PhD degrees in relevant topics, which can be epidemiology, biostatistics, health economics, health informatics, life science subjects, etc.

The Challenges for ACP

Below, we highlight some of the aspects of the challenges the IMGs would need to overcome for a better probability of landing an ACP job in the health and wellness sector. In general, the similar challenges that affect IMGs in their journey toward licensure for becoming a practicing physician impedes their possible success while pursuing an ACP job in the health and wellness sector.

IMGs Are Not Happy or Eager to Choose an Alternative Career

It is important to note that most IMGs have never looked for an alternative career path [64]. Generally, they did not hold any other jobs during their university days, unlike many North American graduates [20]. Their career focus and dream all circled around being and practicing as physicians. For some it is passion; for some, it is a life-long cherished dream. Studies showed that IMGs, in general, have a lack of interest to join an alternate profession and even if they join, they lack a commitment to that career [65, 66]. Many IMGs who are already working in alternative careers want to move back to the original career using that as a stepping-stone [65, 66]. This is understandable given that IMGs have been turned away from their initial career goal and pushed to explore other career paths in a foreign country and in a new professional context, which can be quite daunting. IMGs may not be unwilling to find an alternative career in general; however, they need help and guidance to make informed decisions regarding their future careers [20].

Waiting Too Long to Step Forward for an Alternative Career Build Up

Studies indicate that to excel in an alternative career, IMGs should take this path as early as possible [67]. An article discussed taking up alternate careers by medical graduates mentioned that it is the most common regret of the physicians who chose an alternative career that why they did not leave trying for medical licensure earlier. Waiting too long to step up for an alternative career can deter relocation if they have children and are already settled in a community [68]. A study on an accelerated program for IMGs to become a nurse practitioner indicated that most IMGs in their program had gone after US medical residency for at least 5 years unsuccessfully before considering any alternative options [69].

Lack of Due Diligence in Identifying Suitable Alternative Career Options

Many IMGs do not have a clear idea about what are the possible alternative career options out there [57]. Moreover, they do not know what will be suitable for them [57]. Many career options such as "physician assistant," "diagnostic sonographer" or "pathologist assistant" do not exist in most of their home countries. The variation of job prospects often confuses them. For example, to become a diagnostic medical sonographer, there are no official rules against male candidates. However, according to some reports, this career path is often difficult for male candidates as 85–90% sonographers are female as they are usually needed to evaluate female patients with gynecological, obstetric, or breast problems who often prefer female sonologists [70].

Not Being Able to Accept/Tolerate Rejection or Failure During Alternative Career Building Process

Physicians in any country are usually accomplished individuals and have been at the top of their class from elementary school. They have worked hard and have met with success on most steps of their professional careers [68]. In a new environment, without familiarity of job search techniques and a professional network in the host country, seeking employment is a challenge. Lack of awareness about the labor market is a hindrance, and it is a shock to many IMGs to be rejected repeatedly for non-clinical jobs [57]. Then, to not be accepted into courses leading to an alternative career pathway such as sonography, for example, is very disheartening. While perseverance, tenacity, and relentlessness are key attributes needed to overcome these hurdles, feedback on their applications would be very beneficial to the newcomer. They often are left feeling deflated and make incorrect assumptions as to why they have not been successful in obtaining an interview. It is reported that medical graduates who keep trying for alternative positions eventually were able to secure a non-physician job [68].

Financial Barriers, the Uncertainty of Finding Jobs, and Feeling Too Aged to Start Fresh

Some IMGs expressed that many alternative careers only use a small part of their skills and experience and require extensive upgrading and schooling which is often costly and not possible to bear; particularly, if they have spent savings on the pursuit of becoming licensed with no avail [57]. Moreover, IMGs have expressed the need for near-certainty of finding employment after graduation from programs for alternative careers [67]. Courses that have work placements attached to them are often more beneficial and attractive for this reason. Financial support is scarce and if the jobs are not available, the investment of money and time is simply another unbearable wastage. For a few alternative jobs, IMGs may start from scratch, which is often difficult for the IMGs who moved at an older age and have family responsibilities [57].

Lack of Time to Gain Exposure and Networking

Many IMGs have to do survival jobs to support themselves and their families, which makes it difficult to find time to seek resources including information sessions, bridging or networking programs [20]. Moreover, most non-physician jobs are sought through networking, which takes a big deal of time. It is best practice to save a certain amount of time regularly for exploring the resources and for networking [68].

Not Identifying the Transferable Skill Sets

The most intensive knowledge and skills that the doctors obtain are to diagnose the disease of the individuals and treat patients in clinical settings. They receive tens of thousands of hours of training and experience to master these skills. This training is so specific to this profession that its transferability to other professions is often not perceived by the IMGs [57]. Identification of the transferable skills plays a key role

Table 18.2 Transferable skills of IMGs

Analytical skills	Interpersonal skills
• Critical thinking	• Coordinating
• Decision-making	• Instructing
• Evaluation	• Intercultural skill
• Learning strategies	• Managing conversation
• Operations analysis	• Negotiating
• Problem solving	• Persuading/advising/counseling
• Quality control analysis	• Service orientation
• Researching and investigating	• Social perceptiveness
• Systems analysis	• Working with others
	• Compassion and understanding
	• Empathy
	• Patient advocacy
	• Communication skills
	• Active listening
	• Ability to work in acute, stressful situations
	• Leadership skills
	• Professionalism
	• Ability to teach
Technical skills	**Resource management skills**
• Medical knowledge	• Change management
• Medical terminology	• Crisis management
• Scientific knowledge	• Job task planning and organizing
• Specialty skills	• Management of equipment resources
• Surgical skills	• Management of material resources
• Technical skills	• Management of personnel resources
• Dexterity	• Monitoring
	• Operational planning
	• Projecting outcomes
	• Risk management
	• Strategic planning
	• Talent management
	• Time management
	• Crisis management
	• Patient care
	• Stakeholder management

for successful uptake of alternative careers [20, 57]. A respondent of a study emphasized that the assessment of skills of IMGs should be done systematically in collaboration with potential employers and experts [57]. A list of possible transferable skills of IMGs extracted from various online resources is provided in Table 18.2.

Unfamiliarity with the Job Search and Interview Techniques

Job searching in North America is substantially different from many of the countries from where the IMGs migrate. They may be unfamiliar with North American job search techniques [20, 71]. For example, in the job markets of many of those countries, resumes may include a photo, marital status, or other information considered inappropriate on a North American resume [72]. In North America, job searching requires a combination of certain soft skills that may not be the strongest suit of the IMGs. It requires extensive networking, connections, persistence, openness, and dedication. In-person interviews can sometimes be intimidating to the IMGs who are unfamiliar with the culture of the host countries, while phone interviews can be challenging for language and communication differences [72]. Cultural nuances around eye contact, smiles, voice volume, and handshakes can be important factors in the interview [73].

Gap of Knowledge for the Working Environment

IMGs lack knowledge of the work environment of the alternative professions that dissuades the employers to recruit them [57]. Possible failure to perceive their role and position in a new non-physician healthcare service is an important barrier [74]. Research on IMGs' role as physician assistants (PAs) showed that IMGs have a possible lack of socialization knowledge for PA role and physician-PA relationship [65, 75]. Putting IMGs directly into a new role without acculturation, professional development, and appropriate quality control may lead to negative consequences [66]. Many IMGs do not have adequate training, knowledge, and communication skills to safely work within the Canadian healthcare environment [76].

Language Ability and Cultural Competency

Studies investigated alternative career opportunities for IMGs such as working as a physician assistant (PA) and nurse practitioner (NP) found the language and communication difficulties and a lack of cultural competency act as a barrier for integration into alternative careers for the IMGs [65, 74]. Cultural and language differences may affect patient communication and satisfaction in physician assistant and nurse roles [76, 77]. Moreover, lack of reading comprehension and poor command in English were reported by a study on unlicensed IMGs in a PA program [78].

Experiencing Discrimination in Non-physician Professions

A study on IMGs as physician assistants (PA) found that the IMGs experienced discrimination as IMGs as well as racial minorities in their PA role. This study also found many employers and others in the medical profession do not believe that IMGs working in non-physician health occupations are beneficial to healthcare in the United States [79].

Employers' Reluctance to Recruit IMGs in Alternative Career

Studies showed that potential employers for alternative careers often do not understand why a qualified international medical doctor would want to take an alternate career at a different level. They think perhaps they are overqualified for the position or not prepared for the specific job [80]. Moreover, if the employer hires an IMG without proper training in that specific field, they might fail and there will be negative consequences. A pilot program for IMGs seeking alternative careers found employers' lack of interest in hiring IMGs even for entry-level positions [20]. For example, in a study on programs that allows transition of IMGs to PA, the recruiters were reluctant to accept IMGs as students of the PA program because they are often construed as choosing PA training as a transition stage [75].

Non-recognition of Their Existing Knowledge and Skill Sets at the Alternative Path

The knowledge and skills of IMGs are often not recognized by the body providing potential alternative careers. Often, they require a US or Canadian degree in this field, which is generally unbearable for the IMGs in terms of cost and the fact that their superior knowledge and skills are not given any value [57]. A study interviewed IMGs regarding foreign qualification recognition mentioned that many IMGs expressed their frustration of not having their prior learning recognized, which could ease their entrance into alternative careers [57, 67]. For example, instead of completing a full diploma for being a medical laboratory technologist, physicians feel they should be offered short-term courses or fast-track options [20, 57, 68].

Lack of Job Market Information and Inflexibility

Studies found that *immigrant IMGs* often have no idea of the labor markets before moving to the host country [57]. In a study, key informant respondents from Immigrant Serving Organizations (ISOs) in Canada focused on the issue that IMGs are completely unaware of the local market place and the types of jobs in demand [57]. They suggested that they would like to have information before coming to Canada to avoid relocating once again after arriving [57]. Many IMGs have their children admitted into schools, and it is difficult for them to move once they have settled in a particular location. Adequate labor market information before taking up an alternative career will enable them to choose an appropriate career and if possible, move to a better job market place [68].

Lack of Systematic Support or Non-responsive Programs

There are limited number of career support and bridging programs available across the United States and Canada. However, considering the number of unlicensed IMGs in these countries, they are not sufficient. Moreover, the provided consultations often are neither sufficient, nor appropriate for highly skilled IMGs. It is crucial that those employed in these programs understand the backgrounds of IMGs and the healthcare system. Also, many IMGs do not actively seek assistance. One study investigating the professional journeys of IMGs found that many of those who changed their career path did it on their own without consulting any formal resources or supports. They made their decision following personal reflection and understanding. Blain et al. interpreted that as a result of an "independent" self-image in many physicians, where as seeking information and support from a consulting organization/counsellor could be considered as 'asking for help' which many of these IMGs are not used to and comfortable with [67].

Lack of Opportunities to Connect with Employers and to Showcase IMGs' Abilities

Having local work experience in the United States and Canada is crucial for getting jobs. However, the opportunities for obtaining such experience are very limited for IMGs looking for an alternative career [20, 57]. Finding such an opportunity is imperative to prove the ability to do the respective job particularly for the IMGs. In studies, IMGs urged to make such opportunities available for them that may include work placements, unpaid internships, observerships, and even volunteering opportunities in their field [20, 57]. A pilot program for alternative career struggled to find a practicum work placements and job-shadowing opportunities for IMGs [20].

Lack of Sustained Funding

There are some Immigrant Serving Organizations (ISOs) that help IMGs to integrate professionally. ISO informants of a study stressed that funding is required for continuing and extending their services to the IMGs, as well as for building partnerships and informing people about bridging programs, getting to understand the industry, and maintaining community and employer connections [57, 76].

Overcoming the Challenges

For many IMGs, alternative careers are not their first choice. Despite this, IMGs still need an effective plan to succeed in an alternative career even if it is plan B [68]. It is advised to learn job-seeking methodology, the importance of soft skills, and how to market oneself appropriately for the available opportunities [20, 57]. Often physicians need support in how to describe their previous experiences in relation to the job or pathway they are seeking. A committed approach is required to develop a meaningful and rewarding alternative career. There are a lot of websites across the United States and Canada that offer information about alternative careers. These sites include blogs, community organizations, and immigrant serving organizations. Most of them give the options for an alternative career and some useful information about that career choice such as any degree or certification required or not, average wages, and job prospects. However, there are only a handful of organizations that physically help IMGs to pursue alternative options.

Facilitators That Are Needed to Help IMGs to Overcome the Challenges to ACP

There are not much comprehensive information or focused guidence available on facilitating the integration of alternative career pathways for IMGs. The possible supports are constructed below.

Strategizing Through One-to-One Coaching/Consultation

A pilot career transition program for IMGs in Alberta found that one-to-one coaching sessions can effectively facilitate the professional integration of IMGs [20]. This is particularly needed as even though most IMGs are informed of the myriad of challenges to the licensure pathway upon arrival, they arrive with the hope of making it. They need to be consulted one-on-one with specialists to evaluate their prior learning and experience in order to help them make informed career choices regarding alternative career pathways that take into consideration their prior skill sets and future goals [20, 57]. It is important these coaches are specialists in the area of healthcare.

Profile Promotion and Employer Engagement

Creating a structured professional profile and forwarding this through a supporting organization to potential employers were found quite helpful in a study [20]. Employers were very satisfied with the candidates' biographies they received and expressed the desire to receive more referrals like this [20]. IMGs in a study expressed that employers should know their potential, and on the other hand, IMGs should know the requirements for the job. Employment preparation is needed for both IMGs and employers so that IMGs' intention and preparedness of being in the profession are clear and employers are informed of whom they are hiring. Collaboration with stakeholders, including educators, employers and sector councils, government, regulatory bodies, immigrant-serving organizations (ISOs), for developing and providing support to alternative careers is advised [57].

Skill Building Workshops

Workshops specifically tailored to the needs of the IMGs seeking alternative careers where their skills and knowledge will be best used are imperative [20]. Workshops to increase awareness among IMGs and employers, to develop a career portfolio, engage with mentors, network, and obtain feedback from potential employers, and the introduction of a reflection log all proved to be beneficial in the research [20].

Improve Availability of the Information About ACP Early

IMG participants in a study noted that reliable, complete, and current information would be useful to navigate alternative careers [57]. Information on licensure challenges and alternative careers should be widely available even before arrival. The available information should be accurate and consistent perhaps through a centralized database that IMG-specific organizations, immigrant-serving organizations, and others working in the area of alternative careers could access to ensure consistent, reliable, and up-to-date information [57].

Develop Alternative Career Roadmaps and Tools for Supporting Organizations and IMGs

Many service providers and organizations are working in their own ways with their own resources and experience to help IMGs navigate alternative career paths. However, there is a lack of methodology and tools. It is recommended that a roadmap should be developed to assist counselors to help IMGs navigate career pathways with immigrant-serving organizations as lead stakeholders as they have the most experience with providing different health professionals with alternative career supports [57]. Assessment tools (including self-assessments) should be developed and made available to the IMGs and the employers to recognize prior learning and gaps to plan the next steps to obtain a successful career [57].

Develop a Set of Illustrative Case Studies of IMGs in Different Types of Alternative Careers

Lim Consulting Associates proposed an alternative career model that included illustrated successful stories of health professionals that successfully transitioned to new or unrelated careers [57]. All stakeholders and more importantly IMGs considering alternative careers will benefit from these examples [57].

Targeted Bridging Programs with Workshop Placements

There are only a handful of bridging programs available in the United States and Canada for alternative careers for IMGs. The development of more bridging programs is suggested by the studies for building specific skill sets that will equip the candidates for the new job field [20]. However, a study suggests the length of the program should allow IMGs to work part-time to facilitate living while preparing for alternative careers through skills upgrading [57]. Bridging programs with job shadowing, mentoring, and internships were preferred as they benefit both the employers and IMGs to test the waters [20].

Examples of Alternative Career Support Programs and Processes Currently Existing in the United States and Canada

Surgical Assistant Training

An institution that trains individuals for being surgical assistants who help the surgeons during operation including sponging, suturing, suctioning, electrocautery, and managing wounds conducted a 6-day surgical training for the IMGs [81]. According to their website, international medical graduates qualify to sit for the American Board of Surgical Assistants (ABSA) certifying exam after attending the ACE 6-day Surgical SkillLab™ [81]. Because of IMGs' extensive medical background, they do not require to take the full course of surgical assistant that can be 1-year long. This is a good opportunity for the IMGs who choose alternative careers as an interim step. This will allow them to earn a decent living while preparing for residency as well as create networking opportunities with surgeons, which may facilitate the journey for residency by getting valuable recommendations from US surgeons [81].

Research/Clinical Research

Many IMGs do not have prior research experience and publications. While having research experience facilitates pathways to residency, it may be considered as an alternative career pathway as well. There are a few organizations across the United States and Canada who provide training and certification to the IMGs for clinical research.

A. California Institute of Behavioral Neuroscience and Technology This institute provides online training for learning research methodology, writing, and publishing scientific articles. This institute also provides training for speech pathology and neurolinguistic planning. The institute is not dedicated to the IMGs only, but anyone interested in learning research is welcome. However, IMGs need extensive research training for both improving their chance of getting residency and as an alternative career path. Both of these types of IMGs are learning and being largely benefitted from the institute [82].

B. Certified Clinical Research Professionals Society (CCRPS) Certified Clinical Research Professionals Society (CCRPS) is a not-for-profit professional organization that trains their members in clinical trial research. They provide clinical research professionals who becomes their members with resources, job placement, and support and guidance for resume. They offer a 110-module online clinical research training focused on training physicians and other healthcare professionals willing to work in the clinical research sector. They do not require a prior background in clinical research to be eligible for enrolment, which is an excellent opportunity for many IMGs who do not have prior research experience. Physicians including international medical graduates who were unable to find residency often choose this path. The graduates of the course can enter into the management sector after their first few years. This course comprises a majority of high-yield and low-yield content required in many clinical research positions, which can prepare the IMGs to master the skills required for jobs in clinical research monitoring. This training also allows the physician graduates of the course to later work as principal investigators (with principal investigator training) or in the management sector of pharmaceutical companies, hospitals, and the healthcare industry [83].

C. Internationally Trained Medical Doctors (ITMD) Bridging Program by Ryerson University Ryerson University initiated a pilot program that provides a foundation for an alternative career path for IMGs by teaching and honing the knowledge and skills required for non-licensed health-sector employment. The bridging program for IMGs is a unique initiative designed by the G. Raymond Chang School of Continuing Education at Ryerson University in collaboration with leading health research organizations in Ontario. The ultimate aim of the program is to enable highly qualified, knowledgeable, and skilled IMGs to integrate into the Canadian healthcare workforce through non-licensed healthcare employment. According to an online article, the program attempts to mitigate the barriers for

IMGs to alternative jobs by providing proper assessment of their education and experience, followed by sector-specific training, relevant employment support within top-ranked healthcare facilities in Ontario, and current labor market information [9]. The program consists of a 12-week academic phase followed by a 4-week practicum placement. This program helps IMGs obtain and sharpen additional skills needed to secure positions in health research, health informatics, data analysis, and health management positions in Canada that do not require medical licensing [9, 84].

Health Informatics

A. Health Informatics Master's Program   The University of San Diego, USA, offers an M.S. in Health Care Informatics that is appreciated to be taken by IMGs looking for alternative careers. They highlighted that health informatics is a very fast-growing field due to increasing provision of electronic health records (EHRs) everywhere; and contrary to many alternative jobs for IMGs, health informatics are quite well paid [85]. This job requires the potential candidates to have both health-care knowledge and information technology (IT)-related skills. IMGs get a head start for this field, as they possess extensive medical knowledge and clinical experience. The M.S. in Health Care Informatics at University of San Diego can be obtained online as well as on campus [85].

B. Health Informatics Bridging Program   Another initiative about health informatics in Canada offers a full-time 8-week-long bridging program on Health Informatics that provides the candidates with a real-world experience in this field with practical hands-on labs demonstrated by leading instructors. According to their website, "participants with an interest in the integration of information technologies in the healthcare delivery sector stand to greatly benefit from this program" [86]. Skills for Change organizes this program in collaboration with George Brown College. The college teaches fundamentals of health informatics, while Skills for Change helps IMGs find jobs and develop career pathways through resume writing, profiling, developing market research, networking, and interviewing skills as well as connecting with potential employers and mentors [86].

Naturopathic Medicine Bridging Program for IMGs

This compressed program offered by Canadian College of Naturopathic Medicine (CCNM) provides oppertunity to IMGs to obtain the Doctor of Naturopathy degree in naturopathic medicine in only 2 years instead of 4 years. This program recognizes and accepts previous medical experience and education of IMGs, while providing required learning to become a doctor of naturopathy. However, to become an eligible candidate, IMGs must pass one of the three licensing examinations taken by Medical Council of Canada or USMLE step 1 [87].

International Skills Applied for Geriatrics Bridge Training Program

Geriatrics care can be a good opportunity for the IMGs to utilize their medical knowledge and skills as in an alternative career. This program teaches three academic courses, trains for workplace environment and culture relevant for this job, and communication training. The academic courses are delivered by George Brown College, while JVS Toronto provides other components. They also help IMGs for job search and support, finding job shadowing opportunities, practicum placements, and employer connections [88].

The Bridge to Registration and Employment in Mental Health (BREM) Program

This seems to be another program that could be a good start for the IMGs with experience in mental healthcare. According to their website, The Mennonite New Life Centre of Toronto delivers the program in collaboration with several community-based mental health organizations and settlement agencies. This program has two streams; both of them offer classroom and online training, workshops, practicum placements, and job supports to prepare IMGs to enter the mental health workforce in Canada. Successful candidates will be registered with the College of Registered Psychotherapists of Ontario (CRPO). One stream is called Employment Stream (E stream) that is 9-month long, while the other stream known as Registration and Employment Stream (R stream) provides training for 14 months. In addition to academic training, mentoring, employment support, professional certifications, and placement, the R stream offers help registration with the CRPO and support exam preparation. Eligible candidates have a mental health component during their undergraduate education. Besides, 2 years of work experience in mental health are required for admission. Experience outside Canada or the United States is accepted [89].

Health System Navigator

Working as a health educator or navigator is an achievable alternative career opportunity for IMGs with their knowledge and skills. However, this job may require further polishing of particular soft skills such as presentation skills and interpersonal skills, which can be obtained by short-term training. College Boreal offers a bridging program for being health system navigators for IMGs. This program is 15-week long and offers an additional 8-week internship at College Boreal that will provide training in both English and French. This program is primarily designed for francophone immigrants who are trained in health-related occupation internationally including IMGs. Participants will gain detailed understanding of how the healthcare system in Ontario works and will learn to access community resources [90].

Ultrasound Scanning Evaluation Bridging Program by the Michener's Institute

Diagnostic Medical Sonography uses a great deal of medical knowledge and skills IMGs possess. Besides, many IMGs have degrees from back home or experience working as a sonographer. The following program can recognize their prior learning and experience and bridge that to Canadian context while preparing them to enter into Canadian job market. This program provides an overview of the ultrasound scanning techniques, procedures, and protocols in Canada and prepares the candidates to the standards of Sonography Canada's Canadian Clinical Skills Assessment (CCSA). Simulated laboratory setting will help students learn scanning of abdomen, obstetrical anatomy, pelvic, thyroid, scrotum, lower limbs, and transvaginal sonography. It will also train the students on identifying patients, obtaining informed consent, and maintaining patient safety, hygiene and overall professionalism. Students will also be evaluated for their performance in following procedures regularly. The bridging program takes 1 month to complete and is delivered only at the weekends. Successful IMG candidates will have prior training in sonography and 2 years of relevant experience [91].

Accelerated Programs for IMGs to Become Nurse Practitioners

Florida International University (FIU) offers IMGs an Accelerated Combined BSN/MSN Program for Foreign-Educated Physicians (FEP to BSN [Bachelor of Science in nursing]/MSN [Master of Science in nursing]) program. The accelerated program offers IMGs an MSN degree that allows them to work as nurse practitioners in eight semesters (3 years). There are currently over 200 IMGs enrolled in the FEP to BSN/MSN program [69].

Accredited Programs for IMGs to Become Physician Assistants (PAs)

Unfortunately, some PA schools choose to maintain their distance from IMGs, and some decline applications from IMGs based on some prior research showing IMGs are not good in PA roles. This exclusion fails to recognize that many IMGs indeed are quite successful as PAs [92]. However, MEDEX Northwest, the University Of Washington School Of Medicine's Physician Assistant Program, continues enrolling IMGs in their PA program since the 1990s [92]. The program curriculum emphasize on preparing the candidates for under-served populations. A recent study showed the graduated IMGs doing better performance than traditional PAs [92].

Alternative Careers in Health Promotion and Education for International Medical Graduates (IMGs) Program by Learning Enrichment Foundation, Ontario

This 24-week program initiated by the Learning Enrichment Foundation is intended to enhance employment of IMGs within the healthcare settings as a non-clinician positions in Ontario. This program offers an opportunity to the IMGs for utilizing their medical knowledge and skills in health promotion and education with developing specific essential skills as identified by prospective employers. Courses provided by this program include Public Health and Health Care System in Ontario, Health Promotion and Education Foundations, Business Communication, and Cultural Competence and Careers. Moreover, it offers unpaid work placements, mentoring opportunities, and job search/coaching support [93].

Alberta International Medical Graduates Association's Career Transition Program

Alberta International Medical Graduates Association (AIMGA) is a non-profit organization that helps IMGs seeking licensure and exploring alternative career paths. They piloted a Career Transition Program for IMGs that proved to be a positive initiative in addressing this issue [20]. This pilot has resulted in economic growth for some, the pursuit of alternative pathways for others, new collaborations and capacity building for AIMGA, and opportunities for growth and expansion for future IMGs based on lessons learned throughout this pilot [20]. A total of 22 IMGs participated in the pilot program. IMGs who attempted to become licensed for 3 or more years and have not met with success, were either unemployed or underemployed (i.e., working in a medical clinic or elsewhere and making <$20/h); and wanted to fully participate in the pilot were accepted into the program. Also, IMGs who were not interested in pursuing licensure were included [20].

After recruiting candidates for the program, an orientation was provided (phase 1), a total of eight workshops were developed and delivered in phase 2 of this program. The workshops included an orientation to career transition, determining transferable skill sets for intended alternative careers, a mini alternative career fair, resume writing, networking, what employers are seeking in the Canadian workplace, interview skills, and factors for success [20]. In phase 3, participants had the option to complete a 50-h mentorship placement in order to explore an alternative career of interest to understand its viability, gain practical learning, understand cultural differences, and challenges, as well as obtain feedback, a professional reference, guidance, and networking [20]. Several symposium sessions were conducted providing information regarding alternative career opportunities including Alberta Clinical and Surgical Assistant Program (ACSAP), diagnostic and therapeutic technologies used in the treatment of disease and injury, front-line emergency care, professional assistant programs, information management and training for wellness professionals available at local educational institutions, and what employers want [20]. In phase 4, individual coaching sessions were provided to the IMG participants, which consisted of 4 to 5 h in total for each participant to equip them with the proper tools and resources for finding employment [20]. Workshops with employers took place in phase 5, which included employers from Alberta Health Services and other healthcare organizations, immigrant-serving agencies, and city of Calgary. These workshops aimed at helping healthcare providers to identify the issues and solutions to work more effectively with culturally diverse patients and co-workers [20].

Outcomes from the program (phase 6): Before participating in the program, 17 of 22 of the candidates were unemployed. After participating in the program, 12 had made significant progress, six got jobs, and five got admitted into their desired courses as full-time or part-time students. One participant started her own business. Four of the 17, however, could not be employed yet while one left Canada for personal reasons [20]. Four of the 22 participants reported returning to the pursuit of licensure as they think seeking an alternative career is as hard as pursuing licensure. Five candidates gained volunteer positions following the program [20].

The pilot program learned several important lessons to be considered for facilitating alternative career pathways for IMGs [20]. One-to-one coaching has been found critical to deal with the heightened hopes of many IMGs about licensure and to evaluate their prior learning and experience to make informed career choices [20]. AIMGA also developed a professional profile of each of the candidates as a way to introduce them to employers in their field which acted as a catalyst for getting invitations from potential employers [20]. AIMGA developed ten workshop presentations, a career portfolio, a reflection log, a booklet of weekly readings to correspond with each workshop, which was distributed to create awareness, and a booklet of resources that included both video-mediated and written materials to reinforce the concepts across the ten workshops. The workshops included various guest speakers, which consisted of other IMGs in alternative career pathways as well as mentors from various healthcare backgrounds [20]. The workshops met the program's objective; however, the next step is to develop bridging programs for specific skill buildings to enable the candidates to be competent enough for their intended job field [20]. This pilot program also found IMGs need to be persistent in seeking employment and understand North American ways of job search [20]. Further, even though AIMGA managed to get the support of the Alberta Health Services and other employer organizations to place the candidates in their settings, it was difficult to convince individuals to allow IMGs for job shadowing [20]. Many employers showed interest at first but were committed to other programs and placements or facing shortages due to recent cutbacks. Observership can be a possible alternative for future programs; however, support and connections are needed in this regard. Overall, more work with employers is imperative in the future [20].

Conclusion

Despite the bottleneck situation for IMGs attempting to get into the physician stream in Canada or the United States, we believe that there are untapped opportunities for IMGs to utilize their knowledge and skills in alternative career pathways. Recently, the creation of alternative pathways for IMGs' labor market integration has been gaining momentum. This, in turn, will increase the economic and societal integration of IMGs. Still there is much work that is needed; especially, the exploration of needed skill development, which is very important. Once the different skillsets, which are needed, for improved job market competitiveness, are systematically recognized, we will then be able to create awareness and provide recommendations. Next, appropriate support and training opportunities through practicum placements will be essential. Also, the perceptions of the IMGs also need to be captured through meaningful community engagement where they can play an active role in solution identification and implementation. Engagement with the possible employers will also be a positive step, as this will guide the steps to integration from the employers' perspectives. Academics, support providers, industry stakeholders, and policy makers need to be engaged in this work so that uptake and impact can be ensured.

References

1. National Center for Biotechnology Information: MeSH term. Foreign Medical Graduates. 1970. https://www.ncbi.nlm.nih.gov/mesh/68005550. Accessed 27 Feb 2020.
2. Motala MI, Van Wyk JM. Experiences of Foreign Medical Graduates (FMGs), international medical graduates (IMGs) and overseas trained graduates (OTGs) on entering developing or middle-income countries like South Africa: a scoping review. Hum Resour Health. 2019;17:7. https://doi.org/10.1186/s12960-019-0343-y.
3. Educational Commission for Foreign Medical Graduates (ECFMG). Definition of an IMG. 2019. https://www.ecfmg.org/certification/definition-img.html. Accessed 27 Feb 2020.
4. Sumalinog R, Zacharias A, Rana A. Backgrounder: International Medical Graduates (IMGs) and the Canadian Health Care System: A Joint Project of the Committee on Health Policy and the Committee of Medical Education. Canadian Federation of Medical Students. 2015. http://www.old.cfms.org/attachments/article/1370/BACKGROUNDER%20-%20IMGs%20AND%20THE%20CANADIAN%20HEALTHCARE%20SYSTEM.pdf. Accessed 27 Feb 2020.
5. National Resident Matching Program, results and data: 2019 main residency match®. Washington, DC: National Resident Matching Program; 2019. http://www.nrmp.org/main-residency-match-data/. Accessed 27 Feb 2020.
6. Ranasinghe PD. International medical graduates in the US physician workforce. J Am Osteopath Assoc. 2015;115:236–41.
7. AMA-IMG Section Governing Council. International medical graduates in American medicine: contemporary challenges and opportunities. American Medical Association: Chicago; 2013.
8. MedClerkships: USCE & Residency Consultation. Top 20 US states IMGs practice medicine. 2015. https://medclerkships.com/top-states-img-practice-medicine/. Accessed 27 Feb 2020.
9. Canadian Institute for Health Information. Physicians in Canada, 2016: summary report. Ottawa: CIHI; 2017.

10. The New York Times. Why America needs Foreign Medical Graduates. 2017. https://www. nytimes.com/2017/10/06/upshot/america-is-surprisingly-reliant-on-foreign-medical-gradu- ates.html. Accessed 27 Feb 2020.
11. Organization For Economic Co-Operation and Development (OECE). OECD Stat: health workforce migration: foreign trained doctors by country of origin. 2020. https://stats.oecd.org/ Index.aspx?QueryId=68336. Accessed 27 Feb 2020.
12. General Medical Council. GMC data explorer: list of registered medical practitioners. 2020. www.gmc-uk.org/doctors/register/search_stats.asp. Accessed 27 Feb 2020.
13. Duvivier RJ, Wiley E, Boulet JR. Supply, distribution and characteristics of international medical graduates in family medicine in the United States: a cross-sectional study. BMC Fam Pract. 2019;20:47. https://doi.org/10.1186/s12875-019-0933-8.
14. Yen W, Hodwitz K, Thakkar N, et al. The influence of globalization on medical regulation: a descriptive analysis of international medical graduates registered through alternative licensure routes in Ontario. Can Med Educ J. 2016;7:19–30.
15. Peters J. Highly trained and educated, some foreign-born doctors still can't practice medi- cine in the US. Public Radio International (PRI): The World. 2018. https://www.pri.org/sto- ries/2018-03-26/highly-trained-and-educated-some-foreign-born-doctors-still-can-t-practice. Accessed Feb 27 2020.
16. Paul R. A preliminary report of an environmental scan of human resource practices. Employment Opportunities and Alternate Careers for Internationally Educated Health Professionals in Ontario.
17. McDonald JT, Worswick C. The determinants of the migration decisions of immigrant and non-immigrant physicians in Canada. Hamilton: Program for Research on Social and Economic Dimensions of an Aging Population. 2010. https://socialsciences.mcmaster.ca/ sedap/p/sedap282.pdf. Accessed 27 Feb 2020.
18. Bailey M. STAT. After earning an MD, she's headed back to school – to become a nurse. 2016. https://www.statnews.com/2016/11/28/residency-failed-to-match/comment-page-3/. Accessed 27 Feb 2020.
19. Educational Commission for Foreign Medical Graduates (ECFMG). IMGs continue to show gains in 2019 match: growth in primary-care specialties offers enhanced opportunities. 2019. https://www.ecfmg.org/news/2019/03/15/imgs-continue-to-show-gains-in-2019-match/. Accessed 27 Feb 2020.
20. Alberta International Medical Graduate Association (AIMGA). Career Transition Program for IMGs an exploration of alternative pathways into healthcare. Final report. January 2020.
21. Canadian Resident Matching Service. CaRMS forum data presentation. Presented at CaRMS Forum 2019, Niagara Falls, 2019. https://www.carms.ca/pdfs/2019-CaRMS-Forum.pdf. Accessed 27 Feb 2020.
22. Educational Commission for Foreign Medical Graduates. 2008 Annual report. Philadelphia: Educational Commission for Foreign Medical Graduates; 2009.
23. Boulet J, Swanson DB, Cooper RA, Norcini JJ, McKinley DW. A comparison of the char- acteristics and examination performances of U.S. and non-U.S. citizen international medical graduates who sought Educational Commission for Foreign Medical Graduates certification: 1995–2004. Acad Med. 2006;81(10 suppl):S116–9.
24. Boulet J, Norcini JJ, Whelan GP, Hallock JA, Seeling SS. The international medical graduate pipeline; recent trends in ECFMG certification and residency training. Health Aff (Millwood). 2006;25:469–77.
25. Jolly P, Boulet J, Garrison G, Signer MM. International Medical Graduates: participation in U.S. graduate medical education by graduates of international medical schools. Acad Med. 2011;86(5):559–64.
26. Thomson G, Cohl K. IMG selection: Independent review of access to postgraduate programs by international medical graduates in Ontario. Volume 1: findings and recommendations. September 2011.

27. Ko DT, Austin PC, Chan BT, Tu JV. Quality of care of international and Canadian medical graduates in acute myocardial infarction. Arch Intern Med. 2005;165(4):458–63.
28. Desbiens NA, Vidaillet HJ. Discrimination against international medical graduates in the United States residency program selection process. BMC Med Educ. 2010;10:5. https://doi.org/10.1186/1472-6920-10-5.
29. Nasir LS. Evidence of discrimination against international medical graduates applying to family practice residency programs. Fam Med. 1994;26(10):625–9.
30. Moore RA, Rhodenbaugh EJ. The unkindest cut of all: are international medical school graduates subjected to discrimination by general surgery residency programs? Curr Surg. 2002;59(2):228–36.
31. Woods SE, Harju A, Rao S, Koo J, Kini D. Perceived biases and prejudices experienced by international medical graduates in the US Post-Graduate Medical Education System, Medical Education. 2006. Online, 11:1, 4595. https://doi.org/10.3402/meo.v11i.4595
32. Kuczkowski KM. (Not) "Born in the USA": foreign medical school graduates in the American healthcare system. Sao Paulo Med J [Internet]. 2005;123(3):154–155.
33. Balon R, Mufti R, Williams M, Riba M. Possible discrimination in recruitment of psychiatry residents? Am J Psychiatry. 1997;154(11):1608–9.
34. Hanson CW 3rd, Durbin CG Jr, Maccioli GA, et al. The anesthesiologist in critical care medicine: past, present, and future. Anesthesiology. 2001;95(3):781–8.
35. Atchabahian A. Are "international" medical graduate students second-class anesthesiologists? Anesthesiology. 2002;97(1):278.
36. Minnesota Department of Health. International Medical Graduate. Assistance Program: Report to the Minnesota Legislature. 2016. https://www.health.state.mn.us/facilities/ruralhealth/img/docs/2018imgleg.pdf. Accessed 27 Feb 2020.
37. Nedelman M. 2017. Why refugee doctors become taxi drivers. CNN Health. https://edition.cnn.com/2017/08/09/health/refugee-doctors-medical-training/index.html. Accessed 27 Feb 2020.
38. Association of American Medical Colleges. 2012. A Snapshot of the new and developing medical schools in the US and Canada.pdf [Internet]. https://store.aamc.org/a-snapshot-of-the-new-and-developing-medical-schools-in-the-u-s-and-canada-pdf.html. Accessed 27 Feb 2020.
39. Association of American Medical Colleges. Physician supply and demand through 2025: key findings. 2015. https://www.aamc.org/download/153160/data/physician_shortages_to_worsen_without_increases_in_residency_tr.pdf. Accessed 27 Feb 2020.
40. Traverso G, McMahon GT. Residency training and international medical graduates: coming to America no more. JAMA. 2012;308(21):2193–4.
41. Young S. The problem of unmatched Canadian Medical Graduates: where are we now? UBCMJ. 2019;10(2):53–4. https://med-fom-ubcmj.sites.olt.ubc.ca/files/2019/03/Letter-3.pdf. Accessed 27 Feb 2020.
42. ARMC. Undergraduate Medical Education and Student Affairs Committees. The role of MD programs in transitioning students to residency (position paper). Unpublished.
43. College of Physicians and Surgeons of Alberta. Apply for independent practice. 2020. http://www.cpsa.ca/registration/apply-for-independent-practice/. Accessed 27 Feb 2020.
44. Kamimura A, Samhouri MS, Myers K, et al. Physician migration: experience of international medical graduates in the USA. Int Migration Integration. 2017;18:463–81.
45. Miller RS, Dunn MR, Richter TH, Whitcomb ME. Employment-seeking experiences of resident physicians completing training during 1996. JAMA. 1998;280:777.
46. Med Applications: Medical Coaching by Doctors. CaRMS as an International Medical Graduate (IMG) – part 1. 2020. https://medapplications.com/carms-international-medical-graduate-part-1/. Accessed 27 Feb 2020.
47. FMG Portal. 2018 Trends for non-U.S. IMGs in the match. 2018. https://fmgportal.com/2018-trends-for-non-u-s-imgs-in-the-match/. Accessed 27 Feb 2020.

48. Liang M, Curtin LS, Signer MM, Savoia MC. Understanding the interview and ranking Behaviors of unmatched international medical students and graduates in the 2013 Main residency match. J Grad Med Educ. 2015;7:610–6. https://doi.org/10.4300/JGME-D-14-00742.1.
49. De Silva, R. B. (2014). Theorizing the barriers and facilitators to relicensing and resettling of Albertan international medical graduates (order no. 1569459). Available from ProQuest Dissertations & Theses Global. (1626727091).
50. MedClerkships: USCE & Residency Consultation. How hard is it for International Medical Graduates to match into surgery residency. 2016. https://medclerkships.com/how-hard-is-it-for-international-medical-graduates-to-match-into-a-surgery-residency/. Accessed 27 Feb 2020.
51. Peters C. The bridging education and licensure of international medical doctors in Ontario: a call for commitment, consistency, and transparency. 2013. http://hdl.handle.net/1807/31896. Accessed 27 Feb 2020.
52. Mylonakis E, Mega A, Schiffman FJ. What do program directors in internal medicine think about international medical graduates? Results of a pilot study. Acad Med. 1999;74:452.
53. Zulla R, Baerlocher M, Verma S. International medical graduates (IMGs) needs assessment study: comparison between current IMG trainees and program directors. BMC Med Educ. 2008;8(1):42. https://doi.org/10.1186/1472-6920-8-42.
54. Part HM, Markert RJ. Predicting the first-year performance of international medical graduates in an internal medicine residency. Acad Med. 1993;68:856–8.
55. Bates J, Andrew R. Untangling the roots of some IMGs' poor academic performance. Acad Med. 2001;76(1):43–6.
56. University of Calgary. PGME Clinical Teacher Resources: special considerations and unique cases. 2020. https://www.ucalgary.ca/pgme-clinical-teachers/special-cases. Accessed Feb 2020.
57. Lim Consulting Associates. Foreign qualifications recognition and alternative careers. The Best Practices and Thematic Task Team of the Foreign Qualifications Recognition Working Group. Report: 2013. https://novascotia.ca/lae/RplLabourMobility/documents/AlternativeCareersResearchReport.pdf. Accessed 27 Feb 2020.
58. World Education Services. Who is successful in the Canadian market labour? Predictors of Career Success for Skilled Immigrants. 2019. p. 7. https://knowledge.wes.org/canada-report-who-is-succeeding-in-the-canadian-labour-market.html. Accessed 27 Feb 2020.
59. Neiterman E, Salmonsson L, Bourgeault IL. Navigating otherness and belonging: a comparative case study of IMGs' professional integration in Canada and Sweden. Ephemera: theory and politics in. Organization. 2015;15(4):773–95.
60. Bourgeault IL. Health care brain waste needs a long-term policy solution. 2007. http://www.embassynews.ca. Accessed 27 Feb 2020.
61. Bourgeault IL, Neiterman E, LeBrun J, Viers K, Winkup J. Brain gain, drain & waste: the experiences of internationally educated health professionals in Canada. Ottawa: University of Ottawa; 2010.http://www.threesource.ca/documents/February2011/brain_drain.pdf. Accessed 27 Feb 2020.
62. Batalova J,Fix M, Bachmeier JD. Untapped talent: the costs of brain waste among highly skilled immigrants in the United States. Migration Policy Institute. 2016. https://www.migrationpolicy.org/research/untapped-talent-costs-brain-waste-among-highly-skilled-immigrants-united-states. Accessed 27 Feb 2020.
63. Royal Bank of Canada. Immigrant labour market outcomes in Canada: The benefits of addressing wage and employment gaps. 2011. http://www.rbc.com/newsroom/pdf/1219-2011-immigration.pdf. Accessed 27 Feb 2020.
64. Beran et al. Ego identity development in physicians: a cross-cultural comparison using a mixed method approach. 2012. http://www.biomedcentral.com/1756-0500/5/249. Accessed 27 Feb 2020.

65. Fowkes V, Cawley JF, Herlihy N, Cuadrado RR. Evaluating the potential of international medical graduates as physician assistants in primary care. Acad Med. 1996;71(8):886–92.
66. Jones IW. Should international medical graduates work as physician assistants? J Am Acad PAs. 2015;28(7):8–10.
67. Blain M, Fortin S, Alvarez F. Professional journeys of international medical graduates in Quebec: recognition, uphill battles, or career change. Int Migration Integration. 2017;18:223–47. https://doi.org/10.1007/s12134-016-0475-z.
68. Seak Inc. The biggest mistakes physicians make in transitioning to a non-clinical career and how to avoid them. 2019. https://seak.com/the-biggest-mistakes-physicians-make-in-transitioning-to-a-non-clinical-career-and-how-to-avoid-them/. Accessed 27 Feb 2020.
69. Flowers M, Olenick M. Transitioning from physician to nurse practitioner. J Multidiscip Healthc. 2014;7:51–4. https://doi.org/10.2147/JMDH.S56948.
70. Zegarra M. 7 Things to know before studying diagnostic medical sonographer technology. Florida National University: Academic resources. 2019. https://www.fnu.edu/7-studying-diagnostic-medical-sonographer-technology/. Accessed 27 Feb 2020.
71. Creticos PA, Schultz JM, Beeler A, Ball E. The integration of immigrants in the workplace. Institute for Work and the Economy. 2006. https://zdoc.site/the-integration-of-immigrants-in-the-workplace-institute-for.html. Accessed 27 Feb 2020.
72. Barker C. Barriers to employment and overcoming economic integration challenges for foreign-born workers in Maine. Maine: University of Maine; Spring 5, 2018.
73. Dickstein C, Dorrer J, Love E, Chong T. Building Maine's economy: how Maine can embrace immigrants and strengthen the workforce. Coastal Enterprises; 2016. https://www.ceimaine.org/wpcontent/uploads/2016/03/CEI-Immigration-Report-2016-WEB-PAGES.pdf. Accessed 27 Feb 2020.
74. Grossman D, Jorda ML. Transitioning foreign-educated physicians to nurses: the new Americans in nursing accelerated program. J Nurs Educ. 2008;47(12):544–51.
75. Neiterman E, Bourgeault IL, Covell CL. What do we know and not know about the professional integration of international medical graduates (IMGs) in Canada? Healthcare Policy. 2017;12(4):18–32.
76. Bhimji A. International medical graduates: the Medicentres experience. HealthcarePapers. 2010;10(2):46–9.
77. Howard LW, Garman KA, McCann RE. Another go at the experiment. Public Health Rep. 1995;110(6):668–73.
78. Anderson AL, Gilliss C. Nurse practitioners, certified nurse midwives, and physician assistants in California. West J Med. June 1998;168(5):437–44.
79. Smith MW, Fowkes VK. Unlicensed foreign medical graduates in California: social and demographic characteristics and Progress toward licensure. Med Care. 1983;21(12):1168–86.
80. Nyandat J. Doctors: discover these 8 alternative career paths. MIMS Today. 2016. https://today.mims.com/doctors%2D%2Ddiscover-these-8-alternative-career-paths-. Accessed 27 Feb 2020.
81. Ace Surgical Assistants. Ideal training for Foreign Medical Graduates. 2019. https://www.acesatraining.com/custom-solutions/foreign-medical-graduates/. Accessed 27 Feb 2020.
82. California Institute of Behavioural Neurosciences and Psychology. Learn Course Online. 2020. https://www.cibnp.com/. Accessed 27 Feb 2020.
83. Certified Clinical Research Professionals Society (CCRPS). Clinical research training. 2020. https://ccrps.org/. Accessed 27 Feb 2020.
84. Bhuiyan SU. Ryerson University's internationally trained medical doctors bridging program: preliminary results from a pilot program. Ryerson University and University of Toronto. J Prof Contin Online Educ. 2018. https://journals.library.ualberta.ca/jpcoe/index.php/jpcoe/article/download/35/16. Accessed 27 Feb 2020.
85. University of San Diego. Accelerate your career. Earn your Master's Degree in Health Care Informatics – Online or On Campus. 2019. https://onlinedegrees.sandiego.edu/programs/master-of-science-in-health-care-informatics/. Accessed 27 Feb 2020.

86. Skills for Change. The Health Informatics Bridging Program at Skills for Change provides internationally trained newcomers with a background in healthcare or the IT sector, the knowledge, and experience they need for a rewarding career in the field of Health Informatics. 2019. https://skillsforchange.org/healthinformatics/. Accessed 27 Feb 2020.
87. Canadian College of Naturopathic Medicine (CCNM). CCNM is accepting applications for the two-year bridge delivery program for international medical graduates (IMGs). 2019. https://www.ccnm.edu/future-students/international-medical-graduates. Accessed 27 Feb 2020.
88. JVSTORONTO. ISAGE: international skills applied for geriatrics. 2019. https://www.jvstoronto.org/find-a-job/newcomer-employment-services/. Accessed 27 Feb 2020.
89. Bridge to Registration and employment in Mental Health. 2019. https://brem.bridgingprograms.org/index.php/about-brem/. Accessed 27 Feb 2020.
90. Collège Boréal. Bridging Program – Health System Navigator for internationally educated Francophone professionals. 2019. http://www.collegeboreal.ca/student-services/newcomers/. Accessed 27 Feb 2020.
91. The Michener Institute of Education at UHN. Ultrasound scanning evaluation (BPUS800). 2019. https://michener.ca/program/bpus/. Accessed 27 Feb 2020.
92. Wick KH. International medical graduates as physician assistants. JAAPA. 2015;28(7):43–6. https://doi.org/10.1097/01.JAA.0000466891.23457.b0.
93. Learning Enrichment Foundation. Alternative careers in health promotion and education for International Medical Graduates (IMGs) Program. 2019. http://lefca.org/training/IMGs.shtml. Accessed 27 Feb 2020.

Chapter 19
California Institute of Behavioral Neurosciences and Psychology and Its Role in Helping International Medical Graduates

Syeda Sidra Tohid and Hassaan Tohid

Introduction

Since the beginning of the twentieth century, the concept of "online education" caught the attention of the eyes of the masses across the globe. Thousands of online educational institutes and organizations came to surface in a relatively short span of time. However, it was still a stigma until the end of the first decade of the twenty-first century. Many employers would look at the online degree or diploma of a candidate with doubts and dissatisfaction. However, the way the Internet was growing, it was inevitable that more and more institutes will adopt the online culture of education.

The foundation of the California Institute of Behavioral Neurosciences and Psychology (CiBNP) was another addition to the list of online teaching institutes [1]. Yet we at the CiBNP wanted to do something different; we wanted to have a distinct curriculum and a new concept that had never been done by anyone before. Initially, we did not have any idea of what our unique proposition could be. The name California Institute of Behavioral Neurosciences and Psychology was chosen because one of the founders Dr. Hassaan Tohid was passionate for neurosciences, especially psychology. The name was chosen after a serious brainstorming and thought process. The goal was to create an online teaching and research training institute related to neuroscience which gradually transformed into a general research training institute.

During the first few month, we noticed that the IMGs who apply for US residency each year need to have some publications in order to be more competitive for residency match [2]. We also observed that most IMGs applying for residency match did not have the knowledge of research methodology, research design, writing, and publishing. This is not just confined to IMGs, but overall physicians in the

S. S. Tohid · H. Tohid (✉)
California Institute of Behavioral Neurosciences and Psychology, Fairfield, CA, USA

© Springer Nature Switzerland AG 2021
H. Tohid, H. Maibach (eds.), *International Medical Graduates in the United States*, https://doi.org/10.1007/978-3-030-62249-7_19

USA do not have enough knowledge about research [3]. Moreover, there is a dearth of physician scientists in the USA, which is not a good indicator for a better future of science and the field of research [4]. We also understood that finding appropriate research position was a challenge for IMGs; even a volunteer research position was and is still not easy to find. The students who did find research positions had to travel to join that research position and arrange finances for living and other related expenses. This much of financial expense is not feasible for most IMGs or many IMGs if not most. Due to this reason, many IMGs had to apply for the residency match without research. Under these circumstances, the idea of remote research was a blessing, where students could not just learn to write papers but also get publications along with basic understanding of research methodology. This is how CiBNP research department came into existence.

Therefore, we decided to teach research writing and publishing related to neurosciences (psychology, psychiatry, and neurology). However, the increased demand of IMGs for internal medicine made us change our strategy, and we modified the focus from "neurosciences-only research training" to "general research training for everyone."

This research writing and publishing training was the first course that CiBNP launched, and gradually more courses were incorporated into the CiBNP curriculum related to research due to the increasing demand. The focus now solely was general research for everyone rather than neuroscience only. We decided to keep the name California Institute of Behavioral Neurosciences and Psychology for three key reasons: The first reason was that one of the founders Dr. Hassaan Tohid was fascinated with the field neurosciences including psychiatry, neurology, and psychology. The second reason was that we wanted to keep the memory alive of the same institute that we founded. The third reason was that we still wanted to keep neuroscience-related courses and some courses such as neurolinguistic programming (NLP) and general neurosciences course. Therefore, coaching, such as life coaching, NLP, and public speaking training, remained as one of the components of the CiBNP courses for the general population. However, the CiBNP research training program became popular among the IMGs. Therefore, the CiBNP research department came into existence along with the CiBNP coaching department.

Both departments are still functional with CiBNP research department serving IMGs and helping them get into the US residency programs with research-related courses.

About the Founders

Established in 2016, the California Institute of Behavioral Neurosciences and Psychology also known as CIBNP is an online institute founded by Dr. Hassaan Tohid and spouse Dr. Syeda S Tohid. Dr. H Tohid is an MBBS doctor and a neuroscientist and has been on TEDx talks twice [1]. Dr. S Tohid is a foreign PharmD graduate who entered the entrepreneur world as soon as she stepped in the USA. As foreign graduates in the USA, this duo knew the journey was difficult.

The Challenges

The foundation of CiBNP was not an easy task. We met with many challenges and unexpected hurdles and difficulties. We never imagined it would have been that of a challenge to establish an organization from scratch. The biggest challenge we faced was the lack of capital. We had no money to start business with and run an organization. We had no investors, and we never wanted any investor to help us either. One of the founders Dr. Hassaan Tohid had to carry on his daytime job to make both ends meet while driving Uber on the weekend to save more money to survive and invest in the business. He himself was the first and only teacher and mentor to teach the students, while the wife Dr. Sidra was the key person behind the scenes handling administration, management, and student affairs.

Another great challenge we faced was that no one knew us; it was obvious that as a new organization you are unknown. With little or no knowledge of business, sales, and marketing, we started to our organization. With minimal budget, marketing itself was a challenge, and the challenges did not end here. We faced an extreme lack of trust by the prospects because we were new and the concept of online education itself was not looked at with trust. We were ridiculed and disrespected on social media initially, but gradually with the passage of time, things started to calm down, and we also learned to market, and people started to know us as well. We also did not know the complete paperwork related to business and the minute details of how an organization is run. The challenges to creating social media pages and making them successful along with a professional website with no money were other huge challenges that we faced. With these challenges, the organization has reached at this level where it is today.

An outsider, when hearing about CiBNP, probably thinks, "oh they were lucky," without seeing the background and the hidden problems and challenges we faced in establishing this organization.

Our Story

The story of founding the CIBNP as narrated by the founders themselves:

Starting up in the living room of a one-bedroom apartment in Fairfield, California, punching on some old laptop computers, this young couple started working on their dream of making research easier for foreign graduates. Teaching research writing and training for scientific publishing online was something unheard of in the medical education world, but aiming to make it possible for foreign medical graduates was even more rare.

Facing the criticism from the stereotypical crowd, we decided it was something we want to make happen. Investing our time and effort with almost nothing in our pockets, we started to build our online research writing and publishing training center and came up with a simple but unique logo for our online institute, while saving up money for our basic website and using free social media accounts to spread the word. Together, we taught each other daily by going through and studying several business-related books, and coming from a medical background, this was something that gave us a bittersweet time and which now is a cherished memory.

CIBNP took a kick start within the same year of its coming into being; students came to us with extreme excitement, utter disbelief, and some with plain rudeness. All this because it was something they never expected, specially not in the digital world. As soon as we started getting more students coming to us, we had to come up with a plan on how to manage the online study in a fashion that it benefits the students as well as our lives that just took a start as well. Initially, we two people were CIBNP's administration, production, human resources, customer services, marketing and sales department, and everything in between.

Why CiBNP Came into Existence?

Searching on the Google Search engine about "How to write a research paper" will provide you with several options: established companies that claim to provide the writing experience, opportunities to publish in scientific journals, chance to participate in online research, and much more. However, digging deeper into this pit of information will make your mind boggle. You will go from one platform to another and then back to page one without knowing how to look for something that can help your career.

The California Institute of Behavioral Neurosciences and Psychology (CIBNP) and its founding members knew the struggle of a student who does all the above-mentioned back and forth activities on the search engines, ending up nowhere. The need for this institute became essential when certain colleagues back home shared their experiences of getting scammed by predatory journals and fake companies that promise publications in your name; in return, you pay them a few bucks, which could make sense only if the candidate was actually writing that article/paper that was promised to be published. Many students get scammed by such online companies who ask them for a certain amount of money, claiming that no work is required for the article; they do not tell you what journal the publication is going into, make you and the coauthors pay the amount of money that varies with the financial condition of each of the author, and do not let you select the topic, write the article, or find a journal of your choice but keep everything related to this confidential because "you're getting a publication, how could you complain?"

Unfortunately, as common as they seem, these practices in the academic world are *wrong*. One cannot emphasize enough on how immoral is to take money from a person without his involvement or contribution to the study, promising him the publication that he did not work for. A student with no knowledge about the publication gets in trouble whenever that particular publication or research is discussed in front of him, which many times becomes a decisive factor for the passing of his/her interview and selection.

About the Institute and Its Foundation

The first year for any new organization is difficult. Spreading the word among the interested candidates when you do not know where your market will be found is even more energy consuming. To come up with the idea of teaching scientific writing to students online came with its own challenges. Among the expected challenges were the disbelief from the students, the criticism of the peers, the idea of how no one seems to have done it before, and of course the lack of capital, in fact the capital nowhere to be found.

The shady practices going on over the Internet platform gave us a whole new level of doing something just: the decision to come up with something that would help the international graduates on a level where they no longer feel left out. To stop the students fall prey to the predatory, we came up with this idea of making them learn the skill for which they are ready to pay to be a part of. We came up with a program that will not only help international graduates to learn to write but also to get their piece of writing published in a way that is 100% honest.

What Is Research and Why It Is Important?

The word research is a combination of two words "re" and "search." It simply means searching something again. However, by this definition, it does imply that a second time search is known as research. However, anytime you search anything, it is research.

In terms of science, research is finding an answer to a question or finding a solution to a problem. Although this book is focused on international medical graduates, research is not just confined to medical field. In fact, everything we have today is because of research. We have the Internet because someone decided to research and find an answer how people could be connected and shaped the world we have today. We have computers and cellphones because someone with a similar mind wanted this scientific miracle to happen. Research is present in all fields of the world whether it is engineering, pharmacology, biology, chemistry, physics, mathematics, economics, psychology, literature, or history.

Without research, we would have probably still been living in stone ages with no electricity, airplanes, motor cars, motorcycles, and television sets. The same is true for the medical sciences; without research, medical sciences would not have been where it is today. We now have medications to treat bacteria called antibiotics.

Without which it would have been impossible to treat bacterial illnesses and save people's lives. Similarly, we have vaccines of many life-threatening viruses. Just when COVID-19 pandemic erupted in 2019, we began to realize the importance of vaccines and how lucky we have been to be protected against many other viruses that otherwise would have killed us all or probably wipe out the world beyond exaggeration.

Medical science has realized the importance of research, and the Western world has been very proactive in evolving medical research. The governments of many Western countries are supportive in this regard. For example, in the USA, the Department of Health is very active in helping the National Library of Medicine, and databases such as PubMed and the finding agencies such as NIH exist to assist and expand scientific knowledge for the betterment of society, in a hope to treat many life-threatening diseases. The system not just expects senior medical doctors to engage in some kind of research, but it also expects recent medical graduates to be involved in some kind of research at some level and publish articles to bring some new idea that can revolutionize the world. IMGs coming to the USA already have a disadvantage of being a foreign graduate, must publish some scientific papers, and propose some new idea or question that may help future scientists explore more answers and help the humanity as a whole.

Involvement in research is not just a medical necessity, but it has now become an essential tool for career success as well. University jobs or clinical jobs are dependent on publications. Candidates with more publications tend to get hired easily as compared to their counterparts without any publications. Someone who is a senior licensed physician, a professor at a university or is striving to get into the US residency system tries to get some kind of research experience and publications in order to be more competitive.

Recent data has also shown that American medical graduates (AMGs) and IMGs who match tend to have more publications on average than those IMGs or AMGs who do not have publications.

How Does CiBNP Help IMGs?

Since research experience for IMGs as well as AMGs was becoming increasingly important. We here at the CiBNP realized the importance of publications and research experience. We also realized that it was almost impossible for all the AMGs and IMGs to get research experience because of limited slots and need for research positions and also because many young doctors don't know how to find research positions in the USA.

Preparing for USMLEs, exam application, and the match process itself is hectic and time-consuming. Under these circumstances, finding research position can take considerable amount of time. Now the IMGs are in a situation where one asks: Should I focus on my exams, should I focus on finding clinical experience, should I focus on exam application and personal statement, or should I focus on finding research position? Research position itself is not enough; they are supposed to have some research publications. Therefore, if someone got a research rotation around May or June and he was applying the same year September 15th, it was impossible to get a publication in such a short span of time. Ideally, one had to spend at least a year in a lab to get some publications, but that 1 year also is counted against him because each year the students' year of graduation becomes 1 year older. This confusion deprived so many IMGs and also AMGs from acquiring research experience.

We believed it was a serious problem. Therefore, we brought a solution for everyone to get research publications along with training to write and publish sitting home online. Everything is online nowadays; even the clinical setting is remotely conducted through the Internet. Then why could research not be done remotely? Initially, when we brought this idea, it was received with strange facial expressions, laughter, and mock. However, gradually, it started becoming a norm, and others also followed the same idea, and the concept of online research became popular among the IMGs.

CiBNP provides online research writing and publishing training where we teach students to write and publish and they work on a research project side by side and become a published author while learning side by side.

This concept was driven by the concept of driving schools, where they give you a car to drive while learning. You learn to drive on a real car and on real road, and you become a driver.

The purpose is to make the students independent in research writing and publishing, with a goal that they never need our help in the future again. In fact, they should be able to help others in writing and publishing.

How Is It Done Online?

It is quite natural that a clinical trial is not done online anywhere around the globe. Although it is a high possibility to see clinical trials being done online due to COVID-19, however, it is still very tough. Whoever is collecting data from the patients sitting home can interview the patients, but at least one person needs to be in the proximity of the patient. Therefore, a concept of 100 percent online clinical trial is difficult to achieve. The same is true for other study designs such as cohort studies and case-control studies. To understand the types of study designs, see Fig. 19.1.

We at the CiBNP realized this and decided to just keep those study designs that could be done and published sitting at home online. The study designs that could be done sitting home are systematic reviews, traditional reviews, case reports, or some kinds of cross-sectional studies. However, most of CiBNP students choose to write a systematic review or a traditional review, because it is something that could be done easily sitting home without a need to real patient data and without a need of an IRB approval. Hence, review articles tend to be the best option for IMGs to write at this stage of their career not only because of the feasibility of writing but also because review articles are the kinds of papers that if one chooses to write them,

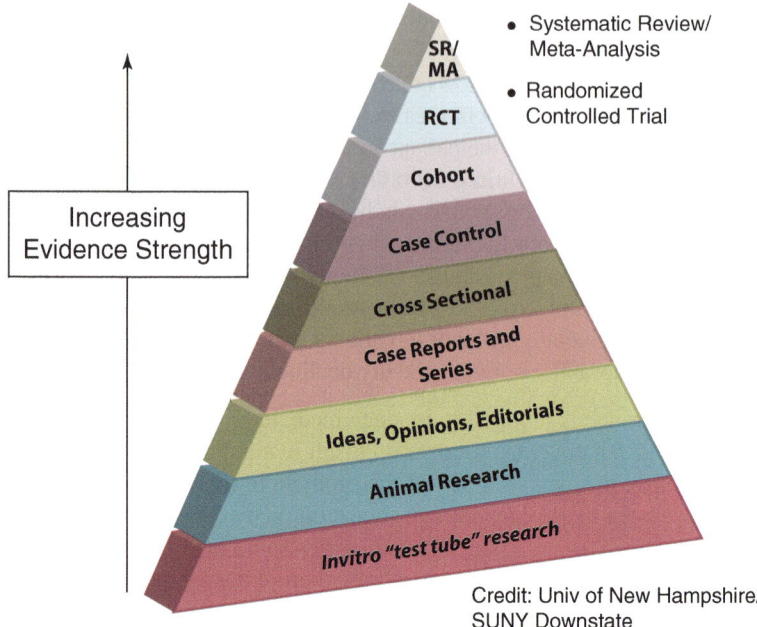

Fig. 19.1 The figure is modified and adopted from the study design pyramid figure by the University of New Hampshire/SUNY Downstate available on Google. The figure shows different kinds of study designs from the weakest to the strongest research evidence. Systematic reviews/meta-analysis are the strongest research evidence, while in vitro "test tube" research is the weakest evidence

then all other kinds of articles become easier to write. Moreover, we look at the study design pyramid, systematic reviews and meta-analysis are on the top of the list with being the strongest research evidence (scientific community accepts them as the highest quality evidence). Thus, CiBNP students learn to write the strongest research evidence that is systematic reviews, and if a meta-analysis is required, it is up to the student to go ahead and do a meta-analysis. Either way, they strengthen their CVs and are more competitive for residency match in comparison to all other candidates applying for residency in the USA, who either have publications such as clinical trials or observational studies or have no publications.

The students learn to collect data using different electronic databases such as PubMed, Medline, PubMed Central, etc. They learn all the prerequisites of data collection and learn to use the search engine to research relevant articles. In the end, they learn to write and then complete their project and then publish their papers. The main goal is to teach students to write, publish, collect data, and analyze, so that they learn all these essential features of any research and also get some publications in the end to be more competitive for the US residency match. This is how CiBNP helps IMGs and trains them for research.

About the Faculty and the Team

The faculty at the CiBNP is comprised of highly qualified scientists and doctors across the globe working in different countries including the USA, Canada, UK, Croatia, and Egypt. The prerequisite of being the CiBNP teaching faculty is to have publications as the first author. The CiBNP faculty members are dedicated, hard-working, and passionate to help students and assist them in research writing and publishing.

CiBNP team also includes dedicated software team to assist in online education system and hardworking accounts, marketing, and administration team.

Our Services

The CiBNP provides teaching services with the following courses:

1. Be a Published Author Program
2. SPSS Statistical Data Analysis Training
3. Research Methodology
4. Introduction to Research
5. Research Proposal Writing
6. Case Report Writing
7. Traditional Review Writing

And some other courses related to career development such as CV Writing, Personal Statement Writing, etc.

CiBNP also provides editing services for our students who find English language difficult to write.

The other courses that CiBNP provides are speech pathology courses and career consultation courses.

Research Courses by CiBNP

The main research-related courses offered by the CiBNP are:

1. Be a Published Author Program
2. SPSS Statistical Data Analysis Program

Both programs are two months in duration.

Be a Published Author Program

The Be a Published Author Program also known as the Two-Month Hands-On Research Writing and Publishing Training Program by the CiBNP is the most popular program by CiBNP among the IMGs. In this distance learning program, the students learn to write and publish research articles in two months of time. The first seven weeks are the writing training, while the last week is the publishing training where the students learn to publish papers. Once the paper they are working on is completed, the paper is submitted for publication to the journal of students' choice.

At the end of the program, the students are awarded certificate of completion and a letter of recommendation depending on their performances. In order to get the certificate and LoR, the students must complete their paper. The certificate and letter are kept on hold until the assignments are submitted. Moreover, the students also receive live Zoom classes each week along with live question answer session with the program director once a week. After each session, the recordings are provided to the students so that they can learn and enjoy the training after the live session as well and keep the study material permanently. The students also receive electronic lecture notes, e-books, exercise books, and hundreds of videos as bonus feature of this program.

SPSS Statistical Data Analysis Training

The software SPSS (Statistical Package for the Social Sciences) is a data analysis tool by IBM. The CiBNP SPSS statistical data analysis training is also a two-month online statistical data analysis training where the students learn data analysis skill on a statistical data analysis software such as SPSS.

Other Courses

The other courses include courses like Introduction to Research, Research Methodology, Research Proposal Writing, Traditional Review Writing, Case Study and Case Report Writing, etc.

Types of Article Writing

As already discussed, according to the study design pyramid, the study designs can be of low- and high-quality evidence. The pyramid keeps in vitro test tube at the bottom, while the systematic reviews and meta-analysis are at the top of the pyramid and are considered as the strongest research evidence by the scientific community. Therefore, CiBNP students learn to write systematic reviews, so that they learn the highest quality evidence. The clinical trials and observational studies are not feasible to be done online anywhere, but the way everything is switching to online mode, we hope to see clinical trials and other study designs being done all around the world. Until then, CiBNP just offers training on certain kinds of articles.

The CiBNP students mainly write the following kinds of articles during the training:

- Systemic reviews
- Traditional reviews
- Case reports

The CiBNP trains the students to write high-quality articles and avoid unethical or wrong doings such as scientific frauds and plagiarism. The CiBNP has a zero-tolerance policy for plagiarism and scientific fraud. All the students are informed that any student found to be involved in plagiarism or any kind of scientific fraud will be reprimanded or expelled from the institute. Therefore, the students who comply with the rules remain cautious while working on their articles.

Mode of Teaching

Teaching is done via live Zoom classes or similar software. The students also receive the recordings of each class after the class. In addition, the students also receive more recorded videos and many other features to enhance the learning process. The other short courses, however, are 100 percent recorded in nature.

Social Interaction Between the Students and Opportunity to Meet New People

The classes during the comprehensive programs are conducted in such a manner that the students are provided with a virtual classroom with Zoom videos with other similar students who are either applying for the US or Canadian clinical residency or are applying for the training programs in the UK. The students are connected with each other on WhatsApp and arrange a student discussion session each week, where they help each other and work with each other so they may coauthor with other classmates. The CiBNP also provides the students from all the groups and batches to interact with each other during the live QA session with the program director. In this way, they can make many lifelong friends from different cultural and ethnic backgrounds.

CIBNP and Its Social Media Platforms

The CiBNP is actively present on all social media platforms like Facebook, YouTube, Instagram, LinkedIn, and Twitter. The CiBNP Facebook group on research writing alone has around 40,000 students as of 2020. The group provides useful information related to research to the members free of cost.

Some of the Publications by Our Talented Students

The CiBNP students have successfully published articles in scientific peer-reviewed PubMed/PMC indexed journals. Some of the publications are as follows:

1. Beriwal N et al. Role of immune-pineal axis in neurodegenerative diseases, unraveling novel hybrid dark hormone therapies. Heliyon. 2019 Jan; 5(1): e01190. Published online 2019 Feb 1. doi: https://doi.org/10.1016/j.heliyon.2019.e01190
2. Ratna Krishnaswamy, Haider Malik, Safeera Khan et al. Anti-CGRP monoclonal antibodies: breakthrough in migraine therapeutics. Migraine therapeutics. 23(3), Published: 13 August 2019. https://doi.org/10.1002/pnp.544
3. Khan, Anser Saeed et al. "Fragile-X premature ovarian insufficiency: a lesser known cause of infertility among Asian women." (2019).
4. Saleem, Hajra et al. "Coronavirus Disease 2019 (COVID-19) in Children: Vulnerable or Spared? A Systematic Review." *Cureus* vol. 12,5 e8207. 20 May. 2020, doi:10.7759/cureus.8207
5. Patel S J, Khan S, M S, et al. (July 21, 2020) The Association Between Cannabis Use and Schizophrenia: Causative or Curative? A Systematic Review. Cureus 12(7): e9309. doi:10.7759/cureus.9309

CIBNP and Its Partnership with Scientific Journal

The CiBNP officially partnered with *Cureus Journal of Medical Science* in 2019 and has an academic channel with *Cureus*. Because of this channel, the CiBNP students can publish their articles in *Cureus* in just few days [5]. The articles go through robust quality assessment before being processed for publication. The CiBNP team and the *Cureus* team work together to make this process faster and easier.

CIBNP and the US Clinical Experience

The CiBNP joined hands with the American Clinical Experience (ACE) in 2019; due to this partnership, CiBNP also provides US clinical experience in different states of the USA. The ACE is also remotely available using telemedicine technology. Many students around the globe are benefitted by with these tele-rotations especially during the pandemic of COVID-19. The students also receive letters of recommendation from the doctors who supervise them.

What Does the Future Hold?

Soon the CiBNP plans to launch more courses on the subjects like psychology, neuroscience, business, and other domains. The CiBNP is actively working on creating new courses on career development for the IMGs and non-IMGs, as well as other professions, with a goal and mission in mind to help and serve millions of students around the globe and help maximum IMGs get high-quality education and remote research and clinical experience at affordable rates.

Why Is CiBNP the Future of Online Research?

The pandemic of COVID-19 has shown to the world that many businesses and companies that we thought could never operate remotely can work remotely 100 percent. This has changed the dynamics of the modern world. Many employees all around the world are solely working from home and utilizing the Internet and Zoom or similar software programs. Until the past decade, the online education was still a stigma, but gradually the online culture took over, and now due to COVID-19 almost all major educational institutes have switched to an online model or if not yet then seriously considered to be online. This clearly shows that the future of education and many professions is distance learning or work from home. The doctors now have begun to realize that the medical consultation can also be solely done online via telemedicine; similarly, the success of CiBNP research writing program has also proven that the future of research will also be online regardless of the study design. The current situation hints us toward a future where we may see clinical trials, animal experiments, and observational studies solely being done online as well. Until then, CiBNP will continue to serve and help physicians and scientists across the globe become astounding research writers and published authors.

Conclusion

The CiBNP continues its mission to serve students online because the concept of distance learning is here to stay. We at CiBNP strive to provide quality education to medical and nonmedical students and specially help IMGs become proficient in research writing and other research-related skills and eventually help them become published research authors. Many CiBNP students matched into the US residency programs and achieved their career goals because of our service. With overcoming every challenge and solving problems associated with running an organization, more challenges and problems are brought to surface, and with dedication, determination, and hard work, we will continue to overcome the challenges and solve problems not only related to running the organization but for the students including international medical graduates (IMGs).

Conflict of Interest The authors Dr. Hassaan Tohid and Dr. Syeda Sidra Tohid are the founders of the California Institute of Behavioral Neurosciences and Psychology (CiBNP). CiBNP is a for-profit organization started in 2016, with an aim of providing quality education online.

References

1. The California Institute of Behavioral Neurosciences and Psychology. Available at https://www.cibnp.com/
2. Rogers CR, Gutowski KA, Munoz-Del Rio A, Larson DL, Edwards M, Hansen JE, Lawrence WT, Stevenson TR, Bentz ML Integrated plastic surgery residency applicant survey: Characteristics of successful applicants and feedback about the interview process.Plast Reconstr Surg. 2009;123(5):1607–17.
3. Rosenberg LE. The physician-scientist: an essential – and fragile – link in the medical research chain. J Clin Invest. 1999;103(12):1621–6.
4. Vidyasagar D. Integrating international medical graduates into the physician-scientist pool: solution to the problem of decreasing physician-scientists in the United States. J Investig Med. 2007;55(8):406–9. https://doi.org/10.2310/6650.2007.00022.
5. The Cureus Medical Journal. Available at www.cibnp.com

Chapter 20
Licensing Requirements by State and Territory for International Medical Graduates

Ai-Tram N. Bui and Vinod E. Nambudiri

Overview of Licensing Requirements for IMGs to Enter an ACGME Residency Program

International medical graduates (IMGs) are a vital part of the US healthcare workforce [1]. All IMGs have to undergo United States Medical Licensing Examinations (USMLEs) and credential verification in order to enter into an Accreditation Council for Graduate Medical Education (ACGME) accredited residency program and obtain medical licensure to practice in the United States [1]. In the United States, the requirements for initial medical licensure are state and/or territory dependent [2]. As an IMG, these licensing requirements may differ and can be challenging to navigate.

The Process for Eligibility to Enter into an ACGME Residency Program

Founded in 1956, the Educational Commission for Foreign Medical Graduates (ECFMG) is an organization that assesses the readiness of IMGs to begin entrance into ACGME-accredited residency programs in the United States [3]. It also serves as an excellent resource for applicants and includes the most accurate

A.-T. N. Bui
Harvard Medical School, Boston, MA, USA
e-mail: ai-tram_bui@hms.harvard.edu

V. E. Nambudiri (✉)
Department of Dermatology, Brigham and Women's Hospital and Harvard Medical School, Boston, MA, USA
e-mail: vnambudiri@bwh.harvard.edu

© Springer Nature Switzerland AG 2021
H. Tohid, H. Maibach (eds.), *International Medical Graduates in the United States*, https://doi.org/10.1007/978-3-030-62249-7_20

requirement information on the certification and licensure process [4]. There are three main steps for IMGs to undergo prior to being eligible to enter ACGME residency programs in the United States: application for ECFMG certification, medical licensing examinations which include the United States Medical Licensing Examination (USMLE) Sequence, and meeting medical education credential requirements [3].

Step 1: Educational Commission for Foreign Medical Graduates Certification Process

In order to be able to apply for and take the USMLE exams, an IMG applicant must submit an application for ECFMG certification. To begin the ECFMG certification process, the applicant must confirm that his or her medical school(s) meets ECFMG requirements listed in the World Directory [4]. Unfortunately, if one's medical school is not listed, he or she is not eligible to apply for ECFMG certification [4].

Step 2: Medical Board Examinations

Once an applicant's ECFMG certification has been accepted, he or she may then apply to take required medical board examinations [3]. The examination requirement includes passing performance on the USMLE board licensing series: Step 1, Step 2 Clinical Knowledge (CK), and Step 2 Clinical Skills (CS) exams. This requirement may differ for Doctor of Osteopathic Medicine (D.O.) applicants who often take either the USMLE or the COMLEX (Comprehensive Osteopathic Medical Licensing Examination) licensing series. To participate in the National Resident Matching Program, it is important to take Step 2 Clinical Skills prior to a specific time line (often December 31 of the year prior to the Match) [3].

Step 3: Medical Education Credentialing

After successful completion of USMLE Step 1 and Step 2 (both CK and CS), medical education credentials must be verified [4]. These include ensuring that an applicant's medical school and graduation year are listed in the World Directory of Medical Schools and that he or she has successfully completed their medical school requirements with credit for at least four credit years of medical school [4]. Moreover, documentation must be submitted for completion of all credits and a receipt of their final medical diploma(s) and transcript(s). Applicants can then successfully enter into and complete an ACGME residency program.

The Requirements of Obtaining an Initial Medical License by State and/or Territory

After completion of residency, IMGs are required to have a medical license granted by a US state or territory to practice medicine independently as a physician [5]. The path of obtaining initial licensure for IMGs can be challenging and complex, with differing requirements per state or territory [5]. Each state may require its own individual applications, and it is important to be meticulous about these requirements for the state one is interested in practicing in. A medical licensure is necessary before a physician can receive hospital credentialing to practice and qualify for medical malpractice insurance [5].

The first step for applicants is the completion of an initial application, which is specific to each state or territory. The completion of USMLE Step 3 or COMLEX Level 3 is also required [2]. The application will require a primary source verification of one's core credentials. Please visit your state's medical licensing board for specific application and licensing requirements [5]. Documents that are usually required include personal contact information, verification of credentials, verification of professional education, curriculum vitae or list of activities, evidence of successful completion of the USMLE/COMLEX series (includes Step/Level 3), and criminal history check, among many other possible documentation requirements [5].

Please see below for the most recent initial licensing requirements by each state and/or territory for eligibility for initial medical licensure [2]. Successful completion of the USMLE Step 1, Step 2 (both CS and CK), and Step 3 exams or COMLEX Level 1, Level 2, and Level 3 is necessary [6]. Some states may require completion of these exams within a limit of attempts or time frame. A minimum number of years of postgraduate training are also required, which may differ for IMGs versus physician graduates of US medical schools. These requirements may be lessened for certain applicants. There is also a time limit for the completion of the entire sequence of the medical licensing examinations. There are several exceptions, particularly for dual-degree M.D./Ph.D. or D.O./Ph.D. applicants.

The Federation Credentials Verification Service (FCVS) is a centralized process and repository of information on applicants. This service is available to all USMLE candidates who complete their Step 3 application. A majority but not all states accept FCVS-verified documents, and using this service may help expedite and centralize credentialing documents [2]. The FCVS may be particularly beneficial for applicants who require licensing in multiple states (e.g., if a physician is planning to practice in two locations in different adjacent states). Listed below are also the states that either currently require or accept FCVS-verified documents.

State-by-State Listing of Licensure Requirements for IMGs

Alabama
- Completion of USMLE exams with up to ten attempts on all exams; up to four attempts at USMLE Step 3 following proof of formal training completion after the third attempt.

- Completion of USMŁE licensing examination sequence within 7 years.
- Completion of COMLEX exams with no limits on attempts.
- Completion of COMLEX licensing examination sequence within no time limit.
- Minimum 3 years of ACGME training.
- FCVS is accepted.

Alaska
- Completion of USMLE or COMLEX exams with up to two attempts per Step/Level.
- Completion of USMLE or COMLEX licensing examination sequence within 7 years.
- Exception for M.D., Ph.D. candidates: can complete USMLE or COMLEX licensing examination sequence within 10 years.
- Minimum 3 years of ACGME training.
- FCVS is accepted.

Arizona (M.D. Applicants)
- Completion of USMLE exams with no limits on attempts.
- Completion of USMLE licensing examination sequence within 7 years for initial licensure; if already licensed, no limits on time.
- Minimum 3 years of ACGME training.
- FCVS is accepted.

Arizona (D.O. Applicants)
- Completion of COMLEX exams, contact state board for information on limits on attempts.
- Completion of COMLEX licensing examination sequence, contact state board for information on time limits.
- Minimum 1 year of ACGME training.
- FCVS is accepted.

Arkansas
- Completion of USMLE or COMLEX exams with up to three attempts per Step/Level.
- Completion of USMLE or COMLEX licensing examination sequence within no time limit.
- Minimum 3 years of ACGME training; exception for those currently enrolled in training program through University of Arkansas for Medical Sciences.
- FCVS is accepted.

California (M.D. Applicants)
- Completion of USMLE exams with up to four attempts at Step 3.
- Passing scores of USMLE licensing examination sequence will be valid for up to 10 years from the month of the examination.
- Minimum 3 years of ACGME training.
- FCVS is accepted.

California (D.O. Applicants)
- Completion of COMLEX exams with no limits on attempts.
- Completion of COMLEX licensing examination sequence with no time limits.
- Minimum 1 year of ACGME training.
- Limited acceptance of FCVS.

Colorado
- Completion of USMLE exams with no limits on attempts.
- Completion of COMLEX exams, contact state board for information on limits on attempts.
- Completion of USMLE or COMLEX licensing examination sequence within 7 years of first examination.
- Exception for M.D., Ph.D. candidates: can complete USMLE or COMLEX licensing examination sequence within 10 years.
- Minimum 3 years of ACGME training.
- FCVS is accepted.

Connecticut
- Completion of USMLE or COMLEX exams with no limits on attempts.
- Completion of USMLE licensing examination sequence within 7 years.
- Completion of COMLEX licensing examination sequence within no time limit.
- Minimum 2 years of postgraduate training.
- FCVS is accepted.

Delaware
- Completion of USMLE exams with up to six attempts per Step.
- Completion of USMLE licensing examination sequence within 7 years.
- Contact state board for information on COMLEX requirements.
- Minimum 3 years of postgraduate training.
- FCVS is accepted.

Washington, D.C.
- Completion of USMLE exams with up to three attempts at Step 3; after three attempts, one additional postgraduate training year is required.
- Completion of USMLE licensing examination sequence within 7 years.
- Completion of COMLEX exams with no limits on attempts.
- Completion of USMLE licensing examination sequence with no time limits.
- Minimum 3 years of postgraduate training.
- FCVS is accepted.

Florida (M.D. Applicants)
- Completion of USMLE exams with no limits on attempts.
- Completion of USMLE licensing examination sequence with no time limits.
- Minimum 2 years of postgraduate training.
- FCVS is highly recommended.

Florida (D.O. Applicants)
- Completion of COMLEX exams, contact state board for information on limits on attempts.
- Completion of COMLEX licensing examination sequence with no time limits.
- Minimum 1 year in an American Osteopathic Association (AOA)-approved program.
- FCVS is highly recommended.

Georgia
- Completion of USMLE exams with up to three attempts per Step exam.
- Completion of USMLE licensing examination sequence within 7 years.
- Exception for M.D., Ph.D. candidates: can complete USMLE licensing examination sequence within 9 years.
- Completion of COMLEX exams with no limits on attempts.
- Completion of COMLEX licensing examination sequence with no time limit.
- Minimum 3 years of postgraduate training if not on list; minimum 1 year of postgraduate training if on list.
- FCVS is accepted.

Hawaii
- Completion of USMLE or COMLEX exams with no limits on attempts.
- Completion of USMLE or COMLEX licensing examination sequence with no time limit.
- Minimum 2 years of postgraduate training.
- FCVS is accepted.

Idaho
- Completion of USMLE exams within two attempts; failure after two attempts may lead to a board interview or further evaluation.
- Completion of USMLE licensing examination sequence within 7 years.
- Exception for M.D., Ph.D. candidates: can complete USMLE licensing examination sequence within 10 years.
- Completion of COMLEX exams with no limits on attempts.
- Completion of COMLEX licensing examination sequence within no time limit.
- Minimum 3 years of postgraduate training; exception for licensing after 2 years if applicant is in good standing with an Idaho residency training program and has signed an agreement to complete residency in Idaho.
- FCVS is accepted; uniform application is required.

Illinois
- Completion of USMLE or COMLEX exams with five attempts on all Steps/Levels combined.
- Completion of USMLE licensing examination sequence within 7 years.
- Completion of COMLEX licensing examination sequence with no time limit.
- Minimum 2 years of postgraduate training.
- FCVS is accepted.

Indiana
- Completion of USMLE exams with three attempts per Step.
- Completion of USMLE licensing examination sequence within 10 years.
- Completion of COMLEX exams with five attempts per Level.
- Completion of COMLEX licensing examination sequence within 7 years.
- Minimum 2 years of postgraduate training.
- FCVS is accepted.

Iowa
- Completion of USMLE exams with six attempts at both Steps 1 and 2, and three attempts at Step 3.
- Completion of COMLEX exams with six attempts at both Levels 1 and 2, and three attempts at Level 3.
- If outside this attempt limit for USMLE or COMLEX, requires 3 years of approved postgraduate training.
- Completion of USMLE or COMLEX licensing examination sequence within 10 years; same requirement for M.D./Ph.D. or D.O./Ph.D. candidates.
- Minimum 2 years of postgraduate training.
- FCVS is accepted; uniform application is utilized.

Kansas
- Completion of USMLE or COMLEX exams with three attempts for Step 3/Level 3.
- Completion of USMLE or COMLEX licensing examination sequence within 10 years.
- Minimum 3 years of postgraduate training; minimum 2 years in an ACGME-approved program.
- FCVS is accepted.

Kentucky
- Completion of USMLE exams with up to four attempts for each Step.
- Completion of COMLEX exams with up to four attempts for each Level.
- Completion of USMLE or COMLEX licensing examination sequence with no time limit.
- Minimum 2 years of postgraduate training.
- FCVS is required.

Louisiana
- Completion of USMLE exams with no limit on Step 1, up to four attempts on Steps 2 and 3.
- Completion of COMLEX exams with no limit on Level 1, up to four attempts on Levels 2 and 3.
- Completion of USMLE or COMLEX licensing examination sequence within 10 years.
- Minimum 3 years of postgraduate training.
- FCVS is required.

Maine (M.D. Applicants)
- Completion of USMLE exams with up to three attempts at Step 3; if more than three, need to request a waiver.
- Completion of USMLE licensing examination sequence within 7 years; if more than 7, need to request a waiver.
- Minimum 3 years of ACGME training.
- FCVS is required.

Maine (D.O. Applicants)
- Completion of COMLEX or USMLE exams with up to three attempts at each Step/Level.
- Completion of COMLEX licensing examination sequence with no limits on attempts.
- Minimum 1 year in an AOA-approved program.
- FCVS is accepted.

Maryland
- Completion of USMLE or COMLEX exams with no limits on attempts.
- Completion of COMLEX licensing examination sequence within no time limit; there may be additional requirements if applicant fails an exam three or more times.
- Minimum 2 years of postgraduate training.
- FCVS is accepted.

Massachusetts
- Completion of USMLE exams with up to three attempts at Step 3.
- Completion of COMLEX exams with up to three attempts.
- Completion of USMLE or COMLEX licensing examination sequence within 7 years.
- Prior to January 2014, 2 years postgraduate training; after January 2014, 3 years postgraduate training.
- FCVS is required.

Michigan (M.D. Applicants)
- Completion of USMLE exams with up to three attempts for each step.
- Completion of USMLE licensing examination sequence within 7 years from the date of first passing any Step of the exam. Must pass Step 3 within 4 years of the first attempt at Step 3 or must complete 1 year of postgraduate training before making additional attempts at Step 3.
- Minimum 2 years of postgraduate training.
- FCVS is accepted.

Michigan (D.O. Applicants)
- Completion of COMLEX or USMLE exams with up to six attempts at each Step/Level.
- Completion of COMLEX licensing examination sequence within 7 years from the date of first passing of any component.

- Minimum 1 year in an AOA-approved program.
- FCVS is accepted.

Minnesota

- Completion of USMLE exams with up to three attempts at each Step; four attempts allowed if current license in another state and current certification by specialty board of American Board of Medical Specialties (ABMS), American Osteopathic Association Bureau of Professional Education (AOABPE), Royal College of Physicians and Surgeons of Canada (RCPSC), and Canadian Family Physician (CFPC).
- Completion of COMLEX exams with up to three attempts per Level.
- Completion of USMLE or COMLEX Step or Level 3 within 5 years of Step or Level 2 or before the end of residency training.
- Minimum 1 year of postgraduate training.
- FCVS is accepted.

Mississippi

- Completion of USMLE exams with up to three attempts at each Step.
- Completion of COMLEX exams with no limits on attempts.
- Completion of USMLE licensing examination sequence within 7 years; no time limit on COMLEX licensing examination sequence.
- Minimum 1–3 years of postgraduate training, contact state medical board for most recent requirement.
- FCVS is accepted.

Missouri

- Completion of USMLE or COMLEX exams with up to three attempts at each Step/Level.
- Completion of USMLE licensing examination sequence within 7 years; no time limit on COMLEX licensing examination sequence.
- Minimum 3 years of postgraduate training.
- FCVS is accepted.

Montana

- Completion of USMLE exams with up to six attempts for Step 3.
- Completion of COMLEX exams with no limits on attempts.
- Completion of USMLE licensing examination sequence within 7 years; no time limit on COMLEX licensing examination sequence; M.D./Ph.D. candidates may possibly be exempt.
- Minimum 3 years of postgraduate training.
- FCVS is accepted.

Nebraska

- Completion of USMLE or COMLEX exams with up to four attempts at each Step/Level.
- Completion of USMLE or COMLEX licensing examination sequence within 10 years.

- Minimum 3 years of postgraduate training.
- FCVS is accepted.

Nevada (M.D. Applicants)
- Completion of all three Steps USMLE exams with up to nine attempts; pass Step 3 with up to three attempts.
- Completion of USMLE licensing examination sequence within 7 years from the date of the first passing any Step of the exam. M.D./Ph.D.: Ph.D. candidates must pass all Steps of the exam within 10 years after the date on which the applicant first passes any Step of the exam.
- Minimum 3 years of postgraduate training.
- Exception: Currently enrolled residents in a postgraduate training program in the United States or Canada who have completed at least 2 years of progressive postgraduate training, pass all three steps, and meet all requirements for an unlimited license in Nevada may be granted an unlimited license. Applicants must also complete in writing to the Nevada State Board of Medical Examiners that they will complete the program and submit satisfactory completion of the program within 60 days of completion of the residency program.
- FCVS is accepted.

Nevada (D.O. Applicants)
- Completion of COMLEX exams with no limits on attempts.
- Completion of COMLEX licensing examination sequence with no time limit.
- Minimum 3 years of postgraduate training; exception is 2 years for residents who sign commitment to practice in Nevada.
- FCVS is accepted.

New Hampshire
- Completion of USMLE or COMLEX exams with up to three attempts at each Step/Level.
- Completion of USMLE or COMLEX licensing examination sequence with no time limit.
- Minimum 2 years of postgraduate training.
- FCVS is required.

New Jersey
- Completion of USMLE with up to five attempts on Step 3.
- Completion of USMLE licensing examination sequence within 7 years.
- Graduates after July 1, 2003: 2 years of postgraduate training with a signed contract for a third year in an accredited program. Graduates prior to July 1, 2003: minimum 3 years of postgraduate training.
- FCVS is accepted.

New Mexico (M.D.)
- Completion of USMLE exams with up to six attempts at each Step.
- Completion of USMLE licensing examination sequence within 7 years.
- Exception for M.D. and Ph.D. candidates: can complete USMLE licensing examination sequence within 10 years.

- Minimum 2 years of postgraduate training.
- FCVS is highly recommended.

New Mexico (D.O.)
- Completion of COMLEX exams with no limit on attempts.
- Minimum 1 year of postgraduate training.
- Completion of COMLEX licensing examination sequence within 7 years of passing the first Level.
- FCVS is highly recommended.

New York
- Completion of USMLE or COMLEX exams with no limits on attempts.
- Completion of USMLE or COMLEX licensing examination sequence with no time limit.
- Minimum 3 years of postgraduate training.
- FCVS is required.

North Carolina
- Completion of USMLE or COMLEX exams with up to three attempts per Step/Level.
- Completion of USMLE or COMLEX licensing examination sequence with no time limit.
- Minimum 3 years of postgraduate training.
- FCVS is highly recommended.

North Dakota
- Completion of USMLE or COMLEX exams with up to three attempts per Step/Level.
- Completion of USMLE or COMLEX licensing examination sequence within 7 years.
- Minimum 30 months of ACGME-accredited training.
- FCVS is accepted.

Ohio
- Completion of USMLE or COMLEX exams with up to five attempts per Step/Level; must pass on the sixth attempt.
- Completion of USMLE or COMLEX licensing examination sequence within 10 years; if there is a good cause for over 10 years, can apply for a possible waiver.
- Minimum 2 years of postgraduate training.
- FCVS is required.

Oklahoma (M.D.)
- Completion of USMLE exams with up to three attempts at each Step (Step 2 = CK and CS).
- Completion of USMLE licensing examination sequence within 10 years.
- Minimum 2 years of postgraduate training.
- FCVS is accepted.

Oklahoma (D.O.)
- Completion of USMLE or COMLEX exams; contact board for more information on attempts.
- Minimum 1 year of postgraduate training.
- Completion of COMLEX licensing examination sequence with no time limits.
- FCVS is accepted.

Oregon
- Completion of USMLE or COMLEX exams with up to three attempts for Step 3/Level 3. Fourth attempt is acceptable after 1 additional year of postgraduate training. Possible waiver of attempt requirement if applicant is ABMS/AOA certified.
- Completion of USMLE or COMLEX licensing examination sequence within 7 years.
- Minimum 3 years of postgraduate training.
- FCVS is accepted.

Pennsylvania (M.D.)
- Completion of USMLE exams with no limit on attempts.
- Completion of USMLE licensing examination sequence within 7 years.
- Minimum 3 years of postgraduate training.
- FCVS is accepted.

Pennsylvania (D.O.)
- Completion of COMLEX exams with no limit on attempts.
- Minimum 1 year of postgraduate training.
- Completion of COMLEX licensing examination sequence with no time limits.
- FCVS is accepted.

Puerto Rico
- Completion of USMLE exams with no limit on attempts.
- Completion of USMLE Step 3 within 7 years of the date of passing Step 1.
- Minimum 3 years of postgraduate training.
- FCVS is accepted.

Rhode Island
- Completion of USMLE or COMLEX exams with up to three attempts at each Step/Level.
- Completion of USMLE licensing examination sequence within 7 years; contact board for information on COMLEX.
- Minimum 2 years of postgraduate training.
- FCVS is required.

South Carolina
- Completion of USMLE or COMLEX exams with up to four attempts at each Step/Level.
- Completion of USMLE or COMLEX licensing examination sequence within 10 years.

- Minimum 3 years of postgraduate training.
- FCVS is required.

South Dakota
- Completion of USMLE or COMLEX exams with up to three attempts.
- Completion of USMLE or COMLEX licensing examination sequence within 7 years.
- Exception for M.D. and Ph.D. candidates: can complete USMLE or COMLEX licensing examination sequence within 10 years.
- Successful completion of residency program.
- FCVS is accepted.

Tennessee (M.D.)
- Completion of USMLE exams with up to three attempts; if fail more than three times, must show ABMS board certification and proof of meeting requirements for Maintenance of Certification to be considered for licensure.
- Completion of USMLE licensing examination sequence within 10 years of the first successful Step, unless applicant qualifies under an exception.
- Minimum 3 years of postgraduate training.
- FCVS is accepted.

Tennessee (D.O.)
- Completion of COMLEX exams with up to three attempts.
- Minimum 1 year of postgraduate training.
- Completion of COMLEX licensing examination sequence with no time limits.
- FCVS is accepted.

Texas
- Completion of USMLE or COMLEX exams with up to three attempts at each Step/Level.
- Exceptions may apply for applicants who held a Texas Physician in Training permit on or before September 1, 2005, or who have been licensed in good standing in another state for 5 years.
- Completion of USMLE or COMLEX licensing examination sequence within 7 years.
- Exception for M.D. and Ph.D. candidates, who are board certified, or who are willing to accept a limited license to practice exclusively in an Medically Underserved Area (MUA) or an Health Professional Shortage Area (HPSA).
- Minimum 2 years of postgraduate training.
- FCVS is accepted.

Utah (M.D.)
- Completion of USMLE exams with up to three attempts for Step 3.
- Completion of USMLE licensing examination sequence within 7 years.
- Exception for M.D. and Ph.D. candidates: can complete USMLE licensing examination sequence within 10 years.

- Minimum 2 years of postgraduate training or 1 year complete, with a second year in the state of Utah in progress.
- FCVS is required.

Utah (D.O.)
- Completion of COMLEX exams with up to three attempts at each Level.
- Completion of COMLEX licensing examination sequence within 10 years.
- Exception for D.O. and Ph.D. candidates: can complete COMLEX licensing examination sequence within 10 years.
- Minimum 2 years of postgraduate training or 1 year complete, with a second year in the state of Utah in progress.
- FCVS is required.

Vermont (M.D.)
- Completion of USMLE exams with up to three attempts for Step 3.
- Completion of USMLE licensing examination sequence within 7 years.
- Minimum 3 years of postgraduate training.
- FCVS is accepted.

Vermont (D.O.)
- Completion of COMLEX exams; no current information on attempts.
- One-year rotating internship or 3-year residency program.
- FCVS is accepted.

Virgin Islands
- Completion of Special Purpose Exam (SPEX) exams and an oral exam with up to two attempts.
- Completion of SPEX licensing examination sequence within 3 years to pass the two attempts; must take oral exam within 1 year after passing the written exam.
- Minimum 6 months of postgraduate training after two attempts for SPEX exam.
- FCVS is required.

Virginia
- Completion of USMLE exams with no limits on attempts.
- Completion of USMLE licensing examination sequence within 10 years; exception for greater than 10 years if applicant is ABMS certified.
- Minimum 2 years of postgraduate training.
- FCVS is accepted.

Washington (M.D.)
- Completion of USMLE exams with up to three attempts for Step 3.
- Completion of USMLE licensing examination sequence within 7 years.
- Minimum 2 years of postgraduate training.
- FCVS is accepted.

Washington (D.O.)
- Completion of COMLEX exams with up to three attempts.
- Completion of COMLEX licensing examination sequence with no time limit.

- Minimum 1 year of postgraduate training.
- FCVS is accepted.

West Virginia (M.D.)
- Completion of USMLE exams with up to six attempts for each Step.
- Completion of USMLE licensing examination sequence within 10 years.
- Minimum 3 years of postgraduate training.
- FCVS is accepted.

West Virginia (D.O.)
- Completion of COMLEX exams with no limits on attempt.
- Completion of COMLEX licensing examination sequence with no time limit.
- Minimum 1 year of postgraduate training.

Wisconsin
- Completion of USMLE or COMLEX exams with up to three attempts for each Step/Level.
- Completion of Step 3 within 10 years of the date of passing Step 1.
- Minimum 2 years of postgraduate training.
- FCVS is accepted.

Wyoming
- Completion of USMLE or COMLEX exams within 7 years; exception for M.D./D.O. and Ph.D. candidates: can complete licensing examination sequence within 8 years.
- Minimum 2 years of postgraduate training; exception of 1 year if applicant has current certification by an American Board of Medical Specialties (ABMS) or American Osteopathic Association Bureau of Osteopathic Specialists (AOABOS/BOC) specialty board, or continuous licensure in good standing in one or more states and/or D.C. for the preceding 5 years.
- FCVS is required.

Helpful Tips for Navigating the Initial Medical Licensure Process by State

The medical licensing process can be lengthy and difficult to navigate [5]. It is important to be aware of the average application processing time by contacting your state's licensing board [2]. It is also wise to update your medical schools and residency training programs of the process so that they can help you with expediting the process [5]. Keeping all verified documents through a centralized FCVS service may also be helpful [5].

Conclusion

While the requirements may be lengthy for both entering into an ACGME residency program and applying for initial medical licensure, it is possible for IMGs to successfully complete this process. It is important to be aware of the differing state- or territory-specific requirements. Oftentimes, these requirements differ for IMGs. With the knowledge of state- or territory-specific requirements, IMGs can be fully prepared to meet necessary requirements and begin practicing medicine as a physician in the United States.

References

1. Ranasinghe PD. International medical graduates in the US physician workforce. J Am Osteopath Assoc. 2015;115(4):236–41.
2. State Specific Requirements for Initial Medical Licensure: Federation of State Medical Boards. Available from: https://www.fsmb.org/step-3/state-licensure/
3. Residency Application Requirements for International Medical Graduates: American Academy of Family Physicians (AAFP). Available from: https://www.aafp.org/medical-school-residency/residency/apply/img.html
4. Requirements for Certification: Educational Commission for Foreign Medical Graduates. Available from: https://www.ecfmg.org/certification/requirements-for-certification.html
5. Navigating State Medical Licensure: American Medical Association. Available from: https://www.ama-assn.org/residents-students/career-planning-resource/navigating-state-medical-licensure
6. Norcini JJ, Boulet JR, Opalek A, Dauphinee WD. The relationship between licensing examination performance and the outcomes of care by international medical school graduates. Acad Med. 2014;89(8):1157–62.

Chapter 21
Sources of Support for IMGs

Michelle S. Lee and Vinod E. Nambudiri

Support systems are especially essential for the transition of international medical graduates (IMGs), who now comprise 26% of the total physician population in the USA [1]. Indeed, IMGs may face many unique challenges in adjusting to medical practice in western cultural settings, including medical knowledge and scope of practice, cultural norms and expectations, language barriers and communication, and individual and personal experiences acculturating to life and work in an unfamiliar society, thus helping with stress management and healthy adjustment [2, 3]. Additionally, the challenges faced may vary dramatically across individuals based on their country of origin, familiarity with the US medical system, prior experiences, and even gender or racial background. Thus, there is clearly a unique role for both formal and informal support networks that can help IMGs navigate the multifaceted and individualized challenges they face.

Cultural Norms and Expectations

International medical graduates may face challenges adjusting to the professional culture and structural hierarchy of the US medical system, which may affect their interactions with colleagues and hospital staff. Unlike US-trained residents, IMGs may not have been socialized to the western "hidden curriculum of medicine," which is defined as "lessons, especially about norms and values, that are embedded in a school's organizational structure and culture but not explicitly intended to be

M. S. Lee · V. E. Nambudiri (✉)
Harvard Medical School, Boston, MA, USA

Department of Dermatology, Brigham and Women's Hospital and Harvard Medical School, Boston, MA, USA
e-mail: michelle_lee3@hms.harvard.edu; vnambudiri@bwh.harvard.edu

© Springer Nature Switzerland AG 2021
H. Tohid, H. Maibach (eds.), *International Medical Graduates in the United States*, https://doi.org/10.1007/978-3-030-62249-7_21

taught, which may be supportive of or contrary to the formal curriculum" [4]. This lack of exposure to the "hidden curriculum of medicine" may unknowingly hamper the clinical or educational performance of trainees, and mentorship can provide a valuable tool to address this deficit.

For example, the US professional culture of medicine includes specific values and practices of feedback, self-directed learning, conflict management, teamwork, and directness and deference that may differ from practices in other countries. Thus, international medical graduates may benefit from additional guidance from both supervisory and peer mentors who can help orient them to the implicit values and attitudes that shape their clinical environment.

In addition, IMGs may benefit from additional programming to help them adjust to cultural differences in the physician–patient interaction. For example, while many countries still define the role of the physician as largely paternalistic, the USA has moved toward a more shared decision-making model that engages patients actively in identifying a treatment choice and in forming a therapeutic alliance [5]. These cultural differences may mean that IMG trainees are not as accustomed to the same level of discussion-based interactions with patients as are expected or commonplace in the US medical system, and failing to undertake such activities may lead to a somewhat negative perception by their patients. However, these cultural nuances are essential for IMGs to understand in order to provide optimal patient-centered care. Indeed, many IMGs undertake their medical education in a cultural environment with "little scope for discussion," which is "further limited by the lack of opportunity to develop patient-centered communications skills in a busy clinical environment" [6]. To this end, programming such as mentorship and workshops may serve a vital role in teaching the trainee communication skills and strategies for their interactions with patients. For example, mentors might be able to provide constructive feedback on the trainees' observed interactions with patients and/or provide opportunities for the trainee to observe his or her own interactions with patients. Additionally, a mentor who is himself or herself an IMG can provide valuable insights on how he or she was able to incorporate learning the style of US clinical encounters alongside learning the practice of clinical medicine. Furthermore, residency programs can have workshops on topics including cultural sensitivity, patient-centered care, and patient–doctor interactions as part of orientation or ongoing curriculum for residents [7].

Career Development

Mentors may be especially helpful to IMGs in guiding their professional trajectory since IMGs may be more unfamiliar with potential career opportunities and navigation of resources in a new medical system. They may also assist in connecting them with other mentors in fields of research or clinical areas of interest, since the IMG may not have a large social network in the USA.

Given the large number of IMGs in the USA, several organizations have developed, which may be particularly of interest to IMGs looking to learn from peers and to advance in terms of career development. First, physicians of many nationalities have organized groups in the USA to provide an outlet for IMG physicians from particular countries to have an affiliated organization. For example, the American Association of Physicians of Indian Origin provides a network for Indian physicians in the USA and can be a valuable resource for mentorship and support for IMGs [8].

In addition, the Internet and social media provides a unique opportunity for IMGs to connect with each other. For example, the Sudanese Junior Doctors' Association in the UK (SJDA-UK) uses social media platforms to provide live videos, interactive sessions, outreach courses, and written advice on immigration to the UK and integration into the National Health Service (NHS) [9]. This platform has become the main resource and point of contact for Sudanese doctors who hope to work in the NHS. The Internet can also be a source of information about advice on applying to residencies as an international medical graduate and lists of opportunities. For example, the American Medical Association (AMA) website includes a list of Observership Programs for IMGs [10].

Other valuable career resources to explore are governmental programs specifically geared toward IMGs. For example, the Minnesota Department of Health has implemented an IMG Assistance Program "to address barriers to practice for immigrant international medical graduates and develop pathways to integrate them into the Minnesota health care delivery system" [11]. This program includes collaborations with nonprofit agencies to assist IMGs with career guidance, exam preparation, and residency applications. IMGs also engage in their Interprofessional Education and Resource Center and Academic Health Center Simulation Center to conduct simulations to help them with professional accreditation and development of clinical skills and patient communication.

Individual and Personal Experiences

Many studies have shown the importance of role models for IMGs who have faced similar circumstances and understand their experience to help reduce anxiety and provide an example of a successful medical career. Mentors, especially those who themselves were IMGs, may be able to provide advice regarding personal experiences and challenges outside of the hospital setting, such as larger acculturation, barriers to gaining employment and length of time living in the host country, and family adjustment challenges [12]. In addition, IMGs are more vulnerable to challenges such as bullying and emotional distress, which are associated with decreased job satisfaction and motivation [3]. Therefore, it is especially important for IMGs to have both supervisory and peer support to monitor their satisfaction and well-being.

Community support and engagement with local communities is also important for IMG success to facilitate social integration and reduce feelings of isolation. Studies have shown that community support helped promote psychological well-being in immigrant populations, and contacts with host support networks had the most significant effect [13, 14].

Communication and Language Skills

IMGs may require support to hone their communication skills to allow for culturally appropriate and professional interactions with colleagues and patients. Indeed, communication is one of the challenges faced by IMGs, with differences in consulting style and cultures impairing interactions with other medical teams in the hospital [15]. Establishing successful communication techniques is important early on in clinical training; interpersonal and communication skills is one of the six accreditation council for graduate medical education (ACGME) Core Competencies upon which all US trainees are evaluated and assessed during their time in training. Tutors can help teach IMGs language nuances, appropriate delivery of speech, and body language to allow for more effective communication. For example, one study by Baker and Robson evaluated a language tutoring program in language training and clinical topics that developed a 6-month program of 15 language training sessions and 6 consultation skills training sessions from experienced general practitioners. Language tutors saw improvements in all areas including pronunciation, understanding, and communication and improvements in consultation skills and language, with 44% of supervisors noticing improvement [15]. Such deliberate training programs can provide IMGs with specific tutoring interventions that can enhance their performance.

Test-Taking Skills

In addition, it is worth examining the role of support for the IMG in the pre-residency application period. Given the role of testing clinical skills and medical knowledge that is assessed in the United States Medical Licensing Exams (USMLEs) may be different from the format or the content presented in medical schools across the world, specific preparation programs for these exams may be particularly beneficial for international medical graduates to explore as they prepare for these important exams. Several test preparation courses – both online and in-person – have emerged including models of longitudinal tutoring over the course of medical education using virtual education remote technologies as well as on-site preparatory courses for hands-on practice of clinical skills prior to undertaking major exams. Tutoring and other career coaching programs targeting these specific exams may be a significant financial cost, but are worth considering for test preparation based on the performance of an individual on practice exams or to build test-taker confidence.

Medical Knowledge and Practices

Both formal and informal mentors may be helpful in ensuring IMGs become familiar with uncommon diagnoses or presentations that may differ from their home country. In addition, they may be able to help guide trainees as to difference in medical practices.

What Is at Stake If IMGs Are Not Provided Adequate Support Systems?

The failure to provide IMGs with appropriate support may jeopardize performance and patient safety. Indeed, research has shown that IMGs are more likely to fail postgraduate assessment and be censured for their fitness to practice [16, 17]. It may also lead to higher rates of dissatisfaction with training and opportunities and a lack of feeling of connectedness [3]. In addition, peer and supervisor support is especially critical since IMGs may face a lack of cultural awareness amongst colleagues and patients, which may lead to a risk of prejudice and discrimination, potentially creating a stressful and hostile environment for the IMG and hindering his or her ability to thrive and learn effectively [18].

Current Models of Support

While formalized support is clearly beneficial for IMGs, the current support structure may be insufficient to meet their needs. Many do not provide sufficient time for supervisors and colleagues to oversee the development of IMGs. In addition, many interventions like induction programs and communication skills courses are implemented at a regional rather than individual level and may not provide continuing support beyond the initial few days and may not be customized to an individual learner's needs. Also, many educators do not have experience with the unique needs of IMGs.

One example of a current support program for IMGs is the Programme for Overseas Doctors (POD) in England, which includes interventions at both the organizational and individual levels, including multiple supervisory and peer mentors [3]. There is a supportive clinical and organizational culture which holds regular meetings to review progress, as well as individual needs assessments to tailor content to the individual and the group, including addressing cultural barriers and communication training. They also administer individual objective structured clinical examination (OSCEs), which are helpful for direct supervision of clinical skills in a controlled setting. Finally, individuals are assigned a tutor who oversees and supports the IMGs, including their clinical performance, well-being, and job satisfaction. The program also emphasized the importance of support in both supervisory and peer mentoring roles. Studies have demonstrated that programs like POD improved the performance of IMGs, including in career progression, fewer complaints, fewer reported errors, and increased retention [3]. In addition, following such interventions, physicians are more likely to feel motivated and confident practicing, with increased happiness and sense of self-worth [3]. This example of a comprehensive mentoring approach can serve as a model for other countries or institutions looking to build a rich training environment for international medical graduate physicians.

Another example of a successful model program is the Clinical Assessment for Practice Program (CAPP) in Canada for family medicine [19]. It is a 12-month mentorship program where a CAPP physician is in active practice and is mentored by an established family physician who provides teaching, supervision, guidance, and regular performance assessment. For example, three physicians might be located in one clinic with a single mentor who spends a significant amount of time mentoring.

Recommendations for a Standardized Program

There is need for a more formal and informal support networks addressing the unique needs of IMGs, through mentoring, supervisory roles, peer mentoring, support in language and medical knowledge, targeted workshops, and engagement with local communities. Interventions at both the organizational and individual levels should be implemented by increasing staff cultural awareness and a supportive culture as well as a sustainable support system. This program should also include frequent reflection and individual needs assessments and feedback to ensure that the IMGs are receiving the individualized support they need.

References

1. American Medical Association IMG Section Governing Council. International medical graduates in American medicine: contemporary challenges and opportunities. http://www.ama-assn.org/resources/doc/img/img-workforce-paper.pdf
2. Triscott JA, Szafran O, Waugh EH, Torti JM, Barton M. Cultural transition of international medical graduate residents into family practice in Canada. Int J Med Educ. 2016;7:132–41.
3. Kehoe A, Metcalf J, Carter M, McLachlan JC, Forrest S, Illing J. Supporting international graduates to success. Clin Teach. 2018 Oct;15(5):361–5.
4. Hafferty F, Gaufberg E, O'Donnell J. The role of the hidden curriculum in "on doctoring" courses. AMA J Ethics. 2015;17(2):129–37.
5. Murgic L, et al. Paternalism and autonomy: views of patients and providers in a transitional (post-communist) country. BMC Med Ethics. 2015 Sep;16(1):65.
6. Rao, Rahul. Improving the coaching and mentoring of IMGs. BMJ. 2014;348:g3424.

7. Chen P, et al. Professional challenges of non-U.S.-born international medical graduates and recommendations for support during residency training. Acad Med. 2011;86(11):1383–8.
8. American Association of Physicians of Indian Origin. 2020. Available from https://www.aapiusa.org
9. Sudanese Junior Doctors Association. 2020. Available from https://www.sjda.uk, Hashim 2018.
10. Observership Program listings for international medical graduates. American Medical Association. 2020. Available from https://www.ama-assn.org/education/international-medical-education/observership-program-listings-international-medical
11. International Medical Graduate Assistance Program: Report to the Minnesota Legislature. Minnesota. Department of Health; 2018. Available from https://www.health.state.mn.us/facilities/ruralhealth/img/docs/2018imgleg.pdf
12. Kehoe A, et al. Supporting international medical graduates' transition to their host-country: realist synthesis. Med Educ. 2016;50(10):1015–32.
13. Aikawa M, Kleyman K. Immigration, coping, and well-being: implications for communities' roles in promoting the well-being of immigrants and refugees. J Prev Interv Community. 2019:1–12.
14. Jasinskaja-Lahti I, Liebkind K, Jaakkola M, Reuter A. Perceived discrimination, social support networks, and psychological well-being among three immigrant groups. J Cross-Cult Psychol. 2006;37(3):293–311.
15. Baker D, Robson J. Communication training for international graduates. Clin Teach. 2012;9(5):325–9.
16. Tiffin PA, Illing J, Kasim AS, McLachlan JC. Annual Review of Competence Progression (ARCP) performance of doctors who passed Professional and Linguistic Assessments Board (PLAB) tests compared with UK medical graduates: national data linkage study. BMJ. 2014;17(348):2622.
17. Tiffin PA, Paton LW, Mwandigha LM, McLachlan JC, Illing J. Predicting fitness to practise events in international medical graduates who registered as UK doctors via the Professional and Linguistic Assessments Board (PLAB) system: a national cohort study. BMC Med. 2017;15(1):66.
18. Romem Y, Benor DE. Training immigrant doctors: issues and responses. Med Educ. 1993;27(1):74–82.
19. Maudsley RF. Assessment of international medical graduates and their integration into family practice: the Clinician Assessment for Practice Program. Acad Med. 2008 Mar;83(3):309–15.

Chapter 22
Thinking Strategically: How "ACE" Helps IMG Trainees

Jonathan Bernad

Respecting the Journey

My father, born in communist Hungary, dreamed to become a doctor in America. At the time, this was seen as unrealistic, even impossible. My entire life is different because he didn't give up, and I was born the son of a doctor in America. I grew up with this story permeating my existence. His hard work and dream shaped a future for me I otherwise would never know. When we help someone today at ACE, we have a deep respect for this journey that our trainees are on: this will not only change the trainee's life but also the life of his or her children. Matching into residency can be life-altering for multiple generations.

Strategy

The process of applying to US residency is straightforward for IMGs. You must be certified by the Educational Commission for Foreign Medical Graduates (ECFMG). In order to be ECFMG-certified, you must graduate from a medical school approved for potential ECFMG certification listed in the World Directory of Medical Schools (https://search.wdoms.org). You must pass your USMLE examinations for Step 1, Step 2 CS* (this does not include Match 2021 due to the unique challenges of Covid-19), and Step 2 CK. After this, you can apply to residency programs using the electronic residency application system (ERAS) in order to participate in the annual National Resident Matching Program (NRMP). Every application in ERAS has a few key components: personal information (which is essentially your CV/resume), personal statement, dean's letter (MSPE), USMLE score reports, ECFMG

J. Bernad (✉)
American Clinical Experience, Los Angeles, CA, USA
e-mail: jon@ace.md; http://www.ace.md

© Springer Nature Switzerland AG 2021
H. Tohid, H. Maibach (eds.), *International Medical Graduates in the United States*, https://doi.org/10.1007/978-3-030-62249-7_22

certification, photo, medical school transcript, and, lastly, letters of recommendation (LORs).

We specifically help with the USCE and accompanying LORs. USCE is included on the CV/resume and can result in LORs that are then uploaded into ERAS as part of each application. LORs are either "waived" or "unwaived" and ideally should be "waived," meaning that the letters are uploaded directly by the doctors and not by the applicants (who waive their right to see the letter). Some programs require three LORs and some require four LORs. Each LOR typically covers a 4-weeks duration.

Emphasis on LORs

The programs we've helped to shape with ACGME-accredited hospital-affiliated doctors are designed to ensure that each participant has an opportunity to demonstrate certain key attributes and that doctors are paying attention to these specific attributes in their performance to increase the chances of strengthening the overall performance and the resulting recommendation letters. While there is no absolute consensus, and different program directors will look for certain aspects within each application, there are some clear guidelines for what will make a stronger residency candidate and therefore what will make for a stronger LOR. Available articles support the anecdotal research we have conducted internally with program directors, doctors who conduct residency interviews, doctors who participate in their residency program search committees, and chief residents who have helped evaluate applicants during interview seasons.

In "The Utility of Letters of Recommendation in Predicting Resident Success: Can the ACGME Competencies Help?" [3], the authors studied the LORs of successful residency applicants admitted to Johns Hopkins University residency in obstetrics and gynecology between 1994 and 2004 to see if they contained the "core competencies" outlined by the Accreditation Council for Graduate Medical Education (ACGME). They found that "[s]uccessful residents had statistically significantly more comments about excellence in the competency areas of patient care, medical knowledge, and interpersonal and communication skills" and conclude that "LORs can provide useful clues to differentiate between students who are likely to become the least versus the most successful residency program graduates. Greater usage of the ACGME core competencies within LORs may be beneficial."

The six ACGME core competencies are used by residency programs to evaluate their residents at different stages of their training. Logically, program directors tend to look for trainees who already possess talent in some of these crucial skills: (1) patient care, (2) medical knowledge, (3) practice-based learning and improvement, (4) interpersonal and communication skills, (5) professionalism, and (6) systems-based practice. We give trainees practical advice on how to demonstrate these qualities during their rotations.

Similarly, in "Dear Program Director: Deciphering Letters of Recommendation" [1], published by the *Journal of Graduate Medical Education*, the authors asked 468 program directors to rate various aspects of LORs to gauge which aspects of the

LOR were most important and to see what phrases were most positively received to create positive impressions of the applicant. A phrase such as "I give my highest recommendation" was more positively seen than other similar phrases. The authors conclude that "[c]ommonly used phrases in LORs were interpreted consistently by PDs and influenced their impressions of candidates." Other important features included the LOR author's depth of interaction with the applicant, specific traits of the applicant, and describing the applicant's abilities. Also, the level of the applicant's involvement in the rotation was ranked as more important than the academic rank of the letter writer. The "work ethic," "trustworthiness," and the trait of being a "team player," "professional," and "compassionate" were all phrases and qualities praised by 96% and above by all the PDs, ranked as more important than such adjectives as "inquisitive."

In "Evolution of Characteristics from Letters of Recommendation in General Surgery Residency Applications" [2], the authors looked at 255 LORs of successfully matched surgery residents at Gundersen Health System in La Crosse, Wisconsin, to find out which qualities were emphasized between 1973 and 2016. They found that "Descriptions of practice-based learning, system-based practice, research, and volunteerism have increased, while professionalism, medical knowledge, and technical skills were consistently described over time."

With these guidelines in place, we recommend that trainees focus on these areas by being mindful of what is considered valuable and prepare and execute those traits during their rotations. For example, it is natural for trainees to want to be the best and outshine others, to exhibit traits akin to a brooding genius that one might find on TV. Instead, we encourage trainees to engage in friendly teamwork, cheerfully greeting every worker they encounter, including secretaries and janitorial staff. Likewise, preceptors check to see if the trainee in question works well with the other trainees in the same rotation or if he or she engages in competitive behavior. By following certain guidelines and thus developing certain important traits, IMGs can better navigate the US healthcare system and achieve their goals.

Even small cultural differences can play an important factor. For example, a person may come from a country where being quiet, modest, and shy is considered signs of intelligence. In a more "American" context, these traits can come across as antisocial, unfriendly, or lacking in confidence. A person's overall performance in a rotation must not be negatively impacted because of these types of misunderstandings.

We educate trainees before each rotation on which features to try to exhibit. Although obvious, the effect is that of a "coach" trying to ensure only the best from each performance.

Preceptors

Importantly, we help facilitate rotations with preceptors who have a special interest in medical education and provide both inpatient and outpatient experience. They are affiliated at ACGME-accredited hospitals and have often trained residents in the past. Some are even former program directors. These doctors know what to look for in strong candidates and can expertly evaluate the performances of candidates in LORs.

One-on-One Guidance

We spend a lot of time fielding questions from IMGs and IMSs. From a broad view, we often talk to international medical students who want to know when they should take electives, what the differences are between certain programs, such as electives and externships, and how to best plan ahead to have a strong application. A common question is when to take the USMLE exams: before or after graduation. They often ask about the importance of research, whether LORs are better on "hospital-letterhead" or "clinic-letterhead," if it's better to take rotations close to the time of residency application, or if rotations should always be in the relevant specialty (e.g., an IM rotation is logical for anesthesiology or neurology applications, but a dermatology rotation would not be as helpful). The advice is never exactly the same for each individual: a whole picture is needed to properly guide someone, as there are many interdependent factors. To take just one example, in the past years, the question of whether someone should wait to take externship rotations when also taking his or her CS exam can depend on whether someone can afford more than one trip to the USA before interview season.

Practical Support

To complete an in-person rotation, a trainee must travel to the city where the rotation takes place. We provide visa assistance and housing options with housing partners who offer safe places with fair rates in close proximity to rotation sites. One interesting development due to Covid-19 is that trainees who cannot travel are now opting to participate in remote research programs and "tele-rotations."

Tele-Rotations

One of the most recent and growing areas of development revolve around "tele-rotations." Via tele-medicine techniques, trainees can participate remotely from across the world. Trainees can stay at home and take histories and even conduct physical exams with the help of a medical assistant who is in the room with the patient. These rotations can also include live lectures, instructional videos, patient discussions, and assignments. Doctors can let trainees access their HIPAA-compliant tele-medicine platforms such as the Epic EMR (electronic medical record) system.

Remote Research

One of the challenges during Covid-19 was seeing how trainees can still stay connected to the US healthcare system and improve their knowledge and CVs without the ability of traveling. Remote research allows trainees to learn about systematic reviews and to be published by PubMed-indexed journals. Our most popular program is currently via a partnership with Dr. Hassaan Tohid and the California Institute of Behavioral Neurosciences and Psychology's "Be a Published Author" course. Trainees referred by ACE receive additional benefits such as extra certificate courses, an extra certificate of publishing training, one extra "research LOR" if requested, and an automatic 50% longer membership timeline to receive help on future papers, have access to online videos, and have the ability to visit live classes.

Locations

ACE primarily helps trainees by placing them into programs that take place in IMG-friendly cities such as New York, Houston, Chicago, and the Washington DC metropolitan area. However, we offer rotations throughout the USA in places such as Miami, Los Angeles, Michigan, Baltimore, and New Jersey.

Countries of Origin

Although we work with trainees who have gone to medical school or live in almost every country in the world, the applicants we work with most regularly come from India and Pakistan. We believe that more trainees apply from these two countries because of various cultural factors including the use of the English language in medical education and a history of successful doctors from India and Pakistan who now work in the USA and stay actively connected to the next generation through structured programs and mentorship to create a sense of community. This includes elder doctors but also current residents who give back to their juniors. Trainees applying from countries such as Russia, Australia, or Mexico tend to be more isolated, applying on their own, and have less encouragement from peers and family.

Challenges

A large challenge that ACE faced was building trust within the IMG community. Much of this is through "word of mouth" whereby one trainee will recommend ACE to his or her colleagues or juniors. In the end, we rely on this form of "advertising" more than Google, Facebook, or Instagram ads. This can happen after someone matches into residency and finishes a rotation or even when someone can't participate in a rotation but receives a 100% refund. There are countless cases as an organization where we tried to do the "right" thing, and this built a larger reputation of trustworthiness. When a trainee can't travel because of visa issues, or has to change plans, we remain flexible and compassionate. Gaining credibility and building relationships with senior-level doctors and hospital organizations in the USA was also quite challenging.

Conclusion

Applying to US residency is incredibly important to one's future. Yet there are few companies or individuals who can reliably assist in this process. Ultimately, the USCE and resulting letters are just one small but important aspect of a residency application. ACE is here to offer advice, support, and guidance to help with this area that can be confusing or bewildering to the IMG community.

Conflict of Interest Jonathan Bernad is the CEO and founder of American Clinical Experience (ACE).

References

1. Stohl HE, Hueppchen NA, Bienstock JL. The utility of letters of recommendation in predicting resident success: can the ACGME competencies help? J Grad Med Educ. 2011 Sep;3(3):387–90.
2. Saudek K, Saudek D, Treat R, et al. Dear program director: deciphering letters of recommendation. J Grad Med Educ. 2018 Jun;10(3):261–6.
3. Shapiro SB, Kallies JK, Borgert AJ, et al. Evolution of characteristics from letters of recommendation in general surgery residency applications. J Surg Educ. 2018 Nov;75(6):e23–30.

Chapter 23
The US Medical Licensing Examination

Ivan Cancarevic

The US Medical Licensing Examination

The US Medical Licensing Examination (USMLE) is a series of exams required for medical licensure in the United States. They consist of USMLE Step 1, USMLE Step 2 Clinical Knowledge (CK), USMLE Step 2 Clinical Skills (CS), and USMLE Step 3. American medical students generally take Step 1 and both parts of Step 2 during medical school, while Step 3 is usually taken in residency. All foreign graduates who wish to obtain residency positions in the United States also need to take these exams. All the exams, except for USMLE Step 2 CS, are scored based on a scale, the details of which are not publicly available. Recently, it has been announced that the USMLE Step 1 will no longer be scored, starting in 2022. The scores on the exams are among the most important aspects of residency application, and any changes to the scoring methods may have profound effects on the applicants. All the exams except for the USMLE Step 2 CS are computer-based exams administered in "Prometric" centers worldwide. The USMLE Step 2 CS is administered at five locations in the United States only as it requires interaction with standardized patients [1].

The USMLE Step 1

The Step 1 of the US Medical Licensing Examination has often been considered the most important and most difficult of the exams. It is usually taken after the first 2 or 3 years of medical school and covers most of the basic, preclinical sciences, such as anatomy, physiology, neuroscience, biochemistry, behavioral science, pathology, pathophysiology, pharmacology, microbiology, and immunology. The questions are

I. Cancarevic (✉)
California Institute of Behavioral Neurosciences and Psychology, Fairfield, CA, USA

© Springer Nature Switzerland AG 2021
H. Tohid, H. Maibach (eds.), *International Medical Graduates in the United States*, https://doi.org/10.1007/978-3-030-62249-7_23

written as short clinical scenarios. Each exam consists of 7 blocks of 40 questions, and students have 1 hour per question block. Being able to answer such a large number of questions from so many disciplines requires good basic science understanding and question-taking skills. The score is reported as a three-digit number, rarely lower than 170 and rarely higher than 270. The minimum passing score changes most years and is currently 194. The average score is around 230, with the standard deviation of 19. Many residency programs have selected a "cutoff" score required to consider an applicant for an interview. With the exam no longer being scored in 2022, it remains an open question which aspect of an individual's CV is going to take its place. The difficulty of the exam and the need for high scores have resulted in the development of a number of courses, question banks, and agencies offering help with USMLE preparation. Scores are generally reported electronically 3–4 weeks after the exam date. It is possible to appeal the score and request a recheck, but it is not possible to find out the correct answers [1].

Preparation

Preparing for the USMLE Step 1 is a difficult task, and many students struggle every step of the way. Developing a good study plan is often as difficult as studying itself as a poorly structured plan may result in spending weeks studying irrelevant, difficult-to-remember material at the expense of what is considered more "high yield." There are no official books to study for any of the USMLE exams and on the USMLE website; the only materials provided are a booklet with the information about the exam and a set of 120 sample questions. As a result of that, a number of private organizations have attempted to create courses which they claim will help students achieve their dream score [1]. The most commonly used book for USMLE Step 1 preparation is called the *First Aid for the USMLE Step 1*. It is updated annually and consists of facts that the USMLE is known to test candidates on, and many consider it to be the most "high-yield book." American medical students usually do not use many additional resources, with many choosing to study solely from the *First Aid for the USMLE Step 1* and a question bank of their choice, most commonly "USMLE World." International medical graduates, on the other hand, rarely use so few resources. There can be many potential explanations of that, including tradition (as many of their peers had followed a different path previously), the time lapse from their preclinical years, and differences in medical school curricula worldwide.

The most famous organization offering USMLE lectures and books is Kaplan Medical. They offer a range of courses, both online and in person, teaching the students the material that the USMLE usually tests on. Their courses are held throughout the United States and even in some other countries where the demand is high. Their courses also offer student visas for those students who wish to study in the United States, and many seize the opportunity to spend the time in the United States, obtain additional clinical experience, and network with American physicians. There are also a number of USMLE tutoring services available, which offer private instruction for students struggling to prepare individually. A cheaper alternative for some students is to choose more typical "review books" that American medical students use to prepare for their medical school exams. Those resources are nevertheless usually accompanied by the *First Aid for the USMLE Step 1* and a question bank. A number of other books and courses are available, but they are not as well known or frequently used.

Another important aspect of USMLE Step 1 preparation is the use of question banks. Question banks are computer programs that generate up to 3000 distinct questions and provide detailed explanations of the concepts necessary to answer them. Most students use them both as study and assessment tools. They are often expensive but with the competitive nature of the exams are likely essential in order to achieve the high score. The most famous question bank is "USMLE World," and it holds an almost sacred status among many students and graduates. The other frequently used question banks are "Kaplan" question bank written by Kaplan Medical faculty and "USMLE Rx" question bank written by the authors of the *First Aid for the USMLE Step 1*. The question banks also provide users with the ability to simulate the real testing environment in the form of timed tests of random topics.

The National Board of Medical Examiners (NBME) provides a number of question forms aimed at assessing the students' progress in their USMLE preparation and providing an estimation of the score the individual would get if they were to sit the USMLE on that day. These forms are also among the most frequently used resources, and students often take many of them before sitting the actual exam. Most reports say that the score estimations are quite accurate so it is common for those who have enough time to choose to delay sitting the USMLE Step 1 until their NBME score estimates are sufficiently high. Interestingly, the software NBME uses to deliver the forms is not representative of the software used on the real USMLE examinations [2].

The USMLE Step 2 Clinical Knowledge

The USMLE Step 2 Clinical Knowledge is an exam largely similar in its outline to the USMLE Step 1. It is also a computer-based test administered in "Prometric" centers around the world. The exam is slightly longer than Step 1 as it consists of 8 blocks of 40 (or slightly fewer) questions. The exam is usually taken by American medical students just before or during their final year of medical school, once they have completed the core clerkships in internal medicine, psychiatry, obstetrics and gynecology, pediatrics, and surgery. Those are also the subjects covered by the exam. Some foreign graduates with recent clinical experience choose to sit USMLE Step 2 CK prior to Step 1 perceiving that taking a more clinically oriented exam would be easier for them. The questions are also written in the form of clinical scenarios, and they are often longer than Step 1 questions. The importance of USMLE Step 2 CK is questionable as not all the applicants report their scores at the time of their application. The score is likely of greater importance for international applicants compared to American applicants. The scoring scale is largely the same as that of Step 1, although the average score on this exam is higher, at around 243, with a standard deviation of 16. Similarly to Step 1, the Step 2 CK scores are also generally reported 3–4 weeks after the test date [1].

Preparation

The way in which students prepare for the USMLE Step 2 CK is much less uniform compared to USMLE Step 1 as there are not as many good resources. A possible reason behind that is the historical perception of the exam as less important. As scoring of Step 1 is phased out, this is likely to change. American students usually use the USMLE World question bank and some dedicated books for individual clinical rotations. It is generally believed that the USMLE World question bank is the single best resource for Step 2 CK preparation and that the content of answer explanations found there is sufficient to achieve a high score on the exam. Overall, recommended study schedules for Step 2 CK are more difficult to find compared to Step 1 study schedules and often less clear.

Nevertheless, a number of other books and courses are also available. They are often used by international medical graduates, especially those who have not practiced medicine recently. Kaplan Medical offers the same set of courses they offer for USMLE Step 1, and many agencies also provide private tutoring. Many students choose to purchase additional books, such as *First Aid for the USMLE Step 2 CK* or the *Master The Boards USMLE Step 2 CK*. The usefulness of these books is debatable. It should also be noted that many believe that the amount of information that students can theoretically be tested on is significantly larger than it was for Step 1. Therefore, often times it is necessary to rely on one's clinical judgment. Besides "USMLE World," "Kaplan" and "USMLE Rx" question banks also exist although they are used much less frequently and considered lower quality than "USMLE World."

Tracking one's progress can again be done through the NBME forms that are available on the NBME website. Unlike the NBME forms for USMLE Step 1, the Step 2 CK forms are not considered as reliably accurate as far as score estimation is concerned, and many students report discrepancies between predicted and achieved scores. The exams provided by the "USMLE World" are often seen as more accurate estimators of the eventual Step 2 CK score. The NBME also provides short exams in individual clinical disciplines, which some find useful [2].

The USMLE Step 2 Clinical Skills

The USMLE Step 2 CS differs from the other USMLE examinations in that it is the only exam that is not computer-delivered, that is not scored, and that is subjectively evaluated. Nevertheless, the passing rate is high. The test can only be taken in

Philadelphia, Chicago, Atlanta, Houston, and Los Angeles, in dedicated exam centers. The exam requires candidates to take histories and perform physical examinations on 12 standardized patients (actors who were trained to simulate conditions commonly encountered in clinical practice). This is followed by writing brief notes and providing differential diagnoses for each of the standardized patients. The candidates are assessed on their communication skills, spoken English proficiency, and ability to complete the clinical encounter and develop an appropriate list of differential diagnoses. The exam usually needs to be booked months in advance, and travel can be difficult and expensive. Since this is the only exam that is graded subjectively, it is also the one that provokes the most anxiety in some takers. For international medical graduates, obtaining the appropriate travel visa can also be an issue. The results are reported based on a schedule provided on the USMLE websites, and many candidates have to wait for a few months to find out whether they have passed the exam. Such a long wait for the Step 2 CS results is a frequent cause of delayed residency applications [1, 3].

Preparation

The preparation for the USMLE Step 2 CS also differs from that for any other exam. Most students believe that the *First Aid for the USMLE Step 2 CS* book is the best book with an overview of the cases they may encounter on the actual exam. The book provides only sample cases, and most students face standardized patients they were not prepared for. The book also provides guidelines on how to manage difficult situations, for example, angry or depressed standardized patients. Additional resources include books written by companies such as Kaplan and text and video resources such as USMLE World.

Many say that the most important aspect of preparation for the USMLE Step 2 CS is having a friend or colleague to play the role of the standardized patients that the test taker can practice with. Going through the sample cases provided in the *First Aid for the USMLE Step 2 CS* or "USMLE World" with a friend acting as the standardized patient is the most frequently recommended strategy. For those who do not have any friends or colleagues they can practice with, many companies offer the option of "hiring a standardized patient" for a fee. In addition, there are a number of companies that offer dedicated USMLE Step 2 CS courses where candidates are taught the necessary communication and physical exam skills and often get to experience a practice exam at the end of the course. It is difficult to judge the usefulness of these courses, although it is plausible that those who have experienced the environment similar to that of the real exam would find it easier to manage the stress of the exam day.

Another unique feature of the exam is the necessity to write notes following each patient encounter, and that usually requires additional preparation. The USMLE provides the note writing form on its website free of charge, and most use it to practice with cases described in the *First Aid for the USMLE Step 2 CS* as the book also gives sample notes. Typing speed is also an important aspect of achieving the passing score on the exam as the time to write the note is limited to 10 minutes. In rare instances, due to failures of the computer systems, candidates may be asked to write by hand, which makes it even harder to finish on time.

The USMLE Step 3

The USMLE Step 3 is the last of the USMLE exams and can only be taken once all the other exams have been passed and the candidate has graduated from medical school. It is a 2-day computer-administered test that can only be taken inside the United States. The results are typically reported 3–4 weeks after the second exam day. The exam consists of question blocks, similar but more clinical and difficult than the ones for Step 2 CK, and a series of "virtual patient encounters" that the test taker solves on the second exam day. An important part of the exam is biostatistics. Although present on all the USMLE exams, biostatistics questions are by far the most relevant and numerous on the USMLE Step 3, and sound knowledge of biostatistics is a requirement to obtain a good score on this exam. Scores on the USMLE Step 3 are lower than on the other exams as the median score is 226 with the standard deviation of 15. The importance of Step 3 score is debatable both in terms of residency applications for international medical graduates and for fellowship applications. The passing result on the USMLE Step 3 is required in order for a candidate to be eligible for the H1-b visa, a form of work visa sponsored by some residency programs. The most frequent form of visa the foreign graduates get, however, is the J-1 exchange visitor visa, and individuals do not need a passing Step 3 result in order to qualify for it [1, 4].

Preparation

The preparation for the USMLE Step 3 is largely similar to that for USMLE Step 2 CK. An important consideration is that most candidates preparing for the USMLE Step 3 are current residents whose work obligations may prevent them from spending extended amounts of time studying for a standardized exam. Many also believe that the fact that most of the USMLE Step 3 questions are internal medicine-based puts residents in other disciplines, especially psychiatry, at a serious disadvantage. The overall study time for this exam is generally shorter than for the others (with the exception of USMLE Step 2 CS).

Most candidates focus primarily on the content in the "USMLE World" question bank. The number of Step 3 questions in the "USMLE World" is lower than the number of Step 1 or Step 2 CK questions. Some students also use additional question banks. The "First Aid for the USMLE Step 3" and "Master the Boards USMLE Step 3" are the most frequently recommended books for USMLE Step 3 preparation. Individual subject books are rarely used. The virtual clinical encounters generally require additional preparation, and USMLE World provides software representative of that on the real exam day. External Step 3 preparation courses are rarer than courses for any of the other exams. The NBME also provides assessment forms for the USMLE Step 3 [2].

References

1. United States Medical Licensing Examination ® [Internet]. [cited 2020 Jul 24]. Available from: https://www.usmle.org/
2. Self-Assessment Services | NBME [Internet]. [cited 2020 Jul 24]. Available from: https://www.nbme.org/taking-assessment/self-assessments
3. CSEC | Test Centers [Internet]. [cited 2020 Jul 24]. Available from: https://www.csecassessments.org/test-centers/
4. Applying for Residency as an International Medical Graduate | NEJM Resident 360 [Internet]. [cited 2020 Jul 24]. Available from: https://resident360.nejm.org/expert-consult/applying-for-residency-as-an-international-medical-graduate

Chapter 24
The Residency Interview

Chau Nguyen, David Dragas, and Ian H. Rutkofsky

Introduction

Congratulations! After applying to ERAS, you have found that you secured an interview and need to find ways to help put your best foot forward to showcase your positive attributes. First impressions are important as this may be one of the deciding factors on how the programs rank you as they would like to ensure that you are a good fit, enthusiastic, knowledgeable, and, most importantly, able to communicate well and work well with others.

It is important to be remembered in a positive light, and this chapter aims to focus on what you can do to help improve your chances of being ranked. The interview helps to display aspects of your personality that are harder to convey in the application package. Preparation is critical, so knowing what to expect before, during, and after the application is essential.

The residency interview lets you showcase your interest in the specialty and the program you applied to. A strong application allows you to get your foot in the door, but at the interview, you now have an opportunity to exhibit qualities not easily conveyed on paper. This also provides an opportunity for you to see and learn from faculty members and current residents at the institution you are applying to. In either case, what is on "paper" may be exceeded from the in-person and closer

C. Nguyen · D. Dragas (✉)
International American University College of Medicine, Vieux Fort, Saint Lucia
e-mail: bnguyen@iau.edu.lc; ddragas@iau.edu.lc

I. H. Rutkofsky
Department of Psychiatry, HCA – Aventura Hospital and Medical Center, Aventura, FL, USA

Department of Research, CiBNP, Fairfield, CA, USA
e-mail: ian.rutkofsky@Hcahealthcare.com

H. Tohid, H. Maibach (eds.), *International Medical Graduates in the United States*, https://doi.org/10.1007/978-3-030-62249-7_24

interaction or, perhaps, the realization that what you see is not what was expected. Nevertheless, the interview is an important aspect of the application. In the 2018 NRMP Program Director Survey, interactions stemming from the interview process were cited as important factors in resident ranking [1]. Before we talk about the nuances relating to the interview, we will first discuss the process that takes place before the interview.

Applying to Programs on ERAS Residency programs will be able to access and review submitted residency applications after the date designated by ERAS. In 2020, because of the COVID-19 pandemic, this date was moved to October from the customary September start date. Programs can review all aspects of documents that have been submitted with the MSPE becoming available 1–2 weeks later. When offers are sent to applicants is dependent on the residency program. Programs may first interview candidates from an affiliated medical school or those having close ties to the region. Be patient; realize that programs can differ in how, when, and who receives interview invitations.

Once selected for an interview, candidates are notified directly through ERAS or the email provided in their ERAS application. Further instructions for scheduling an interview date will be provided. The applicant will be able to see and schedule from available times on the ERAS interview calendar or may need to contact the program with their preferred date(s) from a list provided. Again, there may be variation from program to program concerning scheduling.

You Are Offered an Interview. Now What?

P.S. Treat your interview invitation as the start of your interview. All aspects of communication with the program here on forward may impact deliberations of your application.

If provided with several dates for the interview, considerations when selecting an interview date include, but are not limited to, your current commitments and availability, region, distance, and weather considerations. At the same time, some debate whether it is better to interview early or late in the interview season, weather, and availability to travel are considerations that need to be taken into account, when able. Scheduling an interview earlier in the fall or winter may be something to consider to avoid inclement weather if interviewing in a region known to have winters with heavy snowfall, particularly if you will be flying long distances across the country.

As part of the interview offer, there will be additional information regarding the accommodations and schedule of the interview day. Questions regarding any aspect of the interview can be communicated to the appropriate contact person at the residency program.

Travel and Finances

Travel Depending on the location of the program you received an interview, you would need to travel by land or air. It is advisable to incorporate a margin of error or buffer into your itinerary to account for unforeseeable events: delayed flight, canceled flight, flat tire, engine trouble, and so forth. When flying, try not to book the last flight of the day but perhaps earlier in the afternoon or even the day before to give you time to acclimate. Those traveling across the continental USA may gain or lose as much three hours given the various time zones crossed.

It is best to try to organize your interviews in the same region, whenever possible, to optimize your travel expenses. For instance, if you have an interview in New Jersey, New York, or Pennsylvania, you may fly to one of these states; rent a car; ride a bus, train, and city transportation; or order a shared ride depending on the proximity. Also, this gives you a chance to explore the region and area you are interviewing firsthand and gives you a sense of the culture around you.

If you are on a budget and adventurous and have the luxury to travel from one interview to another without time constraints, you may take a Megabus or a Greyhound. This is an economical route as it may allow you to bring multiple luggage compared to some airlines where additional fees may apply to transport bags. However, be aware that there will be numerous stops on the way, travel time may be longer, and you will have to be more vigilant with your belongings, and the people around you as passengers are constantly boarding on and off the bus.

If you are flying into an airport, you can rent a car upon arrival. Though it may cost more at the airport than off-airport rentals, this is more convenient, especially if you do not know the area very well and have to haul your luggage. However, the best recommendation is to call ahead and reserve a car of your choice due to supply and demand. The easiest is to pay with a credit card. However, if you were to use a debit card, you may need additional requirements such as proof of a round trip airplane ticket. This is the best value considering one-way rideshare such as Uber/Lyft could cost the equivalent of a one-day rental. You could drive to restaurants and groceries, check the surrounding areas, look at your interview site the night before to familiarize yourself with the location of the interview, and store your luggage in the back seat of the trunk.

If you were to go to a metropolitan area, whether you are connecting from an intercity bus, airplane, car, or train, most cities will have their city transportation consisting of busses, shuttles, and rails/trains. This is very cost-efficient, but keep in mind the city's safety, the time of day of traveling, hours of operation, and the number of luggage that you must carry. Additionally, this may also take hours compared to minutes on other forms of transportation. Recommendations are to familiarize the schedule in advance and to download the map into your phone in case phone service or Wi-Fi is not available. It is also recommended to research the peak times thoroughly, possible time delays and detours, cancellations, delays due to mechanical failures, medical emergencies, etc. If you were to choose this form of transportation in the morning, be aware of the stops the night before. The last thing you want to do is miss your ride on the wrong side of the street/track. Also, plan to leave an hour before your interview time. Do not expect to ride to make it on time—plan for unforeseen circumstances as the previous scenarios mentioned. Programs do not want to wait for you when there is a set schedule for the day. You want to stand out, but being late is not one of the reasons to be remembered.

Use this option if your interview is more toward the late morning and afternoon. Otherwise, opt for Uber/Lyft if it is an early interview if the program anticipates you to arrive around 7 or 8 in the morning. Also, research to see if the local area uses Uber/Lyft. They may have their local city rideshares, or you may have to use a taxi service that can be time-consuming and expensive.

Remember, it is best to think of the big picture. You want to arrive at the interview fresh, clean, and stress-free. The anticipation of the interview is stressful enough. It is better to arrive at your interview early and wait an hour in the lobby rather than coming in 10 minutes to spare or, worse, arriving late. You do not want to be in a scenario where you have to figure out how to pay and find parking, detours and delays, missing your stop, or realizing that Uber/Lyft will take 30 minutes from your location to arrive at your interview on time. It is best to have a mindset of preparing for the worse and have a backup plan. This is why the one-hour buffer helps you.

Accommodations Accommodations may or not be provided by the program. As such, it is important to review the interview offer to see the details. If not offered by the program, the program may have "recommended" sites for applicants to book at with a special promotional discount for interviewees. This may be recommended due to the proximity to the hospital/interview site.

However, Airbnb is another excellent option, regardless if you are on a budget. Most of these places are cleaner than the hotels and are more personable. Just ensure that it is near your interview location. Prior to booking, the homes do not list their immediate address until after paying for the site. They will provide the general vicinity/city. It is best to message the host and ask if they are near the hospital, if they offer parking, and if they have nearby public transport if this has not already been listed on their page. You can also read the reviews from previous guests to get a sense of safety, area, transportation, and hosts/hostesses that you will be staying with. Often, the hosts/hostesses have already hosted other applicants. They can also be of a great asset as they know about the area, including the hospital, the culture, and the best places to go. This is great information to implement your interviews as well. Or if you are a private person and/or have limited time to prepare, most hosts will respect that and will give you space. Also, be mindful when you arrive. Remember even though you are paying to stay at their place, they are opening up their home. Be mindful. Pick up after yourself and respect their belongings. Just like the reviews you have read about them, they can also leave reviews about you which may help or break you when trying to find future Airbnb accommodations for interviews in other cities.

Also, do not be afraid to ask. Traveling and finding accommodations can be expensive. If the price point is a little more than your price range, you can always message the host/hostess and explain that you are a medical student or an I.M. graduate student and on a budget and in town for an interview. You can only afford x, y, and z and wonder if they can work with you. This of course is dependent on the hosts/hostesses. The worse they can say is "no," but the best outcome is that they are willing to work with you. Just be thankful for whatever reply they give you and be courteous. Just keep into account that the closest place to the interview site may also save you time and transportation expenses.

If you are involved with a particular religion, sports, or membership with another organization, you may reach out to the contacts to see if they have a spare room or couch to offer. This option may not be best for everyone based on their comfort level.

Of course, you should always reach out to friends, old classmates, and family members who are nearby. After all, they are your biggest cheerleaders, and it would be a great way to help keep your mind off of interviews, or on the contrary, they can help you with your interview process.

Food Food is usually a great topic of discussion during interviews if you have no idea what else to say during those awkward silences. Try to find well-known local restaurants and see what their dishes are well known for. Not only are you branching out, but this could also be used as a conversational piece. Explain your experience and recommend the restaurant if you like it or ask the interviewer for their recommendations. Share the experience if it is a positive one. Perhaps, this may lead to other discussions and unveiling the interviewer's passion which you can then build on which can be a gateway to another conversation. Best websites to check are Yelp where regular people write reviews of their experiences, Google Reviews, Tripadvisor, and HappyCow, just to name a few.

Some Airbnb's will provide a kitchen, and you can do grocery shopping, and some will provide a microwave and mini-fridge. If you have a specific diet, this can also be a better option.

Luggage Storage If possible, you can either store your luggage in a locker at a bus station, airport, trunk of the car, the hospital (ask the clinical coordinator beforehand), the hotel's front desk, or an Airbnb where you can store for an hour or two. Finally, there are apps available that show local businesses that participate in storing luggage.

Interview Preparation

To be your best at the interview requires adequate preparation. Learn as much as you can about the program, its strengths, faculty, and the region it serves. The program may provide information about who will be interviewing you. If not, you can ask the program coordinator if they can provide that information to you. Knowing who will be interviewing you beforehand can be helpful in that it will allow you to review their research history and interests inside and outside of medicine.

Why Is Practice So Important? If you are fortunate to have multiple interviews, you will find that most of the institutions will ask very similar questions and that you are already anticipating their questions. You have said your spiel so many times that it comes second nature, and you are not nervous anymore. For those who only have one or two, the main takeaway point is that, one, you can still anticipate questions and, two, you can practice your spiel with acquaintances, family members, and your pets and record yourself to the point where you already know what you are saying. It may be a daunting task, but you will thank yourself afterward.

You may not be much of a talker and more a listener. However, we can all agree that if you practice your speech and your answers, it sounds more natural and will make you sound polished and articulate, giving the impression you know precisely what you want. Let's face it, in residency, you will have to communicate and present to your seniors, attendings, consultants, med students, observers, and other health professionals, and it is vital to know how to get your message across in a concise manner. They want to see if you can do this. There is also a fine balance to where it does not sound rehearsed. Talk about it passionately as if this is the first time talking about it.

Practicing Interview Questions Practice makes perfect. There are various books, websites, social media groups, and professional organizations that provide information in preparation for the interview including sample questions. Search for a list of questions and think about thoughtful and genuine responses. Do you have any red flags on your application? The interview provides you an opportunity to open up and share additional insight that cannot be conveyed in your application. Additionally, there may be specialty-specific questions typically asked, so be sure to look at any professional association websites and specialty-specific groups online to look at advice for medical students applying to the specialty.

If you have red flags or have to discuss uncomfortable topics, you know this will be inevitable. You have to mentally prepare yourself because if the program is genuinely interested in you, they will need further explanation on concerns they may have. The key is not to avoid this, make light, or defer the question. Accept your shortcomings but also what you have learned from your experiences and what you did to incorporate changes in your life and turn things around. Show how these experiences have helped shape who you are today and why this was a catalyst moment that made you reflect and change yourself for the better. Explain what you can do to benefit the program by previous mistakes and help those that might be going through similar experiences.

Another problem that people often face is at the two ends of the spectrum: they either have problems underselling themselves due to their modesty and humility or can talk about themselves without a problem until the point it may look narcissistic and arrogant. Now is not the time for either of these scenarios. This is the time to talk about your accomplishments, but the keyword is to be tactful and humble. Be proud of your achievements, but do not put other people down. Give thanks to the organization, people, and others who have helped paved the way. Say that it was an enriching and humbling experience that allowed you to do these accomplishments. This shows that you work well with other people and do not have to be in the lime-light, but do not brush off your contributions. Find friends, mentors, acquaintances, and even strangers to hear your answers to give constructive feedback. If you notice a trend in what people say, perhaps reflect on how your actions, tone, and words may give this impression. After all, multiple people who give similar suggestions may see a trend or point out a vibe that you are unaware of. If you do not feel comfortable talking to people you know, you can seek other organizations such as Toastmasters. Here, you will have an opportunity to present prepared or impromptu speeches in front of a supportive audience, receive feedback on speaking and presentation skills, and learn from feedback given to others. This is a great organization to look into as it may polish your interview skills and help overcome nerves with meeting and speaking to groups of people.

You should familiarize yourself with the medical system as some programs are interested in how you approach this. Practice your answers until you answer smoothly without even having to think of your next sentence. However, you do not want to sound monotone as if you are giving this speech for the 20th time.

It is almost guaranteed that you will be asked broad general questions, "tell me about yourself." This is where you can say all the things that were not in your essay that you would have liked to touch base on. Please expand on your answers rather than be minimal. If you have an interesting story on how you want to become a physician, you may use a segue up to this point.

Interviewers have hundreds of people they interview, and to stand out share something personal and unique to yourself that you are willing to share and how it molds you into who you are today to be a well-equipped physician. Be enthusiastic and engaging while giving your story. They will remember how you made them feel such as making them comfortable.

Of course, there may be some curveball questions that they will ask to see how well you think on your feet. Be real. Smile and say, "That is a very interesting or thoughtful question. May I take a moment to think about that?" Do not be uncomfortable if they are sitting and staring at you. Think of a quick and reasonable response. Hopefully, you have prepared yourself with similar questions that you can take a variation of that and incorporate into your answers. Do not ever answer, "I do not know." This just looks like you cannot think under pressure or worse you just gave up and did not attempt. Programs just want to see if you can try to answer and how well you handle yourself.

Some programs may also do an interactive activity to see how well you work with others or how you think. While doing a project, it is important to listen to your teammates and come up with ideas but not necessarily dominate the group, and do not be stressed out or the program can see this. Try to think of innovative ideas to get the project done and contribute. Do not be quiet and stand back. However, if there is a chance that some members are not agreeable, you can take this moment to be a mediator and suggest that you try a certain way first, and if that does not work, you may do an alternative way. Find a place that you are more comfortable with. And show that you are happy to work in a group and boost each other. Do not ever bring anyone down to make yourself look better.

Dress Code Your presentation is an important aspect of your interview because you start making an impression when you first step in the door. You want to dress professionally and be well groomed.

- **Women:**
  - Ideally, if you have a nice business suit, whether it be pants or skirt, this will be the best option. The majority of the interviewees will be wearing this. However, if you are unable to get a suit, navy or blue slacks will be fine with a nice complementing blouse. It goes without saying that you should dress modestly. It is not recommended to wear a low-cut shirt. This will make it awkward for the interviewer to try to avert their eyes elsewhere regardless of their sexual orientation. Also, keep jewelry minimal to accent your wardrobe, but do not be flashy. Try to keep it classy. Also, try to avoid busy and loud patterns. This is not trying to suppress your personality. You can dress however you like once you get into residency, but this is for first-time impressions.
  - Also, be aware that most institutions will do a tour of the hospital/facility so be mindful of that. It is recommended to wear flat shoes and avoid heels if possible. You do not want to feel uncomfortable walking up and down the stairs and slick floors and making the group wait on you to get from point A to point B.
- **Men:**
  - Wear a nice suit if possible. If you do not have a nice jacket, you may wear a nice dress shirt and tie. However, most who do interviews do wear suits. Try to avoid flashy ties with conspicuous brand names or logos. You do not want to give them the impression of being superficial while trying to help the underserved population. Save it for nice occasions or graduation. Also, make sure your shoes are neat and clean.
  - For mustaches and beards. Most interviews do occur during November also known as Movember for those who are bringing awareness to prostate cancer. This can go both ways. This can be a conversationalist piece and a segue why you are passionate about the cause. However, regardless if this is your style or for a cause, try to keep the beard or mustache nicely maintained.
- For both parties, make sure you either iron or steam your clothes the night before the interview. You are representing yourself and you want to look sharp and neat as possible. Try to bring a small carry-on steamer if possible. Most establishments will have an iron at their facility, but if not, at least you have a portable steamer as a backup.

Online Interview Make sure you dress as you would for a real-life meeting. This includes dressing professionally from the waist down. Do not assume you may not need to stand up; it is best to avoid the potential for an embarrassing moment! Dressing professionally shows to others you are serious and that you are not cutting any corners. Make sure you are in an environment that is conducive to your interview. If family members or housemates are home during your interview, make sure that they cannot be heard during your big day. Also, have a nice background to where it is not distracting.

The online interview will likely be heavily utilized in 2020 because of the COVID-19 pandemic, so take extra care in your preparation. The AAMC offers a variety of recourses for online interviews (https://www.aamc.org/what-we-do/mission-areas/medical-education/conducting-interviews-during-coronavirus-pandemic). As mentioned earlier, education organizations such as Toastmasters will help hone communication skills and thinking and answering questions on the spot. Look for additional resources from books to videos online and even courses. Coursera offers several free online courses relating to communication. Finally, practice! Practice recording yourself, reviewing the recordings, and asking for feedback from others. If your interaction with a residency program is limited to the computer screen, make it count!

Interview Day

As mentioned previously, the applicant would also be provided with information about the interview day shortly after receiving an interview. This would possibly include information regarding a preinterview dinner and overview of the interview day which may include morning report, interview schedule, hospital tour, lunch, and city tour. A list of those that will be interviewing you may be included in the interview package. If not, do not hesitate to contact the program closer to the interview date to inquire about the format and who will be interviewing on your interview day.

Interview Dinners They matter. The residents will rank you from the time you step in the door till you leave. We want to see how you interact with each other. Do you share the spotlight or do you constantly turn the spotlight to yourself? Nobody wants to work with someone like that. We want to make sure you are flexible and play well with others. We want to see if you are condescending or helpful and go out of your way to be a team player. We also want to see if you pick up things fast so pay attention to the conversation and jump in when possible, but also make sure you are not overstepping your bounds. Give everybody a fair chance and opportunity to express themselves. Are you a good listener? Do you have insightful thoughts? Do you look interested in our programs by asking us questions?

Be yourself and be cordial to all you meet. For interview dinners, you will meet the residents. Do not dismiss someone you may view as unimportant, and be sure to treat everyone with respect; you never know who will be attending a preinterview dinner. Arrive on time. You may drink socially, but do not get drunk. This is an informal dinner, but at the same time this dinner is very important as they will be ranking you based on your personality and interest in the program and see if you are a good fit with the program and a good fit with the residents. Residents are looking for someone who has similar interests, a team player, easy to get along with, hard workers, and someone they feel they can trust. Though this is a relaxed environment, you must remember that residents are judging you and remember your encounter. Be engaging and ask questions of the program and also questions about their life outside of residency. You do not want not to have any questions and you do not want to ask questions that you can find on the program's website either. Look interested when residents talk to you. Do not look bored even if this is not your number one choice. Also, people may drink during these dinners. This is up to you. Drinking alcohol is not necessarily frowned upon unless you do not know your limit. It also does not look favorably if you spend most of the night with a resident the night before your interviews. The program will hear about it and may think you are not serious.

In the end remember that the residents are watching and judging you. We want to make sure you will fit in and not disturb the balance. We do not want to work with someone who is confrontational and not easy going and quick to temper. We want to be able to count on you. Also, we want to know if you have any similar characteristics, traits, or hobbies aligned with our other colleagues. Be engaged. Follow the pattern.

The Interview The interview is typically conducted with a series of interviews with various faculty members and/or residents. Applicants would be assigned to an order and would meet with each interviewer in the appropriate sequence. Each interview duration will range in time and may depend on the number of interviewers and interviewees.

As you approach your interviewer's room, take a moment to knock on the door before entering the room and greet the interviewer, offering a handshake.

Smile and be engaging. Let the interviewer take the lead. If they want to talk about themselves or the program, sit graciously and attentively. Even though you are a guest, make your interviewer feel comfortable, which will reflect in the conversation as it progresses and in turn that should be reciprocated. Look like you want to be there even though this may not be the program of your dreams. I have often heard that applicants come for an interview and treat the program as it is beneath them. Remember, networking is common so even though you may feel this is the right fit for you, other program directors may know and communicate with one another. Also, even though this may not be your dream program, treat it as an opportunity to practice in preparation for programs you are very interested in. Also, do not be afraid to say what you mean. With this being said, sometimes people are sarcastic and everybody is quick-witted and pick up on tone as well. Others may take things that you say in a joking manner the wrong way, or perhaps they may not share the same sense of humor. Look around the room and eye something that would be a good conversational piece if the interview lags or lulls. Remember you can bring things up. Ask questions and show that you are a good listener by not cutting them off and nodding and smiling, and look like you are really into their stories. This will give the interviewer a feeling that you have bonded. This is great for people who are not much of a talker.

Do not try to speak over an interviewer or try to turn the focus back to you. Wait until your turn. Make sure you can get across the points you want to share in a limited time. This is where practicing is important as mentioned previously. You are only allotted a certain amount of time, and if you have your dialogue prepared in advance, you do not have to worry about forgetting what to say. Also, make sure you ask questions about the programs. Do not ask questions that you can easily find on the website. You can always ask for their advice and experience. Be appreciative and always be a good guest by stating that you enjoyed your day and that you could see yourself at this hospital/program because x, y, and z. Insert what you experience at the dinner, what you and the residents talked about and heard from the tour, and how you would be a good fit in the program, and thank them for taking the time to get to know you.

During an interview, share a personal story that is touching and personal that the program director/interviewer will remember you by. It may not necessarily be related to medicine; in fact, something unrelated will show you to be a well-rounded person.

After your interview, it is good practice to send an email or card and add something personal, such as what you discussed during the interview. Typically, during your interview, contact information will be provided for future correspondence or questions. Do not be shy to ask if none is provided. When you do contact the program, personalize your messages. Do not send generic emails, especially if you are contacting several individuals within the same program. Consider adding a small headshot photo from your ERAS application as part of your signature during email communications so the reader can put your name to a face. When talking to the program directors, they always remember what you said and how you said it. Also, you want to make sure you treat everybody you meet with respect, including the clinical coordinator. They play a huge part. Clinical coordinators remember if you were a difficult person and if you treated them with respect or not. This should be common sense, but you will be surprised by how people act.

If you have special interests in their program, you can always ask for a "second look" where you can visit the program again. This is not always offered, but if you feel it is important to you in deciding if the program is a good fit, reach out and explain to the program.

COVID-19 Considerations The COVID-19 global pandemic has impacted several aspects of a student's experience preparing for The Match, and do not be surprised if that also applies to the residency interview. Depending on the program's location and current cases in the region, programs may opt to conduct online interviews. In this case, the applicant should prepare for the strong possibility of the interview happening online rather than in person. Although not ideal for either party, try to make the most of the situation, making the most of all the individuals you meet and interact with during your interview.

Reference

1. Program NRM, Release D, Committee R. Results of the 2018 NRMP program director survey. Washington, DC: National Resident Matching Program; 2018.

Websites

STAR interview format: https://www.indeed.com/hire/c/info/star-interview-format?aceid=&gclid=Cj0KCQjwgo_5BRDuARIsADDEntTcdiyQVewx93E1NjMN50-Lko1b750ldEJEL_fgbunDPIedLM4nxGEaAq_DEALw_wcB
Coursera: https://www.coursera.org/

Chapter 25
The Match Process and SOAP

David Dragas, Chau Nguyen, and Ian H. Rutkofsky

Introduction

Reaching the application stage of your medical training is a milestone you should take tremendous pride. All your hard work and dedication has led to this point. As you now prepare for the next phase in your training, start thinking about how you will share the story of your journey in medicine. From inspirations in your life that led you to the field of medicine to the accomplishments and challenges you have experienced along the way, applying for residency is your chance to convey to others your interests and passion.

In the United States, the residency application cycle occurs once annually, typically running from September to February, with Match results released to programs and applicants in March. There are nuances to this process that will be discussed in this chapter that include topics such as pre-match and the Supplemental Offer and Acceptance Program® (SOAP®). There are several steps in preparing for The Match. Knowing about the specialty(s) you plan to apply to and the requirements of programs in that specialty are first steps. Ensuring that you have the required documents for a complete ERAS application is the next step. The preparation of your application requires careful thought and consideration in their development. Note that not all materials will be or can be uploaded by you. For example, LoRs will be uploaded by your letter writer through an online ERAS portal. Your school will be responsible for submitting official documents including the medical school

D. Dragas (✉) · C. Nguyen
International American University College of Medicine, Vieux Fort, Saint Lucia
e-mail: ddragas@iau.edu.lc; bnguyen@iau.edu.lc

I. H. Rutkofsky
Department of Psychiatry, HCA – Aventura Hospital and Medical Center, Aventura, FL, USA

Department of Research, CiBNP, Fairfield, CA, USA
e-mail: ian.rutkofsky@Hcahealthcare.com

© Springer Nature Switzerland AG 2021
H. Tohid, H. Maibach (eds.), *International Medical Graduates in the United States*, https://doi.org/10.1007/978-3-030-62249-7_25

transcript and the Medical School Performance Evaluation (MSPE), formerly the Dean's Letter. Additionally, official USMLE score reports and ECFMG certification are requested online via MyERAS and submitted from their respective agencies directly to programs you have applied. Later, in section "Residency Application," we will look in more detail at each of the documents you will need as part of a complete ERAS application. Finally, the application process contains several key dates and deadlines that the applicant will need to be aware of. These key dates are usually similar from year to year, but unforeseen circumstances may lead to changes. Stay up to date on the latest news from the ECFMG, AAMC, and NRMP for the current NRMP Match calendar year. Review their official websites and register for email updates to ensure notification regarding any changes to dates of the application, interview season, Match week, and SOAP®.

Competition in the United States is high, as US allopathic MDs, IMGs, and DOs (Doctor of Osteopathic Medicine) all vie for coveted residency positions. According to the NRMP Results and Data report for the 2020 Match, there were a record number of registrants applying for PGY-1 positions [1]. Knowing specific specialty(s) of interest to you and how IMGs fair in those fields is a great preliminary step to take. Working to ensure a complete and compelling application in time for the start of the application season is a contributing factor to ensure your best opportunities during this process. Preparation in these areas in advance of applying will help alleviate anxieties during this process and maximize success. The goal of this chapter is to provide you with an overview of the process and suggestions in your preparation for submitting your residency application.

By failing to prepare, you are preparing to fail. (Benjamin Franklin)

Learning About Specialties and Training Programs

Preparation will be a recurring theme in this chapter. As we will soon discuss the application procedure, it is important first to ask yourself the question, "what specialty or specialties are of interest to me?" What area or aspects of medicine are you passionate about or fascinate you? If your answer is not certain at this time, that is not uncommon. While some may find a particular calling in medicine before or during medical school while on core or elective rotations, that is not always the case. Your experiences during residency may provide further feedback that you can use in deciding to pursue advanced fellowship training in a subspecialty possibly. Additionally, it is important to be mindful of the various paths you can take after completing a particular residency program specialty. Subspecialty training following completion of residency may be needed to work in a specific area of interest. For example, completing a psychiatry residency and then doing a fellowship in adolescent psychiatry is an example of a pathway you can take based on your career interests and aspirations. There are a variety of free and paid resources that provide a wide range of information on various specialties and subspecialties, including metrics of those successfully matching into training programs. Those interested in the pathways to desired specialties can learn more through a subscription to the AAMC's Careers in Medicine®. This paid subscription provides a detailed overview of over 150 specialties in medicine, including training paths, information on applying, and more. The AMA offers several free resources for students and graduates applying for residency through the Fellowship and Residency Electronic Interactive Database Access (FREIDA™), a residency and fellowship database, and the AMA Career Planning Resource section of their website.

The National Resident Matching Program® (NRMP®) provides several free reports of statistics from the NRMP® Match and surveys of applicants and program directors. These resources offer invaluable information from important factors considered by program directors when offering interviews to an applicant to average board scores of applicants matching into various specialties. Finally, commercial products, such as Match a Resident©, are also available online. These products seek to help applicants find suitable programs to apply to by using applicant metrics, including scores, visa requirements, and year of graduation, compared to program requirements. Most, if not all, of the information that commercial products can offer are publicly available for free. Still, these paid subscriptions may be of benefit to those who do not have time to commit to individually reviewing programs in one or more specialty on FREIDA™ and residency program websites.

Medical School

Your home medical institution should play a pivotal role in your preparation for the residency application, particularly if a significant number of their past graduates have gone on to pursue residency training in the United States. Take advantage of all available resources your medical school provides. Examples of resources include faculty advising, graduate peer-mentorship programs, application workshops, and guideline documents on applying to residency in the United States.

Throughout the preparation process of your application, be sure to seek out feedback from faculty and graduate mentors. Ask them for honest feedback and recommendations to consider to improve the quality of your application. Having an advisor, someone you can occasionally connect with, while preparing your applications and during the residency application is important to gain valued guidance and to help alleviate anxiety. Because of their recent shared experiences of applying to residency and being in the situation you are in now, they more than anyone can provide current and relevant advice and feedback that may be particularly relevant to those that are attending medical school outside of the United States.

Additionally, your medical school will be involved in submitting and preparing various documents for the ERAS application, including an official medical school transcript and the Medical School Performance Evaluation (MSPE), formerly known as the Dean's Letter. Be mindful of deadlines and fees for these documents.

More information will be provided in section "Residency Application" of this chapter.

USMLES

The series of USMLE board examinations are important aspects of medical education in the United States. Passage is required for graduation from medical school. Programs that give scores on the USMLEs are important consideration for applicant selection. Additionally, the passage of the USMLEs is requirement for ECFMG certification, which is required of international graduates.

Because scores are important to the residency application, a plan must be made to ensure adequate study time in preparation for these examinations. Additionally, scheduling will need to be considered. Processing of an application may take weeks before a scheduling permit is issued. With the scheduling permit, the applicant can apply to sit for an examination at a certified testing facility. Having a scheduling permit does not guarantee there will be seating availability if there is a high demand by other test-takers in your region. As residency applications typically begin in mid-September, the months leading up to September can be expected to be competitive for finding positions. Once an examination is taken, results are usually released 3–4 weeks after the examination day for Step 1, Step 2 CK, and Step 3. For Step 2 CS, results are issued according to a reporting schedule available on the USMLE website.

The USMLE Examinations

USMLE Step 1 – Application through ECFMG Interactive Web Application (IWA)
    USMLE Step 2 Clinical Knowledge (CK) – Application through ECFMG IWA
    USMLE Step 2 Clinical Skills (CS) – Application through ECFMG IWA
    USMLE Step 3 – Application through the Federation of State Medical Boards (FSMB)
    N.B. Prospective Step 3 applicants must first have an ECFMG certificate before they can apply for the exam.
    Learn more about each one of these examinations on the Application and Fees portion of the US Medical Licensing Examination® (USMLE®) website: https://www.usmle.org/apply/index.html.

Applying for Step 1, Step 2 CK, and Step 2 CS Application of these exams is through **Interactive Web Applications (IWA)** of the Online Services section of the ECFMG website. As part of the application process, the applicant must submit an IWA application:

- ***Setting up an ECFMG IWA account:*** Detailed instructions for setting up an IWA account can be found on the EFCMG website: https://iwa2.ecfmg.org/gradoverview.asp. The IWA application consists of both an online application and the Certification of Identification Form (Form 186) paper component that is to be mailed to the ECMFG. Both parts must be completed and received by the ECFMG before processing of the application begins. Once processed and accepted by the ECFMG, the Certification of Identification Form remains valid for 5 years, during which time you will be able to apply for USMLE examinations through the ECFMG IWA.

Applying for Step 3:
- ***Setting up an FSMB account:*** Setting up an FSMB account is for those applying for the USMLE Step 3. Applicants will need to complete an online application and submit a Certification of Identity (CID) form requiring a notary stamp.

Location of USMLE Examinations USMLE Step 1 and Step 2 CK can be written outside of the United States at designated testing centers. Fees for examinations conducted outside of the United States depend on the region, with additional information available on the USMLE website. In 2020, the fee schedule for the USMLE is as follows (https://www.usmle.org/apply/index.html). The USMLE Step 2 CS and Step 3 are only offered in the United States, with the USMLE Step 2 CS exam proctored at designated Clinical Skills Evaluation Collaboration (CSEC) test centers. These CSEC locations for Step 2 CS are located in Atlanta, Chicago, Houston, Los Angeles, and Philadelphia.

USMLE Preparation Preparation for these examinations is critical because scores impact evaluation of future residency applications. Surveys conducted by the NRMP of program directors have shown the USMLE Step 1 score is an important factor taken into consideration when offering an interview. Additionally, those seeking an H1-B for residency would require completion of the USMLE Step 3. There exist an immense number of study resources accessible in various formats. Some examples include online question banks, review books, online review courses, apps, etc. While most products are only available for a fee, there exists content available free of charge (OnlineMedEd, Medbullets, etc.).

Study Resources

UWorld Qbank
  AMBOSS Qbank
  Kaplan Qbank
  First Aid for the USMLE series by McGraw Hill
  SketchyMedical
  OnlineMedEd
  Medbullets

Self-assessments: NBME, UWorld, AMBOSS, and USMLE practice questions*
    *USMLE practice material is available for free on USMLE.org. Those already registered for Step 1, 2 CK, or Step 3 and who have a scheduling permit also have the opportunity to register for a USMLE computer-based training practice session. The benefits of doing this are that you will familiarize yourself with the testing facility (bathrooms, lockers, sign-in/sign-out protocol, testing equipment, headphones, etc.) in preparation for your examination. Further details on registering for a USMLE CBT practice session can be found here: https://apps.nbme.org/CBTPSRegistrationWeb/jsp/usmle_CBTPS_registration.jsp.

Clinical and Research Experience

Those not having the US clinical experience (USCE) should pursue clinical and research experiences to include in their application to residency. USCE is helpful to IMGs in that they will allow for familiarization of the US medical system, provide an opportunity to ask for LoRs showing competence and qualities desirable in residency applicants, and offer invaluable networking opportunities.

Finding such experiences can be done in a variety of ways. Contact your home institution for any affiliated programs in the United States and see what clinical sites colleagues from your home institution conducted research. Additionally, there exist paid medical agencies that assist students with finding opportunities in the United States. Finally, if there is a hospital program that you would like to work at, research their website for opportunities and contact the hospital directly with any questions. Costs and prerequisites for application eligibility for clinical and research experiences will vary and need to be reviewed. As with the USMLEs, applying earlier is better to increase the likelihood of placement, because certain programs may have application windows or popular placements may fill up fast.

Residency Application

Application for residency training in the United States warrants careful consideration of important dates stemming from when applicants can apply for the ECFMG Token until the deadline for submitting the NRMP Rank Order List and awaiting Match results. This process requires the applicant to create accounts on various organizational websites. This includes, but may not be limited to the:

- ECFMG to apply for ECFMG certification and apply for your residency token
- AAMC to set up an account and build your Electronic Residency Application Service (ERAS) application and apply to programs
- NRMP to receive your NRMP number that programs will use to rank you and to have your NRMP account where you will be able to locate and rank programs

The ERAS timeline can be viewed on the AAMC website: https://students-residents.aamc.org/applying-residency/article/eras-timeline-img-residency/.

Because of the COVID-19 pandemic, there has been a shift to when programs would be able to review applications. In the 2021 application season, programs will not be able to view applications until October 21, 2020, whereas in previous years, programs would be able to in mid-September. Additionally, it is probable to assume the majority of the residency and fellowship interviews for the 2021 MATCH will be conducted via online video meetings. It is important to have a good Internet connection and a computer with a camera and audio assessable. Other than reducing the risk of COVID-19, additional benefits include saving money on travel and lodging. The downside of interviewing online is that your scope of knowledge may be limited about the hospital or the region the hospital is located.

The official start of the ERAS season begins in June. This is when prospective applicants can create an AAMC account and log in to their ERAS. Later in June (June 23, 2020, of the 2021 cycle), prospective IMG applicants are eligible to apply for a "token" from the ECFMG. This token will allow applicants to create and access the ERAS portal, where applicants will be able to upload and manage various components of their application and have documents uploaded or transferred from their school or LoR references. MyERAS is a centralized location where you can view all parts of your application that will be sent to prospective programs, MSPE, LoRs, USMLE transcripts, photo, and medical school transcript, and where programs will be selected and applied.

P.S. While the NRMP Match is the primary match for the majority of specialties, those applying to ophthalmology or plastic surgery will apply to the SF Match. In contrast, those interested in applying to urology will apply to the Urology Residency Match. The respective websites for the SF Match and the Urology Residency Match are listed at the end of the chapter under Websites.

Registering for a Token As mentioned earlier, to access and prepare an application on the AAMC's ERAS, prospective applicants first need to register and pay for a "token." For international graduates, they will apply and receive their token from the ECFMG:

1. Visit ECFMG.org and sign onto the Online Applicant Status and Information System (OASIS) with your USMLE/ECFMG identification number and password. Those without a USMLE/ECFMG identification number or who are signing onto OASIS for the first time will need to follow instructions on the log-in page to request an identification number or establish an ECFMG Online Services account, respectively.
2. Once logged on in OASIS, click on the ERAS Support Services tab where you will be redirected to the ERAS Token Request page.
3. The cost of the ERAS Token for the 2021 season is 145 USD. This token will be used when registering for the MyERAS account on the AAMC website and is good through the NRMP Main Match and SOAP®.

Research the particular specialty you are applying to see if there are any specific requirements. For example, certain specialties require completion of a transitional or preliminary year before entry into a PGY-2 program. In such circumstances, the applicant would need to apply to two residency type programs: *preliminary* and *advanced*. Additionally, certain specialties such as urology participate in the San Francisco Match. This will include a separate timeline compared to the NRMP Match.

Previously, applicants applying to residency programs in California were required to submit a Postgraduate Authorization Training Letter (PTAL) on ERAS which would be submitted along with the ERAS application. Changes have taken place such that the PTAL is no longer required, starting January 1, 2020, in favor of the Postgraduate Training License (PTL). Additionally, medical schools recognized by the medical board of California have undergone adjustments to include medical schools listed in one of four different directories. More information on the PTAL and recognized medical school can be found on the Medical Board of California's website:

- Senate Bill 798: Changes to Postgraduate Training Requirements: https://www. mbc.ca.gov/Download/Fact-Sheets/SB798PD-FactSheet.pdf
- Medical Board of California Application for a Postgraduate Training License Information and Checklist: https://www.mbc.ca.gov/Download/Forms/ps-ptl-information.pdf

Components of the ERAS Application

- CV
- Letters of recommendation (LoRs)
- Personal statement
- Medical school transcript
- Medical Student Performance Evaluation (MSPE)
- ECFMG status report*
- Photograph

*Due to the COVID-19 pandemic, the USMLE Step 2 CS has been suspended until at least June 1, 2021. As the completion of this exam was important for ECFMG certification, there have been changes implemented by the ECFMG to allow IMGs to pursue ECFMG certification. The ECFMG is providing five different pathways for IMGs to make up for not being able to test for Step 2 CS. Details of the five pathways are found on the ECFMG website: https://www.ecfmg.org/certification-requirements-2021-match/.

Interviews and Pre-match

Residency programs can see and review ERAS applications a period after applicants can submit applicants.

N.B. Unlike previous years where the period before programs can access would be around two weeks, because of the COVID-19 pandemic, applicants in 2020 can submit applications starting September 1. Still, residency programs will not be able to review applications until October 21.

Interviews may be offered at any point after the official start of the application season. Typically, interviews are offered as early as September and may extend into January. Do not be discouraged if you do not get offers at the start of the application season. Programs may prioritize invitations to their medical students or applicants from their region. As the interview season progresses, there may be cancellations made by applicants, and programs would then have spots to offer additional interviews to other applicants.

Criteria for interviews are usually displayed on the program website. Applicants need to review selection criteria for prospective applicants on the program website to see if they meet the requirements for selection criteria. Criteria considered by programs include but are not limited to the year of graduation, letters of recommendation, ECFMG certification, USMLE scores (including Step 1, Step 2 CK, Step 2 CS), a personal statement stating interest in the specialty, and visa acceptable. In addition to admission requirements, there are commonly FAQ sections that address frequently asked questions. Regarding certain components of the application, the program may specify specific requirements. This may include but is not limited to particular USMLE score cutoffs, year of graduation, source of LoRs (letters from faculty in the specialty you are applying to), and whether or not visas are accepted.

Visas for applicants include the J-1 and H1-B visa. Check the website of the program you are applying to see whether they accept applications from those seeking either one of these visas. You can also search for this information on FREIDA™ if the program provides this information.

The Fellowship and Residency Electronic Interactive Database Access (FREIDA™), offered by the American Medical Association (AMA), is a free searchable database that allows applicants to search for particular criteria of programs in the specialty(s) they are seeking to apply. Programs can be searched based on specialty, location (region or state), application info (participation in ERAS, NRMP, etc.), visas accepted (H1-B, J-1), and various metrics provided by the program (total program positions, total first-year positions, %USMD, %IMG, %DO, salary, average hours of work per week, etc.).

Pre-match Some programs may offer pre-match positions before the NRMP Match. Pre-match is an offer for a residency position from a program not participating in the NRMP Match. The program may make an offer following an interview with there being a time limit for which the offer is valid. While you may apply to both pre-match and regular programs participating in The Match, once you receive an offer from a program offering pre-match positions, you will need to decide whether or not to accept. Once accepted, you are no longer eligible to participate in The Match. If you accept a pre-match offer, as a courtesy, you should inform the programs where you have already interviewed and cancel upcoming scheduled interviews and decline any further interview offers. You can find a list of programs of not participating in the NRMP Match on FREIDA™. You apply to these programs through ERAS, as you would programs participating in the NRMP Match.

Month of March and Match

Results of the Match are released in March. On the Monday of Match week, those who matched and did not match are notified of their results via email. Those that match will be notified of the specific residency program they matched on Friday of Match week. Those that did not match will go on to participate in the Supplemental Offer and Acceptance Program® (SOAP®), which will be discussed in the following section. This can be a stressful time if you did not match but do not lose hope. Regroup and prepare to review and apply to programs with openings.

Those who match and require a visa should start the process immediately to allow adequate time for processing. Those applying for a J-1 or H1-B visa will need to contact the appropriate government agency, if necessary, for a statement of need and work in conjunction with the ECFMG and your residency program for processing the visa. The process can take time, so apply early so as not to compromise your ability to travel to the United States for the start of residency training. Of note, those seeking an H-1B visa will require having passed USMLE Step 3 to be eligible to apply.

SOAP

After The Match, there may be unfilled positions remaining at programs, and those programs and applicants who did not "match" will now have the opportunity to take part in the Supplemental Offer and Acceptance Program® (SOAP®). Unlike the regular season, there are some changes in SOAP® that need to be regarded. Included among these is that there is a limit of applications (45) that can be submitted in total. Additionally, applicants are not to initiate contact with the program but instead must wait for the program to initiate contact first. Multiple rounds of offers take place during the week with the number of available positions in each specialty being regularly updated. If an applicant were to receive multiple offers in a given round, they would rank them according to their preference. After SOAP®, the list of remaining positions will be available, and applicants can now reach out directly to programs to share their interests.

Post-SOAP® After the conclusion of SOAP®, a list of programs in various specialties with remaining positions is maintained on the NRMP website and is regularly
updated. Programs may try to reserve positions for unmatched students from their
affiliated medical school. However, it is still possible to match during SOAP®. In
the event you did not match during the NRMP Match or SOAP®, regularly review
the NRMP list of unfilled positions and the AMA's FREIDA™ for vacant residency
positions. If you happen not to MATCH and enter SOAP®, it is important to follow
the guidelines and policy. This includes never emailing the residency programs that
are participating in SOAP®. They must contact you first after you have applied.
Failure to abide by the policy will bar you from entering into SOAP® the subsequent
year as well as getting red-flagged as an NRMP violator in your next application cycle.

July 1: Residency Starts

The official start of residency is July 1. However, programs may request interns to
arrive earlier for orientation programs, including a mini-boot camp review, learning
the EMR, BLS, ACLS certification, etc. This information would be communicated
with the resident from the program office.

Accommodations + Transportation Looking for accommodations and transportation is important factor for those moving to a new city for their residency. As a
general suggestion, it is advisable not to live too far from the training site.
Additionally, it is important to familiarize yourself with the local traffic in the region
you are moving. For example, a 4-mile commute to work may be drastically different based on the city/region and local traffic. Those who do not drive or own a car
will need to live closer to their training site which may mean higher rent. Additionally,
when looking for accommodations, research local crime rates, schools, and other
factors important and relevant to you. Contacting a local real estate agent in the area
is an option to consider allowing for expert advice to guide your decisions.

Addendum: The Match Process and SOAP Chapter

Applying Directly to Fellowship Training in the United States Applicants having postgraduate training and extensive research in their home country that seek
additional advanced subspecialty training in the United States may consider applying directly to fellowship training. Though this may be an arduous process, if certain
application requirements are lacking, the decision to apply should be weighed
against an individual applicant's educational background, achievements, and future
aspirations.

Familiarize yourself with the ERAS fellowship application timeline on the AAMC website, which differs from the residency timeline. Research programs on FREIDA™, identifying programs accepting an H-1B or J-1 visa. When reviewing program websites, note and review both ACGME and non-ACGME fellowship programs offered at an institution. Pay close attention to training requirements and if any non-US training may be taken into consideration and additional requirements for an IMG such as ECFMG certification. Specific application requirement questions should be directed to the fellowship program. Finally, the applicant will need to see if they are eligible for licensure during training in the state the fellowship program is located. Contact the local state medical board with specific questions and inquire if any waivers may exist.

When applying during the current application cycle, the applicant will register for a fellowship token offered from the ERAS® Fellowships Documents Office (EFDO) that is required to begin working on the ERAS application.

Reference

1. National Resident Matching Program. Results and data: 2020 main Residency Match®. Washington, DC: National Resident Matching Program; 2020.

Websites

AAMC's Careers in Medicine®: https://www.aamc.org/cim/
AMA FREIDA™: https://freida.ama-assn.org/Freida/#/
AMA Career Planning Resource: https://www.ama-assn.org/amaone/career-planning-resource
NRMP: https://www.nrmp.org/
Federation of State Medical Boards (FSMB): https://www.fsmb.org/
The United States Medical Licensing Examination® (USMLE®): https://www.usmle.org/
American Urology Association Urology Residency and Fellowship Match: https://www.auanet.org/education/auauniversity/for-residents/urology-and-specialty-matches
SF Match: https://www.sfmatch.org/Default.aspx

Chapter 26
How COVID Threatens IMGs' Residency Training

Shawn Forrester

Introduction

The COVID-19 pandemic has wreaked havoc on our global economies and completely disrupted normative social activities across the world. Recent publications cited COVID's "cytokine storm" as a reason for its severe clinical outcomes [1], but for other reasons, this pandemic, for international medical graduates (IMGs), will create very stormy conditions in the upcoming National Residency Matching Program (The Match ®) and subsequent entry into residency. The most alarming issues facing international medical graduates (IMGs) during this period will be the mounting visa restrictions and travel bans, US Medical Licensing Examinations (USMLE) Step 2 CS suspension, and the retooling of key aspects of the interview and resident selection process. While this article cannot cover the full scope of the problems related to the pandemic, it will highlight these issues as immense priorities shaping the landscape of the US graduate medical education as it relates specifically to non-US foreign medical graduates (or non-US IMGs). The fallout from these challenges will also be briefly discussed, that is, the knock-on effect on the US healthcare system, which is already crippled by the current pandemic, rising healthcare costs, and dwindling resources.

IMGs in the US Healthcare System

It is first and foremost very important to highlight the contributions non-US international medical graduates have historically made to the delivery of US healthcare. Annually since 2010, at least 9330 IMGs have been certified with the Education

S. Forrester (✉)
California Institute of Behavioral Neurosciences and Psychology, Fairfield, CA, USA

Commission for Foreign Medical Graduates (ECFMG) in preparation for The Match® [2]. Statistically, 1 in every 5 PGY-1 residents is a non-US medical graduate. These physicians are more likely to work in clinical specialties such as internal medicine, family medicine or pediatrics, filling lower paying, and labor-intensive specialties less populated by US graduates. On leaving residency, IMG physicians are shunted into areas in dire need of family and geriatric physician services [3, 4]. As such, IMGs who comprise at least 25% of the active physician workforce in nine states (Connecticut, Delaware, Maryland, Nevada, North Dakota, Ohio, Texas, and West Virginia) and 30% or greater in other states (Florida, Illinois, New Jersey, and New York) are a huge complement to the underserved [5]. In general, IMGs residing and working in these regions are more likely to be engaged not only in the large healthcare systems but also in solo practices, directly contacting their patient population with culturally and linguistically appropriated services especially in socio-economically disadvantaged areas and areas with higher elderly populations and vulnerable groups [6–8].

IMGs also make significant contributions to clinical teaching, mentorship, and biomedical research. Data from 2017 suggests that 18.3% of academic physicians in the United States are IMGs and 15.1% of all full professors completed their undergraduate training overseas. In the area of biomedical research scholarship, 18% of all publications are work attributable to foreign medical graduates. They have also been leaders in clinical research acquiring 12.5% of all National Institute of Health (NIH) grants and sponsored clinical trials. This data does not include the crop of foreign medical graduates overseas whose collaborations with US-born physician scientists and researchers contribute to innovations which directly benefit patients in the United States [9]. In the coming years, IMGs are expected to be a valuable resource to the US healthcare system. It is expected that with the general increase in the elderly population (as much as 48%), data provided by the American Association of Medical Colleges (AAMC) predicts a need for 54,100–139,000 physicians by 2030 [10, 11]. Provided US medical education and graduate matriculation, as well as nurse practitioner training and placement, remain stable, the US healthcare system will not be able to meet these demands [12]. As such, non-US international medical graduates will be an even more important for future consideration as a solution to a looming dilemma in the delivery of healthcare.

Since September 2017, there have been a series of executive orders from President Trump affecting immigrant visas from a number of different countries including Iran, Venezuela, Syria, and Yemen [13]. The State Physician Workforce Data Report 2019 revealed a slight decrease in the number of active IMG physicians in 2018, compared to its Physician Specialty Data Report in 2015. These changes following these executive orders may be correlated with the associated restrictions in visa processing. The most recent presidential proclamations motivated by economic recovery in the wake of the pandemic suspend processing of visa categories J-1, H-1B, H2-B, and L which include processing of trainees and interns along with their families [14]. In response to this proclamation, the AAMC has urged the administration to rescind this proclamation, citing that "Over half of the current postdoctoral researchers in this country hold temporary non-immigrant visas and fill a critical need in the U.S. labor market by providing specialized knowledge and skills in the development of innovative and cutting-edge biomedical research." The AAMC went on to reiterate that this proclamation does not help the economy and will seriously harm scientific progress, healthcare access, and the innovation needed to save the thousands of lives lost each year from chronic illnesses (heart disease, cancer, Alzheimer's, and stroke) [15]. Although the proclamations have spawned confusion and anxiety among J-1 exchange participants and delays in visa processing, the ECFMG has reiterated that under the provisions for alien physicians deemed "mission critical to fighting and mitigating the impacts of COVID-19," IMGs attempting to honor their commitments to their respective programs for July 2020 may be exempt from the most recent proclamations [16].

Unmatched IMGs Living in the United States

What will happen in this upcoming 2021 National Residency Matching Program ("The Match") is very uncertain. What is certain is that IMGs living in the United States, all 260,000 of them (Migration Policy Institute analysis of US Census Bureau data), will remain unemployed or underemployed, carrying on in menial jobs. Some have taken to social media platforms such as Twitter® and Facebook® where "unmatchedmd" hashtags can be seen in posts communicating their frustration as trained physicians unable to work in their field. The groundswell of unmatched IMGs is an untapped pool of resources. During this unprecedented pandemic, IMGs seemed to have gotten at least some attention from the Association of American Medical Colleges (AAMC) and lawmakers such as Gov. Andrew Cuomo who made accessions to allow international medical graduates alongside retired physicians to become integrated into the frontline healthcare system during the current pandemic.

In this regard, the dire need to buttress the health services as a result of the pandemic may have been a silver lining for unmatched IMGs living in the United States. Some IMGs were allowed to work in the pandemic getting a proverbial foot in the door to residency. Based on all accounts from IMGs living in New York, the experience may have been more hazardous than it was rewarding. An unofficial number of IMGs took to social media to report retreating from volunteer service after contracting COVID.

The AAMC released its bulletin during this time, reiterating that "The licensure requirements and steps to practice medicine in the U.S. would require you to have additional years of residency training, pass the USMLE exams, become ECFMG certified and apply for licensure within the state that you want to practice medicine." Despite the COVID-related accessions made by lawmakers, there were no new paths created to expedite graduate training and certification of IMGs.

Retooling the Application Process

Many changes have occurred in the wake of this pandemic that will also significantly alter the matching process. The most significant changes are the delays in the *Electronic Residency Application System* (ERAS®) timeline (see Table 26.1), the nationwide closure of Prometric ® test centers, and the suspension of USMLE Step 2 CS for the next 12–18 months [17].

For decades, program directors have relied on USMLE Step 2 credentials as a benchmark for determining clinical competence of all US and non-US graduates. This situation is more problematic for non-US IMGs because without a Step 2 CS pass, IMGs will not be issued their ECFMG certification and will be ineligible to enter the upcoming 2021 Match ®. For the first time in 70 years, the prospect of a matching process devoid of non-US IMGs appears to be a very real possibility. Alternative processes for ECFMG certification at this time are nonexistent. This is especially since the American Medical Association (AMA) withdrew their support for the fifth pathway rendering this alternate avenue useless to final year medical students and unofficial statements. Unofficial statements made by Dr. William Pinsky, CEO of the Education Commission of Foreign Medical Graduates (ECFMG), consolidated this concern when he confirmed that his organization was unprepared [18]. While IMGs were still reeling from the news, others who already passed Step 2 CS will have to wait indefinitely to add vital US clinical clerkship experience to their resume. All clerkships for IMGs have been suspended for an indefinite period creating a situation where IMGs will not only be deficient in valuable prerequisite US clinical experience, but important letters of recommendation may be unattainable as well.

Since ECFMG's initial response, a recourse to ECFMG certification has been devised and promulgated. IMGs will now, without the Step CS examination, be eligible for a temporary ECFMG certificate. Once an IMG is matched into their first

Table 26.1 ERAS 2021 Residency Timeline for IMGs

Date	Timeline
June 8, 2020	ERAS 2021 season begins at 9 a.m. ET
June 23, 2020	ERAS Support Services at ECFMG will begin generating and distributing tokens
September 1, 2020	Applicants may begin submitting applications to residency programs
October 21, 2020	Residency programs may begin reviewing applications and MSPEs are released to programs
January	Urology residency and Military Match results are available
March 15–19, 2020	Supplemental Offer and Acceptance Program (SOAP®) begins on March 15 at 11 a.m. ET National Resident Matching Program (NRMP®) main residency match Results available at 1 p.m. ET
May 31, 2021	ERAS 2021 season ends: MyERAS closes at 5 p.m. ET

Adapted from the Association of American Medical Colleges (AAMC) – July 28, 2020

year of residency, this certificate expires. Those who do not match will have to reattempt certification based on the guidelines at that time. There is a caveat; however, not all IMGs will be eligible for this temporary ECFMG certificate. IMGs who have not taken Step 2CS are eligible if they:

- Meet the general prerequisites for an ECFMG certification (must have completed Step 1 and Step 2CK)
- Have not been sanctioned or barred from ECFMG certification for whatever reason
- Have not been barred by USMLE
- Have not failed or reattempted a step or step component two or more times
- Have not taken or registered for a USMLE step or step component since January 2018

Then eligible applicants must choose to go down one of five (5) pathways (see Table 26.2) to have their clinical competence credentialed [19].

Table 26.2 Pathways and eligibility requirements

Applicants who already have been issued a license to practice medicine without supervision in another country must apply using pathway 1

Pathway 1: Already licensed to practice medicine in another country
Applicant has held a license/registration to practice medicine without supervision in any country at any time on or after January 1, 2015. A provisional license will meet the requirements for this pathway if it permits unsupervised practice. Individuals who hold only a license that requires supervised practice, such as a training license, are not eligible for this pathway. The license/registration does not need to be currently valid
The license/registration has not been subject to disciplinary action

Pathway 2: Already passed a standardized clinical skills exam for medical licensure
Applicant has successfully completed a secure, standardized clinical skills exam in English as a requirement for medical licensure or registration in another country, which is deemed acceptable by ECFMG. This includes such exams as:
General Medical Council: professional and linguistic assessment board (PLAB) part 2
Australian Medical Council: clinical examination part 2 or workplace-based assessment
Medical Council of Canada: qualifying examination part 2 or National Assessment Collaboration Examination
Medical Council of New Zealand: NZREX clinical
Medical Council of Ireland: preregistration examination system (PRES), level 3
Date of examination must be on or after July 1, 2018
In addition to the acceptable exams listed above, ECFMG will consider:
Objective structured clinical examinations (OSCEs) administered as part of the medical licensure or registration process, in any language
Medical school-administered OSCEs that meet the requirements for clinical skills assessment mandated by the appropriate medical regulator for licensure, only if the medical school:
1. Is located in a region/country that is not served by a WFME-recognized accrediting agency; and,
2. Is accredited by an agency that is recognized by the appropriate government agency in that region/country and that is responsible for licensure

(continued)

Table 26.2 (continued)

Pathway 3: Medical school accredited by agency recognized by the World Federation for Medical Education (WFME)
Applicant's medical school must meet one of the following requirements (in addition to meeting all other ECFMG requirements):
Currently accredited by an agency recognized by WFME or accredited by an agency recognized by WFME at the time the applicant matriculated
Date of graduation must be on or after January 1, 2018
An authorized school official must attest to applicant's clinical skills

Pathway 4: Medical school participates in the US Federal Student Loan Program
Applicant's medical school must meet one of the following requirements (in addition to meeting all other ECFMG requirements):
Currently participates in the US Federal Student Loan Program or approved for participation in the US Federal Student Loan Program at the time the applicant matriculated; or
Has a petition for reconsideration in process with the US Federal Student Loan Program
Date of graduation must be on or after January 1, 2018
An authorized school official must attest to applicant's clinical skills

Pathway 5: Medical school issues degree jointly with a US medical school accredited by the Liaison Committee on Medical Education (LCME)
Applicant is a student or graduate of a medical school that grants an MD degree issued jointly with a US medical school accredited by LCME (and meets other ECFMG requirements).
Currently, these include:
  Weill-Cornell medicine – Qatar
  Duke University – National University of Singapore Medical School
Date of graduation must be on or after January 1, 2018
An authorized school official must attest to applicant's clinical skills

Courtesy of the Education Commission of Foreign Medical Graduates (ECMFG), July 17, 2020

At this time, it is uncertain whether or not any further adaptations will be made during the upcoming Match® 2021 season especially in concerning the mechanism by which programs will be able to engage prospective candidates. Social distancing mandates across the United States in the wake of the pandemic obviate the standardized person-to-person interview process in which programs directly engage and evaluate applicants. As of May 11, 2020, however, the newly convened Coalition for Physician Accountability's Work Group on Medical Students in the Class of 2021 Moving Across Institutions for Postgraduate Training released an unprecedented recommendation – virtual interviewing through voice-over IP software. Virtual interviewing recommendations in response to this problem although reasonable may disadvantage IMG candidates. The good thing, in regard to virtual interviews, is that an applicant can accept all interview invitations from the comfort of their own home saving hundreds of dollars they would have normally spent on air-ticketing, accommodations, and ground transport. From that vantage point, it sounds advantageous, but the foreseeable problem is that this system might be biased in favor of top applicants. During the typical interview season, top applicants can receive as many as 10–12 interviews. Other candidates, who might have red flags on their application – a year of graduation over 5 years, a failed exam – may only receive one (1) invite for interview. The foreseeable problem with this upcoming remote interview season is that these underdogs will receive fewer invitations because none of them were declined by the top applicants who were offered them first. Some applicants, IMGs already living in the United States, may be more likely to have in-person interviews. While it is uncertain what will happen in this upcoming Match®, travel restrictions and social distancing directives will certainly disrupt the normative, standardized process and severely hurt IMG's prospects by introducing bias to a system that may already be skewed out of their favor.

The impending changes to the Step 1 score reporting can be highlighted here under this issue of bias. Non-US IMGs on average score 16.1 points higher in Step 1 than their US counterparts [20]. For an IMG, relegating high scores (let's say a 257) to a "pass" doesn't just level the playing field, but it undermines the IMG's talent, hard work, and his/her hard-earned entitlement to a residency spot on the basis of merit over their American counterpart who's score, statistically, is likely to be lower. Whatever way this is interpreted, the IMG's pathway to US graduate medical education gets ever-challenging. Now in the wake of COVID, there are new challenges to be negotiated at least in the next 12–18 months ahead. How indelible these changes will be on the future of graduate medical education in regard to non-US IMGs is uncertain.

References

1. S. F. P. a. Y.-C. Ho. SARS-CoV-2: a storm is raging. J Clin Invest. 2020:2202–3.
2. M. D. Da'Shia Davis. aamc.org/workforce. May 2018. [Online]. Available: https://www.aamc.org/system/files/reports/1/projectedshortageofphysiciansthrough2030sizeofprojectedshortage.pdf. Accessed 24 June 2020.
3. A. o. A. M. Colleges. AAMC.org. November 2019. [Online]. Available: https://store.aamc.org/downloadable/download/sample/sample_id/305/. Accessed 24 June 2020.
4. ECFMG. Standard ECFMG Certificates Issued, 1994-2018. 26 January 2019. [Online]. Available: https://www.ecfmg.org/resources/CertsbyYear1994-2018.pdf. Accessed 25 June 2020.
5. S. M. S. M. F. M. T. A. H. T. R. K. L Gary Hart 1. International medical graduate physicians in the United States: changes since 1981. Health Aff (Milwood). 2007;4(26):1159–69. https://doi.org/10.1377/hlthaff.26.4.1159.
6. M. P. D. F. M. C. L. G. H. Meredith A Fordyce 1. Osteopathic physicians and international medical graduates in the rural primary care physician workforce. Fam Med. 2012;6(44):396–403.
7. M. a. S. L. D. Esther Hing. Role of international medical graduates providing office-based medical care: United States, 2005–2006. February 2009. [Online]. Available: https://www.cdc.gov/nchs/data/databriefs/db13.pdf. Accessed 25 June 2020.
8. D. M. B. 1. A. R. O. 1. A. B. J. 1. Dhruv Khullar 1. U.S. immigration policy and American medical research: the scientific contributions of foreign medical graduates. Ann Intern Med. 2017;8(67):584–6. https://doi.org/10.7326/M17-1304.
9. D. J. Trump. whitehouse.gov. 22 June 2020. [Online]. Available: https://travel.state.gov/content/travel/en/News/visas-news/proclamation-suspending-entry-of-immigrants-and-non-immigrants-who-present-risk-to-the-US-labor-market-during-the-economic-recovery-following-the-COVID-19-outbreak.html. Accessed 25 June 2020.
10. A. o. A. M. Colleges. Association of American Medical Colleges. 23 June 2020. [Online]. Available: https://www.aamc.org/news-insights/press-releases/aamc-statement-presidential-proclamation-limiting-non-immigrant-visas. Accessed 25 June 2020.

11. E. C. o. F. M. Graduates. ecfmg.org. 22 June 2020. [Online]. Available: https://www.ecfmg. org/annc/presidential-proclamation/. Accessed 25 June 2020.
12. A. o. A. M. College. The Complexities of Physician Supply and Demand: Projections from 2018–2033. June 2019. [Online]. Available: https://www.aamc.org/system/files/2020-06/strat-comm-aamc-physician-workforce-projections-june-2020.pdf. Accessed 26 June 2020.
13. U. S. M. L. Examination. Coronavirus Resource Center. 26 May 2020. [Online]. Available: https://covid.usmle.org/announcements/usmle-suspending-step-2-clinical-skills-examination. Accessed 26 June 2020.
14. E. C. o. F. M. Graduates. ecfmg.org. 26 May 2020. [Online]. Available: https://www.ecfmg. org/focus/issue40.html. Accessed 26 June 2020.
15. E. C. f. F. M. Graduates. Requirements for ECFMG Certification for 2021 Match. 18 June 2020. [Online]. Available: https://www.ecfmg.org/certification-requirements-2021-match/. Accessed 26 June 2020.
16. N. R. M. Program. Charting Outcomes in the Match. July 2018. [Online]. Available: https:// www.nrmp.org/wp-content/uploads/2018/06/Charting-Outcomes-in-the-Match-2018-IMGs. pdf. Accessed 26 June 2020.
17. A. C. f. G. M. Education. Data source book academic year 2018-2019. 2019. [Online]. Accessed 27 Aug 2020.
18. W. C. S. S. Radabaugh CL. Long-term potential implications of immigration barriers for medical education. JAMA. 2019:741–2.
19. A. o. A. M. Colleges. aamc-2019-state-physician-workforce-data-report. 2019.
20. A. o. A. M. Colleges. https://www.aamc.org. November 2019. [Online]. Available: https:// www.aamc.org/data-reports/workforce/interactive-data/active-physicians-who-are-interna-tional-medical-graduates-imgs-specialty-2015. Accessed 27 Aug 2020.

Chapter 27
International Medical Graduates and Their Specialties Reviewed

Roohi Afshan Kaleelullah and Kumudhati Tiwari

Introduction and Background

Using the information provided by NRMP's Results and Data 2019 Main Residency Match, we were able to figure out which medical specialties had the highest percentage of US and Non-US IMGs in the positions filled for each specialty from last year's Match ([1], pg.11). As previously mentioned, (ranked in order) pathology, general surgery (preliminary), internal medicine (categorical), neurology (categorical), and family medicine were the most popular specialties for IMGs [2].

The Top Five IMG-Friendly Specialties

Pathology, a Good Choice for IMGs

The current trendsetter among the IMG specialty is pathology. Pathologists study the nature and causes of diseases through microscopic examination and clinical laboratory tests. Pathologists work to diagnose, monitor, and treat diseases. They examine tissues, cells, and bodily fluids – applying biological, chemical, and physical sciences within a lab setting. Pathologists may also examine tissues to determine whether an organ transplant is needed or they may examine the blood of a pregnant

R. A. Kaleelullah (✉)
California Institute of Behavioral Neurosciences and Psychology, Fairfield, CA, USA

The University of North Carolina, Adam's School of Dentistry, Chapel Hill, NC, USA

K. Tiwari
Edison, NJ, USA

© Springer Nature Switzerland AG 2021   411
H. Tohid, H. Maibach (eds.), *International Medical Graduates in the United States*, https://doi.org/10.1007/978-3-030-62249-7_27

woman to ensure the fetus is healthy. They are keen on identifying abnormalities related to certain diseases [3].

Subspecialties of pathology include the following:

- Anatomical pathology
- Blood banking and transfusion medicine
- Chemical pathology
- Clinical pathology
- Genetic pathology
- Forensic pathology
- Cytopathology
- Hematology
- Immunopathology
- Medical microbiology
- Molecular pathology
- Neuropathology
- Pediatric pathology

Pathology continues to get more and more IMG friendly by the day. However, the job market for pathology in the United States is not that great. It is important here to understand that the definitions of a "good job market" differ between an AMG and an IMG. For example, for an AMG, a good job market is defined as high-paying initial jobs (>300 K) in tier-1 cities or near their hometown or any other location with temperatures above 70F during most months of the year. Understandably, these locations are already saturated and more often than not, the AMG pathologists have to relocate to places they do not want to go. Also, pathology is a high-end service and by its inherent nature requires one to subspecialize. It means that AMGs will have to wait one more year to start paying off their huge student loan debt. AMGs are increasingly staying away from pathology residency, which is obvious from the recent NRMP stats. NRMP stats show that 65% of pathology residency positions are filled by IMGs (both US and non-US combined). Most IMGs are okay with the current job market and are having no problems finding employment because most of them are very flexible on geographic location, as well as initial salaries.

Besides, US programs have had very good experiences with IMG residents. Most places have one or two IMG "STAR" residents who had finished their residencies in their home country and are far ahead in the game compared to their peers. These positive attributes in their profile have opened many new avenues for IMG applicants for their future professional advancement.

Pathology Programs and Visas

Sadly, there are only a few programs that sponsor H1b visas, since pathology is a high-end service and most community hospitals are not well-equipped to start and maintain the infrastructure required for a pathology specialty program. This excludes mainly big university programs that do not sponsor H1 visas, even in other specialties. However, it seems J1 visa rejections for pathology programs are much lower, as most of these programs are well-known universities with established results on visa acceptance. Most pathology programs sponsor a J1 visa, and this is problematic because the number of waiver jobs is limited in pathology compared to the primary health care specialties.

Home Country Specialty in Pathology–

Home country specialty is the best credential to have in your profile when applying for a pathology specialty match. The impact is almost equal to having three good US Clinical Experiences (observerships are considered USCE in pathology). However, home country specialty alone is not the one-way "ticket" to securing a solid specialty in the United States.

It has to be complemented with either of the following credentials:

1. Scores above 240.
2. Three, 1-month observerships with good letters. [Well-established programs include Mt. Siani Medical center, Cleveland Clinic – Florida, John Hopkins, Danberry Medical center].
3. Long-term research in pathology and 1/2 observerships.
4. Exceptional research background in pathology.
5. Rare, hands-on pathology experiences in the United States (available only to GC/citizens), such as pathology assistant positions, post-sophomore year, or fellowships that go empty could be filled by IMGs.
6. A related graduate degree from the United States, such as a PhD in pathology, immunology, microbiology, chemistry, etc.

Any of these combined with a home country residency will certainly increase IMGs' chances of a match. The more credentials added, the more the numbers increase (apparently, as high as 41 is documented), but, it also depends on how many programs you applied for in total. There are 150 odd pathology programs and approximately 120 of them sponsor JI/H1 visas; 70–80 is a safe number of applications to residency programs for IMGs.

The basic principles for pathology match are similar to other residences. It is a good time to enter into the pathology residency for an IMG, as it is not very competitive at this time. In 2019, 49.21% of pathology positions were filled by IMGs. As the job market continues to improve, the balance will shift to the other side in due time. The IMGs who have established their careers in pathology show no regrets on their choice of specialty.

The pathologists seeking jobs will find that a more competitive job market is pushing salaries up over $300,000 per year on average. Also, most new jobs come with a hiring bonus and funds for the relocation of as much as $12,000 and continuing medical education of $3500. AmeriPath and Pathology Service Associates are the two companies that are narrowed down in managing group practices of hiring pathological talents [4].

General Surgery (Preliminary)

The second most popular specialty of IMGs in the United States is general surgery (preliminary). Physicians specializing in surgery can choose to become general surgeons or pursue a subspecialty in a specific area of the body, type of patient, or type of surgery. General surgery provides a wide range of life-saving surgeries, such as appendectomies and splenectomies. They receive broad training in human anatomy, physiology, intensive care, and wound healing [3].

The Association of American Medical Colleges and American College of Surgeons outline many surgical subspecialties and areas of practice, including the following:

- Colon and rectal surgery
- General surgery
- Surgical critical care
- Gynecologic oncology
- Plastic surgery
- Craniofacial surgery
- Hand surgery
- Neurological surgery
- Endovascular surgical neuroradiology
- Ophthalmic surgery
- Oral and maxillofacial surgery
- Orthopedic surgery
- Adult reconstructive orthopedics
- Foot and ankle orthopedics
- Musculoskeletal oncology
- Orthopedic sports medicine
- Orthopedic surgery of the spine
- Orthopedic trauma
- Pediatric orthopedics
- Otolaryngology
- Pediatric otolaryngology
- Otology and neurotology
- Pediatric surgery
- Neonatal
- Prenatal
- Trauma
- Pediatric oncology
- Thoracic surgery
- Congenital cardiac surgery
- Thoracic surgery-integrated
- Vascular surgery

Usually, surgery programs will take IMGs as preliminary interns, in a way of "testing" their knowledge, clinical abilities, etc., for one year. If they do a good job, they either apply again and then match for the categorical slot or they are transitioned to a categorical position as a second-year resident. The competition experienced by IMGs when applying for a 5-year categorical position in general surgery is overwhelming. Applicants are often left unmatched, and applying for a 1-year preliminary surgery position is an attractive option as a way to gain experience and strengthen applications for a categorical position the following year. However, completion of a preliminary surgery year does not always guarantee the candidate a categorical position in the future, and accepting this position can be risky. The preliminary position is essential to training programs to balance work-hour restrictions and personnel requirements. In return, these positions can be valuable such that they provide experience and a path toward a career in surgery. However, the position has been referred to as a "dead-end" for those looking to continue in general surgery. Preliminary general surgery dropped from the fifth position up to second due to its increasing demand among IMGs, as opposed to internal medicine, which has many more slots compared to general surgery. In 2019, 42.69% of general surgery (preliminary) positions were filled by IMGs. General surgery will continue to remain a very competitive field, and non-US citizen applicants must utilize the opportunity to adapt themselves to the US system and keep an open mind toward other surgical specialties ([5] pg.704–742).

The small number of IMGs matching into general surgery (GS)-categorical positions can be explained by the program director's perceptions of these candidates. Moore and Rhodenbaugh published a study showing that a majority of GS residency program directors believe that IMGs are subject to discrimination during the candidate selection process. They also reported that 20% of the Program Directors that responded, felt severe pressure to rank American graduates above IMGs who were more qualified.

A stipend is provided for all the 5 years as competitive in that region. Depending on the university they choose, the numbers may vary [6]. As of July 1, 2019:

- PGY-1 – $56,262
- PGY-2 – $60,767
- PGY-3 – $63,193
- PGY-4 – $65,728
- PGY-5 – $69,16

Internal Medicine (Categorical)

The third most popular specialty of IMGs in the United States is internal medicine (categorical). Internal medicine is practiced by a physician who treats diseases of the heart, blood, kidneys, joints, digestive, respiratory, and vascular systems of adolescents, adults, and the elderly to provide long-term care, comprehensive care in hospital settings, and offices. Because they undergo primary care training on internal medicine, these physicians also address disease prevention, wellness, substance abuse, and mental health [3].

Subspecialties of internal medicine include the following:

- Advanced heart failure and transplant cardiology
- Cardiovascular disease
- Clinical cardiac electrophysiology
- Critical care medicine
- Endocrinology
- Diabetes
- Metabolism
- Gastroenterology
- Geriatric medicine
- Hematology
- Oncology
- Gynecology
- Maternal-fetal medicine
- Female pelvic medicine and reconstructive surgery
- Reproductive endocrinology and infertility
- Infectious disease
- Interventional cardiology
- Nephrology
- Pediatric internal medicine
- Pulmonary disease
- Critical care medicine
- Rheumatology

Basic training in internal medicine is 3 years of residency (termed "categorical" training) following medical school. Followed by the completion of 3 years of training, residents are eligible for board certification in internal medicine. About half of the country's internal medicine residents choose to practice general internal medicine. General internists are capable of functioning in many different roles. For example, many focus on ambulatory practice and may serve as primary care physicians, adding patients longitudinally for their ongoing medical care. Others may spend the majority of their time caring for hospitalized patients in the role of hospitalist (over 90% of hospitalists are general internists). However, many general internists care for both ambulatory and hospitalized patients in a very wide variety of practice models [7].

Others choose to pursue additional training beyond the basic 3 years of residency training, subspecializing in a particular area of interest within internal medicine.

Internal medicine training may also be combined with training in another specialty, leading to board certification in both fields. These *dual training programs* are generally structured to be shorter than the time it would take to complete an independent residency in both fields, and graduates of these programs are particularly qualified to care for patients in both areas of focus. Examples include internal medicine and pediatrics, emergency medicine, and psychiatry. This serves as a boon for pursuing this specialty.

Internists may also develop specific skills in other areas of interest, although individuals may achieve qualifications in these areas from backgrounds other than internal medicine. Examples include geriatrics, sports medicine, hospice and palliative care medicine, and sleep medicine [8].

Internal medicine specialty is the most filled slots among other specialties. In 2019, 40.59% of internal medicine positions were filled by IMGs. The shortest residency duration is 3 years to specialize in general internal medicine. The job market is very welcoming toward this specialty. Depending on the universities, the FMGs choose, the numbers may vary. The average stipend for a resident year-wise is as follows:

- PGY1 – $54,864
- PGY2 – $57,548
- PGY3 – $60,199

Neurology (Categorical)

The fourth most popular specialty of IMGs in the United States is neurology. Neurology is a specialty in the medical field about nerves and the nervous system. Neurologists diagnose and treat diseases of the brain, spinal cord, peripheral nerves, muscles, autonomic nervous system, and blood vessels. Much of neurology is consultative, as neurologists treat patients suffering from strokes, Alzheimer's disease, seizure disorders, and spinal cord disorders [3].

Subspecialties of neurology include the following:

- Brain injury medicine
- Child neurology
- Clinical neurophysiology
- Endovascular surgical neuroradiology
- Hospice/palliative medicine
- Neurodevelopment disabilities
- Neuromuscular medicine
- Pain medicine
- Sleep medicine
- Vascular neurology [9]

Preparing for a neurology match needs some specific skills and experiences as compared to the traditional categorical specialties.

- To begin with, neurology is a subspecialty compared to other broad specialties such as internal medicine, which can be multidisciplinary. Neurology means narrowing the career path. This is what the FMGs will be doing for the rest of their lives; hence, *commitment and passion* are keys [10].

- Second, a strong neurology applicant will have a good academic record in general. *Neurology-specific experience* in terms of electives, or observerships, will suffice for an IMG to become a stronger applicant. In most universities, neurology exposure is limited to a couple of weeks to attain more relevant experience from these electives and research [11].
- Finally, there is this focus on *research*. The majority of neurology programs are university based and they encourage research. While there are some community programs with neurology residency, most applicants nowadays do research as well, to strengthen their application [12].

Neurology residents work hard, probably harder compared to other medical specialties (nonsurgical) to make sure the FMGs hard-working nature and ability to stretch that extra mile are reflected in their application and during the interviews. The reviewers and interviewers are looking for this trait [13].

Neurology programs are looking for your interest in the field and your fit for the program. The rate of IMGs pursuing a 1–2 year of fellowship followed by the specialty is remarkably higher. Neurology is a small but growing specialty. In 2019, 34.51% of neurology positions were filled by IMGs. The average salary of a neurologist is $243, 105 USD. The estimates are according to April 1, 2017 [14].

Grad Level

1. $52, 474
2. $54, 341
3. $56, 265
4. $58, 867
5. $61, 887
6. $64, 408
7. $66, 498
8. $70, 762

Family Medicine

The fifth and final most popular specialty of IMGs in the United States is family medicine. Family medicine focuses on integrated care and treating the patient as a whole. Those practicing family medicine treat patients of all ages, provide comprehensive health care, and treat most ailments.

Subspecialties of family medicine include the following:

- Adolescent medicine
- Geriatric medicine
- Hospice/palliative medicine
- Pain medicine
- Sleep medicine
- Sports medicine [15].

Family medicine is for any residency candidate dedicated to long-term primary care and close relationships with patients. Family medicine is one of the most flexible medical specialties when it comes to USMLE exam scores, and is one of the largest, most IMG-friendly medical specialties. However, family medicine is not a specialty to be taken lightly. Program directors in family medicine programs are looking for residency applicants with a background and visibly deep interest in family medicine practice [10]. This dedication can best be demonstrated throughout the residency application. Residency candidates looking to apply to family medicine residency programs should focus on getting family medicine experience and specialty-specific Family Medicine Letters of Recommendation to prove they are truly invested in the specialty. It is also important to have a well-written Family Medicine Personal Statement, which shows an applicant's personal connection to primary care and their Family Medicine experience.

In 2019, 29.08% of family medicine positions were filled by IMGs ([16] pg. 743–773).

The estimate depends on the universities location and with respect to 2019–2020, the range is as follows:

- PGY-1 $57,470
- PGY-2 $59,548
- PGY-3 $61,737

Less IMG-Friendly Specialties

Although pathology, general surgery, internal medicine, neurology, and family medicine are the top socialites for IMGs, there are other *less IMG-friendly* specialties they may choose to pursue [17].

These specialties include the following:

- Allergy and immunology
- Anesthesiology
- Dermatology
- Diagnostic radiology
- Emergency medicine
- Internal medicine
- Nuclear medicine
- Obstetrics and gynecology
- Ophthalmology
- Pathology
- Pediatrics
- Physical medicine and rehabilitation
- Preventative medicine
- Radiation oncology
- Surgery
- Urology, as well as the subspecialties of each of these specialties [18].

Allergy and Immunology

Specialists in allergy and immunology work with both adult and pediatric patients suffering from allergies and diseases of the respiratory tract or immune system. They may help patients suffering from common diseases such as asthma, food and drug allergies, immune deficiencies, and diseases of the lung. Specialists in allergy and immunology can pursue opportunities in research, education, or clinical practice [19].

Anesthesiology

Anesthesiology is the branch of medicine dedicated to pain relief for patients before, during, and after surgery. The American Board of Anesthesiology outlines the following subspecialties within the field in the following areas of care:

- Critical care medicine
- Hospice and palliative care
- Pain medicine
- Pediatric anesthesiology
- Sleep medicine [20]

Dermatology

Dermatologists are physicians who treat adult and pediatric patients with disorders of the skin, hair, nails, and adjacent mucous membranes. They diagnose everything from skin cancer, tumors, inflammatory diseases of the skin, and infectious diseases. They also perform skin biopsies and dermatological surgical procedures.

Subspecialties within the dermatology field include the following:

- Dermatopathology
- Pediatric dermatology
- Procedural dermatology [21]

Diagnostic Radiology

Physicians specializing in diagnostic radiology are trained to diagnose illnesses in patients through the use of X-rays, radioactive substances, sound waves in ultrasounds, or the body's natural magnetism in magnetic resonance images (MRIs).

They can also pursue a subspecialty in the following areas:

- Abdominal radiology
- Breast imaging

- Cardiothoracic radiology
- Cardiovascular radiology
- Chest radiology
- Emergency radiology
- Endovascular surgical neuroradiology
- Gastrointestinal radiology
- Genitourinary radiology
- Head and neck radiology
- Interventional radiology
- Musculoskeletal radiology
- Neuroradiology
- Nuclear radiology
- Pediatric radiology
- Radiation oncology
- Vascular and interventional radiology [22]

Emergency Medicine

Physicians specializing in emergency medicine provide care for adult and pediatric patients in emergencies. These specialists provide immediate decision-making and action to save lives and prevent further injury. They help patients in the prehospital setting by directing emergency medical technicians and assisting patients once they arrive in the emergency department [23].

Emergency medicine is also home to several subspecialties, including the following:

- Anesthesiology critical care medicine
- Emergency medical services
- Hospice and palliative medicine
- Internal medicine/critical care medicine
- Medical toxicology
- Pain medicine
- Pediatric emergency medicine
- Sports medicine [24]

Genetics

A medical geneticist is a physician who treats hereditary disorders and diagnoses diseases that are caused by genetic defects. Medical geneticists may provide patients with therapeutic interventions and specialized counseling. They also educate patients and their families on their diagnosis to cope up with their genetic disorder. Medical geneticists conduct cytogenetic, radiologic, and biochemical testing and scientific research in the field.

Medical geneticists house several subspecialties within the field, including the following:

- Biochemical genetics
- Clinical cytogenetics
- Clinical genetics
- Molecular genetic pathology [21]

Nuclear Medicine

Physicians who practice nuclear medicine are called nuclear radiologists or nuclear medicine radiologists. They use radioactive materials to diagnose and treat diseases. Utilizing techniques such as scintigraphy, these physicians analyze images of the body's organs to visualize certain diseases. They may also use radiopharmaceuticals to treat hyperthyroidism, thyroid cancer, tumors, and bone cancer [25].

Obstetrics and Gynecology

Obstetrician/gynecologists (OB/GYNs) care for the female reproductive system and associated disorders. This field of medicine encompasses a wide array of care, including the care of pregnant women, gynecologic care, oncology, surgery, and primary health care for women [26].

Ophthalmology

Physicians specializing in ophthalmology develop comprehensive medical and surgical care of the eyes. Ophthalmologists diagnose and treat vision problems. They may treat strabismus, diabetic retinopathy, or perform surgeries on cataracts or corneal transplantation.

There are several subspecialties within the ophthalmology field, including the following:

- Anterior segment/cornea ophthalmology
- Glaucoma ophthalmology
- Neuro-ophthalmology
- Ocular oncology
- Oculoplastics/orbit
- Ophthalmic plastic and reconstructive surgery
- Retina/uveitis
- Strabismus/pediatric ophthalmology [27]

Pediatrics

Physicians specializing in pediatrics work to diagnose and treat patients from infancy through adolescence. Pediatricians practice preventative medicine and also diagnose common childhood diseases, such as asthma, allergies, and croup [28].

They may work as a primary care pediatrician treating an array of ailments, or narrowing their scope of practice in one of the following subspecialties:

- Adolescent medicine
- Child abuse pediatrics
- Developmental-behavioral pediatrics
- Neonatal-perinatal medicine
- Pediatric cardiology
- Pediatric critical care medicine
- Pediatric endocrinology
- Pediatric gastroenterology
- Pediatric hematology-oncology
- Pediatric infectious diseases
- Pediatric nephrology
- Pediatric pulmonology
- Pediatric rheumatology
- Pediatric sports medicine
- Pediatric transplant hepatology [29].

Physical Medicine and Rehabilitation

Physicians specializing in physical medicine and rehabilitation work to help patients with disabilities of the brain, spinal cord, nerves, bones, joints, ligaments, muscles, and tendons. Physiatrists work with patients of all ages and design care plans for conditions, such as spinal cord or brain injury, stroke, multiple sclerosis, and musculoskeletal and pediatric rehabilitation [30]. Unlike many other medical specialties, physiatrists work to improve patient quality of life, rather than seek medical cures.

Subspecialties in this field include the following:

- Brain injury medicine
- Hospice and palliative medicine
- Neuromuscular medicine
- Pain medicine
- Pediatric rehabilitation medicine
- Spinal cord injury medicine
- Sports medicine [31]

Preventive Medicine

Physicians specializing in preventive medicine work to prevent disease by promoting patient health and well-being. Their expertise goes far beyond preventive practices in clinical medicine, covering elements of biostatistics, epidemiology, environmental and occupational medicine, and even the evaluation and management of health services and health care organizations. The field combines interdisciplinary elements of medical, social, economic, and behavioral sciences to understand the causes of disease and injury in population groups.

Subspecialties within preventive medicine include the following:

- Aerospace medicine
- Medical toxicology
- Occupational medicine
- Public health medicine [32]

Psychiatry

Physicians specializing in psychiatry devote their careers to mental health and its associated mental and physical ramifications. Understanding the connections between genetics, emotion, and mental illness is important while psychiatrists also conduct medical laboratory and psychological tests to diagnose and treat patients [33].

Subspecialties within psychiatry include the following:

- Addiction psychiatry
- Administrative psychiatry
- Child and adolescent psychiatry
- Community psychiatry
- Consultation/liaison psychiatry
- Emergency psychiatry
- Forensic psychiatry
- Geriatric psychiatry
- Mental retardation psychiatry
- Military psychiatry
- Pain medicine
- Psychiatric research
- Psychosomatic medicine

Another notable change observed in 2018 was that *psychiatry became less IMG friendly* than it had been in the past. Interestingly, since the 2016 NRMP Match, the IMG friendliness of psychiatry dropped to 16.22 percent from 21.4 percent.

Step 3 (noted above) is an absolute requirement only at the 15–20 institutions that sponsor H1b, for the simple reason that they feel safe to start the H1 process having already completed Step 3. A few programs even cancel the offered interviews if Step

3 is not completed, but that is only in rare cases. Finishing Step 3 before starting residency is universally advised by all program directors [34].

Radiation Oncology

Physicians specializing in radiation oncology treat cancer with the use of high-energy radiation therapy. By targeting radiation doses in small areas of the body, radiation oncologists damage the DNA of cancer cells, preventing further growth. Radiation oncologists work with cancer patients, prescribing, and implementing treatment plans while monitoring their progress throughout.

Radiation oncology houses a few subspecialties, including the following:

- Hospice and palliative medicine
- Pain medicine ([35], pg.774–819).

Urology

Urology is the health care segment that cares for the male and female urinary tract, including kidneys, ureters, bladder, and urethra. It also deals with male sex organs. Urologists have knowledge of surgery, internal medicine, pediatrics, gynecology, and more.

Within urology, there are several areas of subspecialty, including the following:

- Pediatric urology
- Urologic oncology
- Renal transplant
- Male infertility
- Calculi
- Female urology
- Neurourology [36].

Your choices are anything but limited when it comes to medical specialties and subspecialties. Selecting a specialty that challenges you, aligns with your career goals, and provides your desired lifestyle are all important aspects you need to take into consideration.

IMG-Friendly Trends

Not only must IMG residency applicants research individual residency programs, but they should also be aware of state limitations and the overall IMG friendliness of whole states. Learning more about IMG-friendly states can help IMGs better focus their research and resources [37].

The top 12 states which are IMG friendly to name are *New York, Michigan, Florida, Pennsylvania, New Jersey, Texas, Illinois, California, Ohio, Massachusetts, Maryland,* and *Georgia.*

According to March 2019 General statistics, an idea of the number of IMGs matched in the specialty is provided.

2997 US IMG (57.1% match rate)

4028 Non-US IMG (56.1% match rate) [38].

The top five countries from where the IMGs originate are as follows:

- India – 19.9%
- Philippines – 8.7%
- Mexico – 5.8%
- Pakistan – 4.8%
- Dominican Republic – 3.3% [39].

Compared to the 2017 NRMP Match, there were some surprises in the 2018 NMRP Match. One such surprise was that preliminary general surgery went from the fifth most popular to the second most popular specialty among IMGs. However, the same five specialties (pathology, general surgery, internal medicine, neurology, and family medicine) did not change from 2017 to 2018. Another notable change observed was that *psychiatry became less IMG friendly* than it had been in the past. Interestingly, since the 2016 NRMP Match, the IMG friendliness of psychiatry dropped to 16.22 percent from 21.4 percent [40].

Other IMG Factors

Beyond statistics, there are other factors IMG residency candidates should consider when choosing medical specialties. First being, specialty-wise USMLE score expectations. Some specialties are more competitive and have increased expectations of residency candidates. For example, general surgery programs typically require higher USMLE scores than psychiatry. Second, previous work and clinical experiences matter to a great extent. All specialties like to see some evidence of commitment and a deep interest in the specialty [41]. Going above and beyond is a necessary trait. Specialties such as Family Medicine highly prefer to see some history of Family Medicine experience to prove your dedication, interest, and commitment. Having specific supporting documents is another fantastic way to prove your interest and dedication to a specialty. You should work hard to obtain specialty-specific Letters of Recommendation and a Personal Statement for each specialty you plan on applying to. Finances are also something to seriously consider because applying to residency can be very expensive. The suggested minimum applications for IMG candidates are 100 programs per specialty, which can add up to thousands of dollars very quickly. Make sure you assess your specialty decision carefully to make the best use of your resources and finances. Program choices and opportunities are also very important for IMGs. Your choice may depend on how large the specialty you choose is and the number of programs you qualify to apply to based on your professional credentials and each program's application requirements. If you pick too narrow a specialty, you may need to prepare a backup specialty just in case. Choosing a specialty will take time, care, dedication, and consideration. While some specialties are less competitive than others, no one specialty is a guaranteed "In." No matter which specialty you pick, you will still have to put lots of hard work and effort into your ERAS Application materials, program research, and beyond [42].

If you are an international medical graduate, picking which medical specialties to apply to starts with first learning which medical specialties are the most IMG friendly. First, however, it is good to review some general match statistics to understand the big picture.

Licensing Fee
All Medical Board Licensing Fees and USMLE Step III application fees are paid by the University.

Vacation
Four weeks of paid vacation are offered per year. Additional leave for illness, family medical emergencies, or maternity/paternity may be taken according to the written policy.

Insurance Coverage
Health insurance with Blue Cross and disability plans are available to resident physicians and their dependents, as well as dental and vision coverage provided as an employee benefit with NO COST to the resident or his/her dependents.

Life Insurance
There is a $40,000 life insurance plan for the resident physician, which includes a double indemnity clause of $80,000, and is provided by the university at no cost to the resident. Malpractice insurance is also provided by the university.

Match 2019 General Statistics

30,538 PGY-1 Positions Filled

17,763 US Senior (94.3% Match Rate) 674 US Graduate (43.8% Match Rate) 5076 Osteopathic (81.4% Match Rate) 2997 US IMG (57.1% Match Rate) 4028 Non-US IMG (56.1% Match Rate)

Discovering which medical specialties are the most IMG friendly requires a deep and thorough analysis of NRMP Match Data. The IMG percentage was calculated by adding together the US and Non-US IMGs who obtained a residency position in the specialty, and calculated what percent of the total positions filled were IMGs.

For example, in Emergency Medicine there were 2458 Total Positions Filled

- 112 Positions Filled by US IMGs
- 27 Positions Filled by Non-US IMGs

- 139 Total Positions Filled by IMGs
- 5.66% of Positions Filled by IMGs

This process was repeated for all of the medical specialties to uncover the most IMG-friendly specialties.

Importance of USCE/Research to Match

I feel that some US Clinical Experience is more important than research when it comes to IMGs matching for residency. USCE makes its students more acquainted with the practice of pathology in the United States compared to research, which is mostly bench work. Moreover, the letters of recommendation obtained from a daily sign-out session are more residency oriented, while the research letter may make you seem more like a Ph.D. applicant. In pathology and all other specialties, research should only be sought after you have finished at least three observerships of 4 weeks each and secured three US letters for the sign-out experience [43].

Most applicants are home country trained in pathology, but there are about 30–35% of young graduates applying directly after completing medical school. Also, it should be noted that many applicants apply to pathology only as a backup to internal medicine. In addition to the IMG pathologists, even the other two categories can match if they get those abovementioned three observerships and obtain good letters. Compared to trained pathologists who usually do observerships as a colleague to the junior faculties and do well in their rotations, the other two categories of students do not seem to match. However, this game is fair. Many programs prefer only young graduates with good scores. Also, many programs entertain a diverse subset of applicants. In the words of one PD during the interview season, "Do not think that because three out of six of you are already trained pathologists, the rest of them are already out of the race. We have called you for an interview as we know that each one of you is special in your way. While half of you are vastly experienced, the other half has great scores and are young and we need both kinds of residents to make our program rich." [44].

An inexperienced medical student in a pathology rotation can still get a good letter of recommendation. They need to be sincere and show up on time, dress well, and behave with the techs, residents, fellows, and attending. A golden tip is to accept that you know nothing, be curious, willing to learn, and ask questions [45]. If an attending shows you angiosarcoma, for example, go home and read up about angiosarcoma at night and come back again with a few genuine questions to discuss with the resident or fellow (and be sure you are not asking something silly). Not only does this show that you are attentive during sign-out, but also that you are truly intrigued and went home to study more. It shows you are genuinely curious, willing to share information, and ask questions. You don't have to be a good pathologist to be a pathology resident, you have to be a good, sincere student (this applies to all specialties) and be sure you are interested. You must try to understand what kind of people they are looking for and see if you fit. Pathologists are clichéd to be the doctors that do not interact with people, but this is simply not the case. Although pathologists do not speak with patients regularly, they do speak with clinicians very often. If you come across as someone who can express themselves well over the phone, during an academic discussion, or in written format (like this paper), you are a personality that would fit quite well in the pathology department. Pathology is all about how well you communicate what you see to the clinicians. Communication skills are key to both good rotation and interviews [46].

Attempting to finish a pathology residency in your home country to improve your chances for a pathology match is an extreme step. Although it gives you a good backup plan, it takes away 3 precious years of GC application from you, especially if you know that there are ways to match without home country residency.

Other Important Trends IMGs Should Be Aware Of

A recent trend among non-visa-requiring candidates is to look for pathology assistant jobs. This is the strongest hands-on grossing experience that anyone can have in the United States as an IMG. J2/L2 EADs can also be employed in these positions. Also, doing all of your pathology USCE at one institution or state may be considered a lack of flexibility, and it is preferable to do at least one rotation in an IMG-friendly place such as NY. The job market is getting much better and this is reflected by the increased numbers of job postings on websites such as pathology-outlines.com and sudden fellowship position openings in off-seasons that depict that those who secured a job left their second scheduled fellowship [47].

Conclusion

The overall match rate for all specialties for non-US citizen IMGs in 2015 was 49.5%. The competition experienced by IMGs when applying for a 5-year categorical position in general surgery is overwhelming [48]. Applicants are often left unmatched and applying for a 1-year preliminary surgery position. This is an attractive option as a way to gain experience and strengthen applications for a categorical position the following year. However, sadly, completion of a preliminary surgery year does not always guarantee the candidate a categorical position in the future. Accepting this position can be risky. The preliminary position is essential to all training programs to balance work-hour restrictions and personnel requirements. In return, these positions can be valuable in that they provide experience and a path toward a career in surgery. However, the position has been referred to as a "dead-end" for those looking to continue to general surgery in the future [49].

Although several residents are IMGs, the number of US medical graduates accepted to categorical positions far exceeds the IMG. In the 2015 match, 121 out of 1085 IMG applicants matched categorical surgery. There were a total of 1219 categorical positions filled, of which 1101 (90%) were filled by American graduates and 121 (10%) by IMGs (both US citizens (n = 71, 5%) and non-US citizens (n = 50, 4%). The majority of categorical positions completed a preliminary year. The small number of IMGs matching into general surgery (GS) categorical positions can be explained by the program director's perceptions of these candidates. Moore and Rhodenbaugh published a study showing that a majority of GS residency program directors believe that IMGs are subject to discrimination during the candidate selection process. They also reported that 20% of the Program Directors that responded felt severe pressure to rank American graduates above IMG's who were more qualified.

Several other factors for IMG applicants to overcome include obtaining high scores on the USMLE Step 1 and 2 and making an exceptional impression on interview day [50].

In conclusion, matching for residency programs can prove to be more difficult for IMGs in the United States, but it is not impossible. The future looks bright for IMGs in the United States especially for the top five IMG specialties including pathology, general surgery, internal medicine, neurology, and family medicine.

References

Book Chapter or Article Within a Book

1. Aggarwal R, Levounis P. Graduate Medical Education, and Career Paths. In: Rao NR, Roberts LW, editors. International Medical Graduate Physicians. Cham: Springer; 2016. p. 11–25. https://pubmed.ncbi.nlm.nih.gov/27683436/. https://doi.org/10.1007/978-3-319-39460-2.

Website

2. Top 5 Most IMG Friendly Specialties 2019 Match. https://blog.matcharesident.com/top-5-img-friendly-specialties-2019-match/
3. 4 medical specialties among the friendliest for IMG PGY-1 matches. https://www.ama-assn.org/residents-students/specialty-profiles/4-medical-specialties-among-friendliest-img-pgy-1-matches

Article Within a Journal

4. Genzen JR. An overview of United States physician training, certification, and career pathways in clinical pathology (laboratory medicine). https://pubmed.ncbi.nlm.nih.gov/27683436/
5. Mittal VK, Lax EA. Hurdles in US Surgical Training for International Medical Graduates. https://doi.org/10.1007/s12262-016-1517-7.

Website

6. A non-US citizen international student's chances of matching in surgery. https://medclerkships.com/a-non-us-citizen-international-students-chances-of-matching-in-surgery/

Article Within a Journal

7. Chadaga AR, Villines D, Krikorian A. Medical student preferences for the internal medicine residency interview day: A cross-sectional study. https://doi.org/10.1371/journal.pone.0199382.

Website

8. (Residency program requirements for international medical graduates). https://www.ama-assn.org/education/international-medical-education/residency-program-requirements-international-medical.
9. Neurology. https://residency.wustl.edu/choosing-a-specialty/specialty-descriptions/neurology/.
10. Graduate Medical Education. https://health.uconn.edu/graduate-medical-education/neurology-residency-program/program-overview/

Article Within a Journal

11. Scheitler KM, Lu VM, Carlstrom LP., Graffeo CS, Perry A, Daniels DJ, Meyer, FB. Geographic distribution of international medical graduate residents in U.S. Neurosurgery Training Programs. https://residency.wustl.edu/choosing-a-specialty/specialty-descriptions/neurology/, https://doi.org/10.1016/j.wneu.2020.01.201.
12. Chandra AB, Wadhwa MG, et al. The path to U.S. neurosurgical residency for foreign medical graduates: trends from a decade 2007–2017. https://doi.org/10.1016/j.wneu.2020.02.069.

Website

13. Neurology. https://www.matcharesident.com/our-specialties/Neurology
14. How hard is it to get in a neurosurgery medical residency in the US as an IMG?. https://www.quora.com/How-hard-is-it-to-get-in-a-neurosurgery-medical-residency-in-the-US-as-an-IMG

Article Within a Journal

15. Duvivier RJ, Wiley E, Boulet JR. Supply, distribution and characteristics of international medical graduates in family medicine in the United States: a cross-sectional study. https://doi.org/10.1186/s12875-019-0933-8.

Website

16. Family Medicine. https://residency.wustl.edu/choosing-a-specialty/specialty-descriptions/family-medicine/.

Article Within a Journal

17. Nguyen VAT, Könings KD, Wright EP, et al. Why do graduates choose to work in a less attractive specialty? https://doi.org/10.1186/s12960-020-00474-y.

Website

18. The Ultimate List of Medical Specialties and Subspecialties. https://www.sgu.edu/blog/medical/ultimate-list-of-medical-specialties.

Article Within a Journal

19. Yu JE, Kumar A, Bruhn C, Teuber SS, Sicherer SH. Development of a food allergy education resource for primary care physicians. https://doi.org/10.1186/1472-6920-8-45.
20. Ortwein H, Knigge M, Rehberg B, Hein OV, Spies C. Validation of core competencies during residency training in anaesthesiology. https://doi.org/10.3205/000146.
21. Oliver B, Macri CJ, Friedman AJ. Genetics education in US dermatology residency programs: a survey-based study. https://doi.org/10.4300/JGME-D-16-00881.1.
22. Hawnaur J. Diagnostic radiology. https://doi.org/10.1136/bmj.319.7203.168.
23. Dagher GAL, Ali C, et al. The International Medical Graduate and Emergency Medicine. https://doi.org/10.1016/j.jemermed.2019.10.023.
24. Hoelle RM, Vega T, et al. Emergency medicine residency programs: the changing face of graduate medical education. https://doi.org/10.5116/ijme.5a47.8274.
25. Arevalo-Perez J, Paris M, Graham MM, Osborne JR. A Perspective of the future of nuclear medicine training and certification. https://doi.org/10.1053/j.semnuclmed.2015.10.003.
26. Kristin J, Hung AC, Tsai TRB, Johnson RP, Bangsberg DR, Kerry VB. The scope of global health training in U.S. obstetrics and gynecology residency programs. https://doi.org/10.1097/AOG.0b013e3182a9c1c8.
27. Yousuf SJ, Kwagyan J, Jones LS. Applicants' choice of an ophthalmology residency program. https://doi.org/10.1016/j.ophtha.2012.07.084.
28. Osta AD, Barnes MM, et al. Acculturation needs of pediatric international medical graduates: a qualitative study. https://doi.org/10.1080/10401334.2016.1251321.
29. Jimenez-Gomez A, FitzGerald MR, et al. Performance of international medical graduates in pediatric residency: a study of peer and faculty perceptions. https://doi.org/10.1016/j.acap.2018.07.006.
30. Tolu S, Rezvani A, Gürcan, Atci A, et al. Factors influencing subspecialty training and career choices: a national survey of physical and rehabilitation medicine residents. https://doi.org/10.5606/ArchRheumatol.2019.6742.
31. Jani AA, Trask J, Ali A. Integrative medicine in preventive medicine education: competency and curriculum development for preventive medicine and other specialty residency programs. https://doi.org/10.1016/j.amepre.2015.08.019.
32. Wells EV, Sarigiannis AN, Boulton ML. Assessing integration of clinical and public health skills in preventive medicine residencies: Using competency mapping. https://doi.org/10.2105/AJPH.2012.300753.
33. Sockalingam S, Thiara G, et al. A transition to residency curriculum for international medical graduate psychiatry trainees. https://doi.org/10.1007/s40596-015-0389-7.
34. Elkady R. Early career international medical graduate psychiatrists. https://doi.org/10.1016/j.jaac.2019.07.409.
35. Spraker MB, Nyflot MJ, Hendrickson KRG, et al. Radiation oncology resident training in patient safety and quality improvement: a national survey of residency program directors. https://doi.org/10.1186/s13014-018-1128-5.

36. Halpern JA, Al Hussein Al Awamlh B, et al. International medical graduate training in urology: are we missing an opportunity?. https://doi.org/10.1016/j.urology.2016.03.063
37. Ahmed AA, TingThomas HW, et al. International medical graduates in the US physician work-force and graduate medical education: current and historical trends. https://doi.org/10.4300/JGME-D-17-00580.1.
38. Gauer JL, Jackson JB. The association of USMLE Step 1 and Step 2 CK scores with residency match specialty and location. https://doi.org/10.1080/10872981.2017.1358579.

Website

39. Residency Match for IMGs. https://www.usmlesarthi.com/sarthiresidencymatchservices.html.

Article Within a Journal

40. Hau DK, Smart LR, DiPace JI, Peck RN. Global health training among U.S. residency special-ties: a systematic literature review. https://doi.org/10.1080/10872981.2016.1270020.
41. Mitsouras K, Dong F, Safaoui MN, Helf SC. Student academic performance factors affect-ing matching into first-choice residency and competitive specialties. https://doi.org/10.1186/s12909-019-1669-9.

Complete Book

42. Raghav GSM, Ramaswamy BSB. BhagavanSwathi Beladakere Ramaswamy RGSM, edi-tor. International medical graduate and the United States medical residency application. Champions: Springer. https://doi.org/10.1007/978-3-030-31045-5.

Article Within a Journal

43. Stadler DJ, Archuleta SC, Joseph Ibrahim H. Successful international medical education research collaboration. https://doi.org/10.4300/JGME-D-18-01061.
44. Rezhake RH, Zhao SY, Qian Y. Impact of international collaborative training programs on medical students' research ability. https://doi.org/10.1007/s13187-016-1134-y.
45. Archuleta S, Chew N, Ibrahim H. The value of international research and learning in graduate medical education. https://doi.org/10.4300/JGME-D-19-00478.
46. Chakraborty RR, Mobeen H. The pivotal role of the international medical graduate. https://doi.org/10.1542/peds.2018-1189.
47. Katakam SK, Frintner MP, Pelaez-Velez C. Work experiences and satisfaction of international medical school graduates. https://doi.org/10.1542/peds.2018-1953.

Website

48. International medical graduate. https://en.wikipedia.org/wiki/International_medical_graduate#United_States.
49. Post-Match SOAP. https://blog.matcharesident.com/category/www-electronicresidency-com/.
50. NRMP® Advanced 2017 Main Residency Match Data. https://blog.matcharesident.com/nrmp-advanced-2017-main-residency-match-data/.

Chapter 28
The Book *First Aid* and USMLE/ Scholar-RX: How They Have Been Instrumental in Serving International Medical Graduates?

Hassaan Tohid

Introduction

The USMLE is a tough exam and obviously needs robust preparation. The exam has totally three parts: Step 1, Step 2, and Step 3. The USMLE Step 1 exam is primarily focused on the basic concepts that medical students usually develop during their medical school preparation. Step 2 on the other hand is divided into two parts: Step 2 clinical knowledge (CK) and Step 2 clinical skills (CS), and Step 3 has its own unique way of testing clinical decision-making and concepts [1]. If we combine all of these three exams, it is a lot of information and a lot of topics that international medical graduates (IMGs) must read, understand, and remember in order to be successful in these exams. Reading and learning every single thing about medicine is not humanly possible, nor it is logical to read all the medical school curriculum books in a short span of time.

Therefore, the students rely on review books and Question Banks (online questions) to practice and simulate the real exam because the USMLE is a computer-based exam and needs the students to answer all the required questions in a short span of time on a computer screen. Therefore, there was a huge need of better review books and Question Banks that could help the students acclimatize with the real exam. There had been veracious books by various publishers and organizations; however, the emergence of the book *First Aid* turned out to be a cornerstone in the preparation of the exam, especially for Step 1. The book was an immediate hit and was easy to use and easy to understand mainly because of the high yield topics it covered. The *Step 1 First Aid* book covered all the high yield topics in a concise and easy to understand manner.

H. Tohid (✉)
California Institute of Behavioral Neurosciences and Psychology, Fairfield, CA, USA

© Springer Nature Switzerland AG 2021
H. Tohid, H. Maibach (eds.), *International Medical Graduates in the United States*, https://doi.org/10.1007/978-3-030-62249-7_28

One of the book editors and co-authors Dr. Tao Le later expanded the concept of *First Aid* and initiated a digital platform for IMGs and medical students to prepare for the exam [2]. In this chapter I will highlight how *First Aid*, Dr. Tao Le, and USMLE/Scholar-RX have been phenomenal in serving IMGs.

First Aid the Book

If we ask any international medical graduate (IMG) or American medical graduate (AMG) which book should be used to prepare for USMLE Step 1 exam, the unanimous answer that almost all IMGs will provide is *First Aid*. IMGs all around the world, whether in Canada, Mexico, South America, Europe, or Asia, are aware of *First Aid*, the book which is published by McGraw-Hill.

The book *First Aid* was written around 30 years ago by Vikas Bhushan, then student at University of California, San Francisco (UCSF). Later on, the book editorial board was joined by the current CEO of Scholar-RX Dr. Tao Le. Dr. Le had a mission and goal in mind to further spread the invaluable knowledge by the book *First Aid* and complement the mission of Vikas Bhushan of educating the IMGs and helping them prepare for the USMLE. Very soon the book *First Aid* became one of the most reliable and most popular books among the IMGs for USMLE preparation. The book covers high yield topics for the USMLE preparation and almost every year a new edition is published by McGraw-Hill Education. As of 2020, the 30th edition is currently used by the students all over the world.

According to the website www.firstaidteam.com, the initial story of the book is as follows, exactly in the words of the authors:

> We lived in San Francisco and Los Angeles during medical school and residency. It was before the Web, and before med students could afford cell phones and laptops, so we relied on AOL e-mail and bulky desktops. One of us would drive down to the other person's place for multiple weekends of frenetic revisions fueled by triple-Swiss white chocolate lattes from the Coffee Bean & Tea Leaf, with R.E.M. and the Nusrat Fateh Ali Khan playing in the background. Everything was marked up on 11- by 17-inch "tearsheets," and at the end of the marathon weekend we would converge at the local 24-hour Kinko's followed by the FedEx box near LAX (10 years before these two great institutions merged). [3]

Scholar-RX and Its Mission

Once the book *FIRST AID* was a big hit and became popular among the IMGs and AMGs, Dr. Tao Le decided to take the *First Aid* knowledge to a new level. Hence, the organization USMLE/Scholar-RX was founded.

Mission

The mission of Scholar-RX was the same to serve millions of IMGs and help them get great scores and be more competitive for residency match by utilizing the technology and Internet.

Service

The company Scholar-RX is founded by Dr. Tao Le and provides services to IMGs through their online platform known as USMLE-RX.

Difference Between **First Aid***, Scholar-RX, and USMLE-RX*

This is one of the most confusing questions for many students about the difference between the three: *First Aid* the book, Scholar-RX, and USMLE-RX.

Now let us understand the structure:

- The *First Aid* is the name of the book published by McGraw-Hill Education. The first edition was published 30 years ago, the 30th edition came out in 2020. The first author of the book was Dr. Vikas Bhushan, who was a medical student at UCSF as stated before, when he wrote the book. Dr. Tao Le, the founder of Scholar-RX, joined the editorial team of the book with Dr. Bhushan and since then the book became famous with the two editors/authors: Dr. Tao Le and Dr. Vikas Bhushan.
- Scholar-RX is a company founded by Dr. Tao Le with a mission to digitize the knowledge of *First Aid* for medical students around the globe.
- USMLE-RX is a digital platform created by Scholar-RX organization, keeping the topics of *First Aid* book into consideration. The USMLE-Rx platform contains Question Banks called Qmax, and Bricks as online tools for IMGs to prepare for the exam.

The Interview of the *First Aid* Author and the CEO of Scholar-RX Dr. Tao Le

To understand further how *First Aid* and Scholar-RX have been instrumental in serving IMGs, I had a privilege to interview Dr. Tao Le. I am grateful to Dr. Le for his time for recording this interview with me.

The interview is as follows:

Me:

How does First Aid/Scholar-RX *help IMGs?*

Dr. Tao Le:

That's a great question ..., First Aid is partially written by IMGs, if you look at the authors and the various contributors over the years including under special acknowledges you see that there are many IMGs that are involved in the book from small contribution to the co-editing of the publication over the years and you know we believe that makes the publication helpful for more IMGS because it captures the perspective of IMGs ... a you know and what their learning needs are a and the how best to address them so you know that's one way the book helps IMGs and the other way obviously the way the book is structured it is very well organized in to various sections and subsections that are easily integratable how IMGs generally have to prepare for the exam regardless of whether they umm are under graduate medical education training was many years ago whether they are still going through the table of contents helps it organize ... makes it very easy for them to map it what they can previously learn and then take a going forward you know when they have to prepare for obviously USMLE.

Me:

Why do you think the First Aid/USMLE-RX *is one of the most popular books and the tool for USMLE preparation for IMGs?*

Dr. Tao Le:

I think First Aid *and USMLE-Rx rose to prominence because we were one of the very first people to be able to really master and harness the power of crowd of students and IMGs ... And I can remember we were working on the book and making critical decisions to you know don't have at least on paper any particular qualification other than they are very intelligent and they are very hardworking ... the original book was developed by the medical students at the UCSF and of course UCSF is a top tier medical school and students there are very very intelligent but none of them had ... you know doesn't necessarily had any prior advanced degrees, none of them had prior teaching experience, or authoring experience, or faculty experience. I was the part of the early authors' team, we worked really hard at the very beginning set the right system, the right set of processes it allows students and IMGs to get involved and really productively harness that power and energy to create something that would be truly useful. And would be able to rapidly (inaudible) ... over time has made it very useful because you again if you look at when the book first came to prominence in early 1990s, books back then were not revised on a regular basis even books today you know are not typically revised on a regular basis ... every three year. If a book is successful it is typically revised every three years. We wanted our first major book be revised annually ... we were able to keep up with the rapid changes in the USMLE and we were agile and we take feedback directly from IMGS and students so we can rapidly adjust what's going on and because of that we have managed to stay current and not just current but even ahead of where in some cases where the USMLE is going and that has ensured our relevance.*

Me:

First Aid *is the book and USMLE-RX is a Question Bank, how did this Question Bank come into action? As we know it is also an extremely popular tool now?*

Dr. Tao Le:

Yeah, a great question … we the authors had always been interested in technology and power of the Internet to transform medical education. We got involved as early as late 1990s in education technology initiatives and so forth but it took us till early 2000s … 2003–2004. We were able to focus it into a specific technology initiative and that was USMLE-RX Questions. And again it used a lot of same principles and core values as First Aid *and that is student and IMG driven, very much peer to peer, how to gather information and we basically used student IMGs power to do kind of rapid survey the education landscape (in audible)… identified that we can address as a Question Bank and then be able to develop high quality questions and explanations in an easy to use platform and we were able to then launch it into mid-2006 or so and then again we were using the same principles rapidly to iterate that with student and IMG feedback … almost on a daily basis we were taking feedback and making adjustments to questions with our student IMG authors and a large team of faculty advisers and reviewers who would keep it current.*

Me:

Is First Aid *and Scholar-Rx the same entity or they are sister organizations? How is the functionality?*

Dr. Tao Le:

They are sister publications. First Aid USMLE Step 1 *and the* First Aid *Series were published by McGraw-Hill, so they are my publishers. I authored* First Aid*, I also obviously have a role in Scholar-RX to oversee the entire operations in working with other like-minded editors and really organized it with the editors and the authors using the same principles of* First Aid *to develop that platform … We studied and developed our own technology because at that time there were not many people that developed these kinds of platform again because I have a kind of background in technology. I had access to good developers who were able to build the platform from scratch to deliver the Question Banks but again USMLE-RX and* FIRST AID *use a lot of same methodology from that stand point they share a lot of the same genes.*

Me:

How does the future for First Aid*/Scholar-RX look like?*

Dr. Tao Le:

Yeah great question … as you are already aware, USMLE is going pass/fail in Step 1, we still think that even with USMLE going pass/fail that there is absolutely a need of FIRST AID*.* FIRST AID *has grown from being more than just obviously a book for USMLE preparation, it has become a* de facto *curriculum outline in some parts of the world including in the US as well and so we think that we have obligation to keep it updated and the students and IMGs continue to depend on it for not only for USMLE preparation but for their course focus as well. I mean keep in mind even the USMLE exam going pass & Fail it is a challenging exam, it's a very hard exam, for everyone including IMGs, we feel that we still have critical role in guiding IMGs and students through this challenging process. We will continue to keep the book current evolve it rapidly to meet the changing needs of students to keep ahead* *where the exam is going obviously as you are aware. In addition to going pass/fail there will be over the time … we expect adding more patient communication items. Every 2-3 years there is a major change or there are different types of changes, we will keep that current with new topics. Obviously, right now the hot topic is COVID-19 that surely will be tested on the exam very soon, so we will be getting COVID-19 into the book well before the USMLE actually starts testing about it. In the future, we continue to hope to coordinate with what we were doing between* First Aid *as a book and Scholar-RX. USMLE-RX is a digital platform the two platforms continue to complement each other very nicely so that IMGs and students can use* First Aid *for test preparation but for broader resources and support with regards to curriculum preparation and to learning the foundations of biomedical science that they can count on Scholar-RX to bring to them to the table and engage in a digital way and then to be able to integrate that to* First Aid, *such that the student & IMGs can go back and forth between course work after school prepare for USMLE seamlessly right. So, you have this whole ecosystem both tangible and digital and they can back and forth integrate test preparation and broaden study to become a well-rounded compassionate patient-centered physician.*

Me:

What would have been different if there were no First Aid*?*

Dr. Tao Le:

That's a great question, we really don't know haa (laughter), would somebody have created another First Aid *eventually may be but nobody knows, but certainly there would have been another test preparation resources, but honestly nobody knows … Its hard to imagine the world without* First Aid, *what would students have done without* FIRST AID. *Fortunately, we are glad we don't have to speculate.*

Me:

What is the unique proposition for First Aid, *Scholar-RX?*

Dr. Tao Le:

I think that it remains relevant even numerous resources that they can help IMGs and students these days. First Aid *remains relevant because of its laser focus is on USMLE preparation and being extremely high quality, very succinct, and very adaptable. Also, that it has been iterated enough rapidly enough that you know IMGs and students can feel very comfortable. All the major concepts that can possibly be tested on USMLE are essentially covered in the book, one way or the other. Its not to say that some minor stuff don't make it antsy, but all the major themes, major concepts are covered in* First Aid *and that's incredibly hard to do in a 700-800 page book considering how vast the field of medicine is.*

Me:

I believe the unique proposition you have is, that you are ahead of times, like you just mentioned about COVID-19. There is no announcement yet but you are proactively thinking about bringing COVID-19 in the new edition of the book.

Dr. Tao Le:

Thank you and we agree. We try to think about where the USMLE gonna be not just where they are now you do take a risk obviously because occasionally you can predict you can be wrong in your prediction but we have been very fortunate that most of our predictions have been accurate in terms of where the trends have been going with USMLE.

Me:

What message would you give to the IMGs in the end?

Many IMGs who went into the field, they are not doing it for money, they are not doing it for fame, easy life style, they are doing it because they truly care about other human beings, about each other, about society. IMG physicians and the physicians that I know are some of the most outstanding people I have ever met. They truly think about everybody. Therefore, I encourage IMGs to continue to pursue those dreams … to dream at the higher level, about what they can do for others, for society, those who are underprivileged, for those who are underserved. And I think if they work hard enough and prepare well enough truly, they can find their path and be able to fulfill those dreams and be able to be really beacons for humanity.

Acknowledgments   I thank Dr. Tao Le, MD, the CEO and Founder of USMLE/Scholar-RX, for recording the audio interview with me.

Conflict of Interest   Dr. Hassaan Tohid served as a Course Director of Psychiatry for *First Aid*/USMLE-RX.

References

1. Who is USMLE? United States Medical Licensing Examination (USMLE). Available from https://www.usmle.org/about/
2. The Scholar-RX Story. Scholar-RX. Available from https://scholarrx.com/about/
3. The First Aid Team-For All Your First Aid Need and USMLE-RX Updates. Available from https://firstaidteam.com/2019/12/27/now-available-the-30th-anniversary-edition-of-first-aid-for-the-usmle-step-1-2020-edition/

Chapter 29
Visa Hurdles Faced by IMGs

Gokul Ramani and Ian H. Rutkofsky

Introduction

The visa process is a significant milestone in the journey toward an international medical graduate's (IMG) medical career in the United States (US). Most physicians apply for multiple visa status changes throughout their career, ranging from visitor visas such as the B1/B2 to work visas like the H1B. Table 29.1 summarizes the common visa types used by IMGs (Table 29.1). From medical school to residency, obtaining the right travel and work documentation is an early step [1]. More than 25% of applicants are IMGs and play a crucial role in the US healthcare system [2]. The following texts summarize common visa scenarios, so that readers can make an informed decision and construct realistic timelines to achieve the best outcomes in their medical careers. The vast majority (~90%) enter on a J1 exchange visa sponsored by the Education Commission for Foreign Medical Graduates(r) (ECFMG) (Table 29.2) [3, 4]. Immigration-related information is beyond the scope of these texts which were primarily drafted to help medical students and graduates start a residency training. There are many more complex visa and work document types including the O1 visa [5, 6]. The authors recommend expert immigration advice for all immigration and visa-related issues. Few tips for success have been included in Table 29.3.

G. Ramani (✉)
Jacobi Medical Center/Albert Einstein College of Medicine, Department of Internal Medicine, Bronx, NY, USA

I. H. Rutkofsky
Department of Psychiatry, HCA – Aventura Hospital and Medical Center, Aventura, FL, USA

Department of Research, CiBNP, Fairfield, CA, USA

© Springer Nature Switzerland AG 2021
H. Tohid, H. Maibach (eds.), *International Medical Graduates in the United States*, https://doi.org/10.1007/978-3-030-62249-7_29

Table 29.1 Visa types

Visa type	Purpose	Maximum duration	Limitations	Common uses	Notes
B1/B2	Tourist/business	6 months, Visa validity variable	No employment	Electives Interviews	Cannot work
J1	Residency/ fellowship or research	7 years	No employment outside program or network	Residency Fellowship Research	Dependent visa: J2 Bond+ J2: Employment through Employment authorization document (EAD)
H1B	Fellowship or employment	6 years	Renewal limitations Narrower fellowship options H2: No employment	Residency Fellowship Employment	Dependent visa: H2 No Bond
O1	All the above	3 years initially, renewed annually, unlimited extensions	O3 No employment	Same as H1B and J1	Dependent visa: O3

Table 29.2 Top countries with exchange physicians

Country	Number of physicians
Canada	2539
India	2453
Pakistan	1182
Saudi Arabia	422
Lebanon	391
Jordan	391
Venezuela	248
Nigeria	229
Colombia	197

Source: Data: ECFMG Database, January 9, 2020 [4]

Table 29.3 Tips

Plan timelines early
Apply early
Be honest
Combine multiple USMLE objectives together
Make a clear decision about the visa type preferable to you; consider USMLE Step 3 early
Believe in yourself
Confidence is key

Consular Experiences

The process of applying for a visa is available online and all applicants must familiarize themselves with the process prior to sending the application. Various forms you may encounter are summarized in Table 29.4. You are to fill out a DS-160, pay the required fees, select an interview slot via the consular website unique to your country, and apply for the visa type [7]. The B1/B2 application and interview process is available online (Table 29.5). Consulates have a system in place to allow for an emergency interview, provided you can offer sufficient evidence to support your case. Should you experience delays to start due to a delay in obtaining an interview date on time, this may be used, especially for the J1 or H1B class. After your interview, your visa status can be tracked/viewed online, on the Consular Electronic Application Center (CEAC) website and the USTravelDocs website (Table 29.5).

Medical students are better off applying when still in medical school or in internship which in many countries is a part of their medical curriculum. Some students extend their internship or graduation date which is used by many applicants to take up clerkships which can only be taken up by medical students and is better for entry. Medical school is also a tie compelling you to return so it is better to plan this ahead.

When interviewing for J1, applicants must be clear to the consular officer that their intention is "post graduate medical education" only and that they would when they complete their training [8].

The H1B visa process starts shortly after the match. Certain programs have a designated lawyer who will help the process, which may span a variable amount of time. The authors recommend "premium processing" to avoid any delays in getting the visa [9]. The cost of premium processing may be borne by the program or the applicant depending on the program. In common scenarios, for example, if the lawyer sends the documents by the end of May, approvals are appreciated in 1–2 weeks followed by a consular interview. Emergency appointments may be needed, and programs offer support in the form of a letter requesting the need for an emergency appointment, since you are working in healthcare and this is a safety issue.

At the end of the interview one of three scenarios may happen. The most favorable outcome is if they approve your visa, they take your passport and give you an acknowledgment that your visa was approved. The other scenario is if your visa is refused, whereby they will give your passport back to you at once [10]. The other

Table 29.4 Various forms		
	I-94	Admission record, accessible online
	DS-160	Initial visa application form
	DS-2019	Exchange visitor and sponsor verification form
	I-20	Exchange student and sponsor verification form
	I-797	H1B petition approval form

Table 29.5 Resources

Presidential proclamation	https://www.ecfmg.org/annc/presidential-proclamation/
ECFMG	https://www.ecfmg.org
DS-160	https://travel.state.gov/content/travel/en/us-visas/visa-information-resources/forms/ds-160-online-nonimmigrant-visa-application.html
USTravelDocs	https://www.ustraveldocs.com
HRSA Shortage areas	https://data.hrsa.gov/tools/shortage-area/by-address
ECFMG Accreditation 2023	https://www.ecfmg.org/accreditation/
NRMP Match Data	https://www.nrmp.org/main-residency-match-data/
Deferred Inspection Sites	https://www.cbp.gov/contact/ports/deferred-inspection-sites
State Department: B1/B2	https://fam.state.gov/FAM/09FAM/09FAM040202.html
Visa Status Check	https://ceac.state.gov/CEACStatTracker/Status.aspx
I-94 Online	https://i94.cbp.dhs.gov/I94/
O1 Visa	https://www.uscis.gov/working-in-the-united-states/temporary-workers/o-1-visa-individuals-with-extraordinary-ability-or-achievement

uncommon scenario is they take your passport but tell you that your case requires "Administrative Processing" [11]. Both these situations are summarized below.

Denials Denials under section 214(b) are common occurrences even amongst physicians. The rate of denials can be country-specific or individual-specific. Everyone is seen as a potential immigrant even while you are applying for a nonimmigrant visa such as the J1 [10]. The denial scenarios discussed below are regarding B1, J1, and F1, and not on H1B or O1 denial.

Proof of ties is usually carried to the interview to support an applicant's case. Such proofs may be physical ties such as property (owning a home or other immovable assets), bank statements, letter of support from a family member, occupational ties such as employment in a country outside of the US if the applicant is currently employed (you may carry a letter from your employer and your salary attestations), or social ties such as friends and family including spouses if married [10]. Students may not have all these ties and rely more on social ties and invitation letters; however, denials are still common among medical students, and having more ties and proving intent to return to your home country is important. Having return tickets when entering the country is also a tip from some applicants.

A denial does not have to be permanent. An applicant can re-apply soon after; however, it is best to address the reason for denial before applying again. In certain situations, the consular officer may not tell you the reason for denial at once, the applicant must ask why he or she was refused, and the officer has an obligation to tell you if you ask. Appropriate steps could be taken to change the circumstances that leading to the denial (such as not having enough ties).

Administrative Processing A common concern among applicants who have their interview is "administrative processing." These may appear in at least two scenarios: one when the candidate was granted a visa to enter. In that scenario, the visa status briefly changes to "administrative processing" until delivery, which is normal. The other is if the consular officer says the application is going to undergo "administrative processing." This may happen to anyone irrespective of the visa class including the H1B or O1. This may not even be related to any candidate-specific factor; certain times this occurs randomly. This is an uncertain situation, and it is difficult to predict the exact timelines of when you will know the outcome [11].

Borders

The Customs and Border Protection (CBP) officer will decide the right entry type [12]. Hospitals offering externships supply an invitation letter or cover letter that will help support your entry. The B1/B2 visa is used by medical students to begin their clinical electives. The CBP officer will decide if you qualify for a B1 or a B2 [13]. The cover letter from the hospital should have the duration of the rotation in it. Medical students enter on a B1 for their electives or clerkships, while others may enter on a B2 for observation in a hospital. B1 is a business visa, and certain letter of invitation would specifically mention the right entry type. No financial payment is allowed from the hospital.

Entering on an H1B is straightforward; the authors recommend carrying the original I797 to present to the CBP officer. No travel validation is necessary prior to travel.

Entry on a J1 is also straightforward. Travel validation is needed, and the authors recommend applying for travel validation in advance with the ECFMG. It may take a few days for the travel validated DS-2019 to arrive, and the authors recommend uploading a shipping label from OASIS to expedited delivery if necessary.

The F1 entry is like entering on a J1 except that you present the I-20 form along with your passport. The I-20 has three pages; it is wise to carry all the sheets. Like the DS-2019, travel validation with the sponsoring agency might be necessary.

If the I-94 has an error, the applicant must contact the nearest United States citizenship and immigration services (USCIS) deferred inspection site closest to you to get it corrected (Table 29.5).

Secondary Screening

Most physicians can effortlessly pass through immigration. You will be asked questions and to present documents. Rarely, you may be subjected to secondary screening if anything on your profile raised a red flag, or even at random. The flag could be a similar name or a high-risk travel destination or if the CBP officer is concerned that you are managing your finances internally in the US. You should carry sufficient proof that you can support yourself or a family member supports you. They could ask the same questions repeatedly as it was in one of the residents we interviewed. Again, being honest and straightforward with the officer is important. Certain physicians get pulled to secondary screening due to reasons ranging from the CBP officer not being convinced if you qualify for the visa type you are applying for, to issues relating to documents, amongst many others. The authors wish to let the readers know that you may not have the right to privacy during the screening process: your phone, tablet, laptop, and other electronic devices (which are considered "closed containers" for the purposes of customs searches of items entering the US) and your social medial activity could be detained and searched during the time of the examination. According to one resident who was interviewed, the CBP officer appeared to be less informed about residency interviews or residency training process in general. The Supreme Court has ruled that no suspicion (probable cause) is necessary for search at borders such as international airports (United States v. Ramsey 1977) [14].

Overstaying a B1/B2 or returning to the US soon after exit could result in getting pulled into secondary screening as well. The authors recommend combining multiple United States Medical Licensing Examinations (r) (USMLE) exam steps with each entry and plan with a timeline to avoid getting flagged for visa abuse when on the tourist visa. It is important to carry all necessary proof of funds.

Electives

Most applicants start preparing their application by obtaining clinical experiences as a medical student. Most programs that invite students to rotate, allow so under a B1/B2 visa status [15]. Certain programs offer electives on an F1 visa.

As a medical student, you will still have an educational tie with your medical school which would compel you to return, which could supply added advantage. Most candidates often use this opportunity to complete their USMLE Step 2 USMLE Clinical skills (CS) examination. Electives offer a comprehensive clinical experience that would give the applicant an opportunity to gain clinical skills necessary to take the USMLE Step 2 CS examination. The clinical experience is only for "observational" and for no payment or compensation in return. Tables 29.6 and 29.7 summarize the rules of entry. You may be needed to pay a fee for your experience; however, you may not receive monetary compensation or take part in patient care. Most students and graduates combine USMLE milestones such as either taking the STEP 2 CS or taking the STEP 3 at the same time as the electives to minimize time in the US or minimize travel.

Table 29.6 B1 and B2 visa entry types [15]

B1: Clause	Description
9 FAM 402.2-5(E) [3] (U) Clerkship	Medical Clerkship: An alien who is studying at a foreign medical school and seeks to enter the United States temporarily in order to take an "elective clerkship" at a U.S. medical school's hospital without remuneration from the hospital. The medical clerkship is only for medical students pursuing their normal third- or fourth-year internship in a U.S. medical school as part of a foreign medical school degree. (An "elective clerkship" affords practical experience and instructions in the various disciplines of medicine under the supervision and direction of faculty physicians at a U.S. medical school's hospital as an approved part of the alien's foreign medical school education. It does not apply to graduate medical training, which is restricted by INA 212(e) and normally requires a J-visa.)
9 FAM 402.2-5(E) [3] (U) Business or other Professional or Vocational Activities	An alien who is coming to the United States merely and exclusively to observe the conduct of business or other professional or vocational activity may be classified B-1, provided the alien pays for his or her own expenses. However, aliens, often students, who seek to gain practical experience through on-the-job training or clerkships must qualify under INA 101(a) [16](H) or INA 101(a) [15](L), or when an appropriate exchange visitors program exists (J). Provided certain requirements are met, interns at embassies, consulates, miscellaneous foreign government offices (MFGOs), missions to international organizations, or international organizations may qualify for A-2, G-1, G-2, G-3, or G-4 visas. See 9 FAM 402.3-5(D) [1] and 9 FAM 402.3–7(B).
9 FAM 402.2-5(F) [3] (U) Medical Doctor	A medical doctor whose purpose for coming to the United States is to observe U.S. medical practices and consult with colleagues on latest techniques, provided no remuneration is received from a U.S. source and no patient care is involved. Failure to pass the Foreign Medical Graduate Examination (FMGE) is irrelevant in such a case.

Source: Department of State Foreign Affairs Manual [15]

Table 29.7 B1 clerkship clause

B1: Clause	Description
9 FAM 402.2-5(E) [3] (U) Clerkship	Medical Clerkship: An alien who is studying at a foreign medical school and seeks to enter the United States temporarily in order to take an "elective clerkship" at a U.S. medical school's hospital without remuneration from the hospital. The medical clerkship is only for medical students pursuing their normal third- or fourth-year internship in a U.S. medical school as part of a foreign medical school degree. (An "elective clerkship" affords practical experience and instructions in the various disciplines of medicine under the supervision and direction of faculty physicians at a U.S. medical school's hospital as an approved part of the alien's foreign medical school education. It does not apply to graduate medical training, which is restricted by INA 212(e) and normally requires a J-visa.)

Source: Department of State Foreign Affairs Manual [15]

Residency Interview

You can enter the country on B1/B2 to "negotiate a contract," which means, legally speaking, you can enter the country on a B1/B2 visa and take part in interviews. The duration of which you can enter will be decided by the CBP officer at the border. Table 29.8 summarizes the rules for entry for residency interviews [15].

Residency and Visa: Maintenance of Visa Status

The two most popular visa types for residency are the J1 and the H1B. Around 12,000 J1s are issued each year to residents from various countries (Fig. 29.1) (Table 29.2) [4, 17]. A contract or job offer for residency is necessary to apply for both and have their own unique advantages and disadvantages as summarized below and in Table 29.1. An informed decision is to be made before opting for either of the visa options. The authors recommend expert immigration advice.

J1 Visa

J1 visa is also program-friendly; hospitals can bring in residents easily since ECFMG facilitates the processing and most of the paperwork [4]. The application for the visa will require issuance of a Statement of Need from the government of your home

Table 29.8 Residency interview entry on B1/B2 [15]

9 FAM 402.2-5(B) (U) Aliens Traveling to United States to Engage in Commercial Transactions, **Negotiations, Consultations, Conferences**, Etc. (CT:VISA-999; 01-24-2020)	**Negotiate contracts. Participate in scientific, educational, professional, or business conventions, conferences, or seminars**

Source: Department of State Foreign Affairs Manual [15]

Fig. 29.1 ECFMG J1 sponsorships trend. (Source: ECFMG Database ECFMG March 2020) [4, 17]

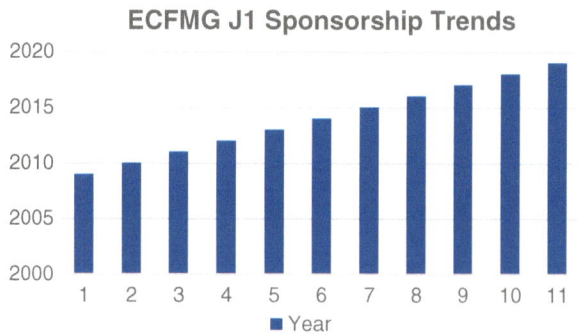

country. You may enter 1 month prior to the start date said on the DS-2019. If you aspire a fellowship, J1 has way more options than the H1B. The application process is considered by more candidate as heavy since the applicant must take more steps in the application process. The timelines are predictable when compared to H1B. There are more fellowship options available to J1 applicants since more programs accept J1 than the H1B, especially for competitive fellowships.

Limitations

Under section 212(e) of the Immigration and Nationality Act (INA), visa holders must return to their home countries for 2 years unless they are able to waive off the home-country requirement [8].

J1 Maintenance of an Active Visa Status: The DS-2019

Renewing a J1 visa during residency is a process that must be done annually. After every July, you are issued a new DS-2019 with which you may exit the country after you receive a travel-validated DS-2019 [18]. After the visa stamp expiration (at the end of 1 year, usually expires after June), to re-enter you must apply for a new visa (at the consulate of your country of residence), except if traveling to certain countries (e.g., Canada and Mexico) for a certain number of days depending on circumstances. The authors focus on most common scenarios and recommend expert advice prior to embarking on travel with expired visas. The authors recommend that you apply for an interview with the consulate well in advance, at once upon arriving to an overseas country by filing the DS-160 early. Sometimes, national holidays (both US and local) may result in embassy closures and significant delays in processing. The DS-2019 must be renewed yearly. This requires a fee payment as well as a form to be filled. You may be asked to upload copies of the arrival form, copies of your passport, and forms from your program. The authors recommend travel validating the DS-2019 early if international travel is expected. Additionally, certain documents such as the I94, contract, and letter from program will have to be uploaded yearly to OASIS and your health insurance information will have to be updated in OASIS on an annual basis [16].

J1 Wavier: The National Interest Waivers

To waive the J1, the first step is to find an employer willing to sponsor the wavier in a wavier eligible area, which is decided by the qualifying Healthcare Professional Shortage Area (HPSA) or a Medically Underserved Area (MUA). Next step is to find a state or federal agency to sponsor the National interest wavier (NIW). These agencies are the State Department of Health for CONRAD-30 (limited to 30 sponsorships per state) or any of the following federal agencies:

(a) The Veterans Affairs Hospital (unlimited number of waivers allowed).
(b) Delta Regional Authority (DRA – along the Mississippi river delta) for both primary care and specialists.
(c) Appalachian Regional Commission – mainly primary care waivers.

The applicant will need to then involve an immigration attorney who will help with the steps moving forward. Depending on the agency applied to, approvals could take a few weeks to months, after which the application is forwarded to the Department of State (DOS) a federal agency which then forwards it to USCIS, which can take a few weeks to issue an approval notice called the I-612, with which you can file for H1B visa conversion.

H1B

Taking the USMLE Step 3 prior to applying to residency has the advantages that one can apply for an H1B visa. This visa type has traditionally been the visa type of choice if one were to eventually settle in the US. The maximum duration for the visa is 6 years, which makes training in certain programs or advanced training difficult if beyond that period. Applicants rank H1B programs higher and are attractive to IMGs. Certain forms must be filled by the applicant and a lawyer assists in filing the documents. The process of applying for the H1B is considered comparatively difficult with respect to the J1. The processing center approves the petition in around 2 weeks via premium processing. The DS-160 is filled and you go to the interview to your consulate. In busy consulates or during peak travel times of the year, the consulate can get busy and the wait times to get an interview can be exceptionally long and will need to be factored when applying. Above it all, certain visa applicants may need administrative processing which can take weeks to finish, further delaying start dates. Applicants may request for an emergency appointment with sufficient evidence such as the start dates in the contract. Please note, under H1B, you may enter 10 days prior to start date not including the orientation in most situations. In all cases, the authors recommend keeping your program updated over emails or the telephone.

The H1B is valid for a period of 6 years. Training in certain programs or even advanced trainings such as fellowship will require a visa of even longer duration. In certain situations, the H1B might be right. Take the example of an IMG medical student who just matched into an Internal Medicine program (3 years duration) and now wishes to apply to Cardiology which is a 3-year training. The duration of residency and fellowship combined is 6 years which is right for the H1B. However, certain added training, such as a year as Chief Resident, would extend the training period to 7 years. In this situation, it is best to speak with your program as well as the immigration attorney to formulate a plan well in advance in order to avoid immigration hassles. H1B wages could be lower than J1 according to our independent interviews [19].

H1B Maintenance It is easier to support an H1B compared to a J1. Applicants may leave the country for vacation and re-enter without needing to visit the consulate yearly for a new stamp for each DS-2019 like the J1. Travel validation is unnecessary.

All applicants we interviewed who were on H1B were satisfied with the absence of the 2-year home-country requirement or the wavier requirements. The authors recommend taking the USMLE Step 3 in advance and to have the scorecard ready by the time it is match day if H1B aligns well with your goals, while being mindful about fewer fellowship options.

F1 Student Visa

F1 visas are student visas offered to take up training in the US [8]. Certain medical classes for the USMLE or CS classes offer F1 visa sponsorship to take up the course. F1 is valid till the duration of the course; there may be mandatory live classes required to support the visa. The F1 is not a valid visa for residency training, although it could open opportunities for clinical electives or observation in addition to taking up USMLE such as CS and Step 3. Applicants may stay for up to 60 days after completion of the course.

O1 Visa

The O1 visa is an uncommon visa type focused on outstanding achievements recorded in one's professional area of expertise [6]. It is a nonimmigrant visa and requires demonstration of exemplary work in the field of choice. The visa is easily renewed and is an emerging visa type among applicants as they advance in their careers. The process involves the program filing at least 45 days before the stated start date and the application involves an immigration lawyer.

Changing from an F1 to an O1 requires a wavier; recommendation cannot be done within the United States and must be done abroad. The authors recommend discussing with your fellowship program about the O1 visa application and recommend considering premium processing to speed up the application process. The general criteria for an O1 visa are summarized in Table 29.9.

Table 29.9 Evidentiary criteria for O1-A

Evidence that the beneficiary has received a major, internationally recognized award, such as a Nobel Prize, or evidence of <u>at least (3) three</u> of the following:
Receipt of nationally or internationally recognized prizes or awards for excellence in the field of endeavor
Membership in associations in the field for which classification is sought which require outstanding achievements, as judged by recognized national or international experts in the field
Published material in professional or major trade publications or major media about the beneficiary related to the beneficiary's work in the field for which classification is sought
Original scientific, scholarly, or business-related contributions of major significance in the field
Authorship of scholarly articles in professional journals or other major media in the field for which classification is sought
A high salary or other remuneration for services or that the beneficiary will command a high salary or other remuneration for services as evidenced by contracts or other reliable evidence
Participation on a panel, or individually, as a judge of the work of others in the same or in a field of specialization allied to that field for which classification is sought
Employment in a critical or essential capacity for organizations and establishments that have a distinguished reputation

Source: USCIS O1 [5]

Special Circumstances

COVID-19 Pandemic and Travel Restrictions

June 22, 2020, Presidential Proclamation: President Trump issued the "Proclamation Suspending Entry of Aliens Who Present a Risk to the U.S. Labor Market Following the Coronavirus Outbreak." However, the alien physician category and any foreign national accompanying or following to join such alien are omitted from the suspension and are, therefore, exempt from the provisions of the proclamation. For more information, please refer to Table 29.5 [20].

Presidential Proclamations Resulted in "Enhanced Vetting" of Certain Nationals

1. On September 14, 2017, the President issued a proclamation titled "Enhancing Vetting Capabilities and Processes for Detecting Attempted Entry into the United States by Terrorists or other Public-Safety Threats." There were certain countries that the President deemed necessary to impose restrictions. However, on November 17, 2017, the US Court of Appeals for the Ninth Circuit granted a stay order for the Presidential Proclamation, prohibiting the implementation of certain clauses. Nationals of eight countries are still subject to certain travel restrictions (Table 29.10). Individuals with visas issued prior to the proclamation were not affected [21].

Table 29.10 Nationals with travel restrictions over 2017 Presidential Proclamation

Country	Nonimmigrant visas	Immigrant and diversity visas
Chad	No B1, B2, and B1/B2 visas	No immigrant or diversity visas
Iran	No nonimmigrant visas except F, M, and J student visas	No immigrant or diversity visas
Libya	No B1, B2, and B1/B2 visas	No immigrant or diversity visas
North Korea	No nonimmigrant visas	No immigrant or diversity visas
Syria	No nonimmigrant visas	No immigrant or diversity visas
Venezuela	No B1, B2, or B1/B2 visas of any kind for officials of the following government agencies: Ministry of Interior, Justice, and Peace; the Administrative Service of Identification, Migration, and Immigration; the Corps of Scientific Investigations, Judicial and Criminal; the Bolivarian Intelligence Service; and the People's Power Ministry of Foreign Affairs, and their immediate family members.	No restrictions
Yemen	No B1, B2, and B1/B2 visas	No immigrant or diversity visas
Somalia		No immigrant or diversity visas

Source: The White House. 2020. Proclamation on Improving Enhanced Vetting Capabilities and Processes for Detecting Attempted Entry [10, 15, 21]

Summary

In summary, physicians have a wide variety of visa and immigration options to choose from during their training. Each visa has a specific purpose, and the authors recommend the readers to familiarize with each type. Early timeline planning is crucial. Taking the USMLE Step 3 early opens opportunities to obtain an H1B. The authors recommend expert immigration advice in all situations about visas and immigration.

References

1. Travel.state.gov. 2020. Update on visas for medical professionals. [online] Available at: https://travel.state.gov/content/travel/en/News/visas-news/update-on-h-and-j-visas-for-medical-professionals.html. Accessed Aug 2020.
2. Ranasinghe PD. International medical graduates in the US physician workforce. J Am Osteopath Assoc. 2015;115(4):236–41. https://doi.org/10.7556/jaoa.2015.047.
3. ECFMG. 2020. Resources: data – ECFMG J-1 visa sponsorship. [online] Available at: https://www.ecfmg.org/resources/data-sponsorship.html. Accessed Aug 2020.

4. ECFMG Database, January 9, 2020 – Ecfmg.org. 2020. Number of exchange visitor physicians sponsored 2009–2019 calendar years. [Online] Available at: https://www.ecfmg.org/resources/EVSPData_EVs_09-19_6.1.20.pdf. Accessed 27 Aug 2020.
5. USCIS O1. 2020. O-1 Visa: individuals with extraordinary ability or achievement. [Online] Available at: https://www.uscis.gov/working-in-the-united-states/temporary-workers/o-1-visa-individuals-with-extraordinary-ability-or-achievement. Accessed Aug 2020.
6. Fam.state.gov. 2020. 9 FAM 402.13 ALIENS OF EXTRAORDINARY ABILITY O VISAS. [Online] Available at: https://fam.state.gov/fam/09FAM/09FAM040213.html. Accessed Aug 2020.
7. DS160. 2020. DS-160: frequently asked questions. [Online] Available at: https://travel.state.gov/content/travel/en/us-visas/visa-information-resources/forms/ds-160-online-nonimmigrant-visa-application/ds-160-faqs.html. Accessed Aug 2020.
8. J1/F1 Fam.state.gov. 2020. 9 FAM 402.5 (U) STUDENTS AND EXCHANGE VISITORS – F, M, AND J VISAS. [Online] Available at: https://fam.state.gov/FAM/09FAM/09FAM040205.html. Accessed Aug 2020.
9. USCIS. 2020. H1B premium processing. [Online] Available at: https://www.uscis.gov/forms/all-forms/how-do-i-request-premium-processing. Accessed Aug 2020.
10. Travel.state.gov. 2020. Visa denials. [Online] Available at: https://travel.state.gov/content/travel/en/us-visas/visa-information-resources/visa-denials.html. Accessed Aug 2020.
11. Travel.state.gov. 2020. Administrative processing information. [Online] Available at: https://travel.state.gov/content/travel/en/us-visas/visa-information-resources/administrative-processing-information.html. Accessed Aug 2020.
12. CBP. 2020. Border crossing. [Online] Available at: https://www.cbp.gov/travel/international-visitors/applying-admission-united-states. Accessed Aug 2020.
13. CBP. 2020. B1 Or B2. [Online] Available at: https://www.cbp.gov/faqs/what-b1-b2-or-b1b2-visa-how-can-i-find-out-what-visa-type-i-have. Accessed Aug 2020.
14. Elsevier Connect. 2013. What are your rights at airport screenings and checkpoints?. [Online] Available at: https://www.elsevier.com/connect/what-are-your-rights-at-airport-screenings-and-checkpoints. Accessed Aug 2020.
15. US Department of State: Foreign Affairs Manual B1/B2 Fam.state.gov. 2020. 9 FAM 402.2 (U) TOURISTS AND BUSINESS VISITORS AND MEXICAN BORDER CROSSING CARDS – B VISAS AND BCCS. [Online] Available at: https://fam.state.gov/fam/09FAM/09FAM040202.html. Accessed Aug 2020.
16. J1visa.state.gov. 2014. [Online] Available at: https://j1visa.state.gov/wp-content/uploads/2014/10/Subpart-A-Federal-Register-publication-8893_PublishedFR_10-6-2014.pdf. Accessed Aug 2020, 60304 Federal Register/Vol. 79, No. 193/Monday, October 6, 2014/Rules and Regulations, Section 62.14.
17. ECFMG. 2019. ECFMG fact card. [Online] Available at: https://www.ecfmg.org/forms/fact-card.pdf. Accessed Aug 2020.
18. ECFMG. 2020. Travel validation of J1. [online] Available at: https://www.ecfmg.org/evsp/applicants-current-travel.html. Accessed Aug 2020.
19. Fam.state.gov. 2020. 9 FAM 402.10 (U) TEMPORARY WORKERS AND TRAINEES – H VISAS. [Online] Available at: https://fam.state.gov/fam/09FAM/09FAM040210.html. Accessed Aug 2020.
20. The White House. 2020. Proclamation suspending entry of immigrants who present risk to the U.S. labor market during the economic recovery following the COVID-19 outbreak | U.S. Embassy In Armenia. [Online] Available at: https://www.whitehouse.gov/presidential-actions/proclamation-suspending-entry-aliens-present-risk-u-s-labor-market-following-coronavirus-outbreak/. Accessed Aug 2020.
21. The White House. 2020. Proclamation on improving enhanced vetting capabilities and processes for detecting attempted entry | The White House. [Online] Available at: https://www.whitehouse.gov/presidential-actions/proclamation-improving-enhanced-vetting-capabilities-processes-detecting-attempted-entry/. Accessed Aug 2020.

Chapter 30
International Medical Graduates and the US Clinical Residency Match: The Editors' Perspective

Hassaan Tohid

Introduction

It is normal to assume that not all international medical graduates (IMGs) will match and get residency in the United States (US). However, the IMGs applying for match can still at least increase their chances of matching drastically if they follow certain ideas and suggestions mentioned in this chapter.

It is also not uncommon to see many IMGs becoming depressed and anxious because of the match process. Even the best students with unusually high scores on the USMLEs suffer from this issue of extreme anxiety, stress, and the fear that comes because of uncertainty. One of the most common reasons for these issues is a lack of awareness and proper guidance for these IMGs who apply for a match. Once matched, this stress is resolved, but serious issues arise if these students do not match. If they do not match, these signs of temporary anxiety and fear may become serious issues such as generalized anxiety disorder (GAD), major depression (MD), or some other serious behavioral issues.

Once the United States medical license examinations (USMLEs) are done, if the students match, that is wonderful. However, if they do not match, instead of getting disappointed and depressed, the students should remember that there are other options available for them. If they want to remain in the US and they did not match, then they can use a strategy of changing their field. However, if changing the field is not an option, then they can still be clinicians in the US of different kind. However, if they desperately want to be a physician and have not matched in the US, then there are some other strategies they can adopt. I will highlight these strategies and options in this chapter.

H. Tohid (✉)
California Institute of Behavioral Neurosciences and Psychology, Fairfield, CA, USA

© Springer Nature Switzerland AG 2021   457
H. Tohid, H. Maibach (eds.), *International Medical Graduates in the United States*, https://doi.org/10.1007/978-3-030-62249-7_30

The Helpful Strategies That IMGs Must Develop

There are two types of strategies IMGs can adopt:

- Strategy of changing their mindset.
- Strategy of taking certain actions toward their career goals.

Everything starts with mindset; therefore, the first three strategies are associated with mindset change, while the rest are about taking certain actions.

Strategies of Changing the Mindset

Responsibility

Developing a strong sense of responsibility is the foremost strategy every IMG should have. It is merely a state of mind but can have drastic consequences in one's life. There are two types of people around the world: the blamers and the ones who take responsibility of everything they do. The IMGs must develop an attitude of taking absolute responsibility. Anything that they have right now, they are responsible for. The same is true for all of us. If we are not satisfied with our career and consider it is a mess, then we are responsible. No one else is to blame. If our health is deteriorating, then only we are responsible, no one else is. If our finances are messed up, we should remember that it is no one else's responsibility to fix our finances. Our situation will improve only if we increase the level of responsibility we take in each aspect of our lives.

The opposite of responsibility is blaming. It is rightly said that a successful person takes responsibility of everything in his/her life, while an unsuccessful person blames others. Therefore, the best strategy is to stop blaming and think, "Where have I messed up? What did I do wrong? How can I fix it? And how can I improve my CV? And how can I be successful in my career?"

Attitude

If there is one thing that can have the highest impact on anyone's life is the right attitude. Most people do not get rejected or fired from jobs because of lack of skills or knowledge, but actually because of a bad attitude. The IMGs must learn to work hard on improving their attitude.

It is not easy if we habitually have a bad attitude, but anything can be learned with practice and patience. The IMGs must learn positive mental attitude and should also learn how to stay positive in adversity, learn how to remain happy (most of the time), and not to complain. Employers do not like complaining, they like gratitude, so always be grateful. Once you are a grateful person, it is evident in your personality and cannot remain hidden. All of these are signs of people with positive mental attitude.

The strategy to develop positive mental attitude begins with contemplation. If we remain in pre-contemplation stage of behavior change and assume that we have no room for improvement and there is nothing wrong with us, then we do not work on changing ourselves. However, the moment we realize that we all are human beings and make mistakes and have a lot to learn and improve, then we work on our attitude. Improving attitude is a life-long process, and we must be mindful of the idea that too much of negativity around us has the potential to affect our attitude.

Change the Destructive Thought of What People Think

One of the most destructive thought processes is what others think about us. Many IMGs remain under unnecessary stress of what others will think about them. They have strange anxiety or unknown fear that if they do not take their USMLE around the same time as their peers, it will be disastrous because then everyone around them will probably laugh at them. Thus, IMGs should not worry about what people will say; instead, they should run at their own pace. They should remember that they are not in a competition with anyone, but themselves. They should just think about whether they are better than what they were last year. The approach should be "deaf to the world"; no one's comments should matter to them and their plans. If students do not think about what other people think about them, they will release themselves from a huge unnecessary burden. They will feel more relaxed and happier. USMLE is a tough exam and needs focus; therefore, without being happy and relaxed, it is extremely difficult to achieve the goal of passing the exam.

Strategies of Taking Certain Action

Integrity

The IMGs must remember the power of being honest. They must never lie on their CVs or personal statements. Every single point mentioned on their CV, resume, or personal statement should be backed up by evidence. A slight misrepresentation or lie on the CV can damage their careers. They should consider that if they lie about something on their CV, and they are caught in that lie, what will be the consequences? If it is caught by the residency director during the interview, then they lose any chance of matching in that particular program whatsoever.

Self-Improvement

One of the best ways students can raise their chances of matching and get clinical residency is the phenomenon of self-improvement. IMGs should emphasize on learning more and more. This learning does not have to be related to their field of medicine. In fact, they should learn about the US healthcare system, health insurance, and the US culture and political system as well. However, the most important area of development they should focus on is communication. They should learn to write, speak, listen, and read well. These are extremely important areas of personal development and are often ignored. If students can just continuously work on the way they talk and listen, they can impress the interviewers during their interviews. Many IMGs complain that they had great scores and got interviews yet were not matched. Under these circumstances, many times, the hidden reason is weak communication skills. Therefore, this aspect of self-improvement and personal growth should never be ignored.

Clinical Experience

The IMGs must find some US clinical experience as soon as they arrive in the US after graduation. This experience can be of any kind, whether it is volunteering, observership, or externship. Clinical experience opportunities can be easily found online nowadays or by using personal connections. This experience is one of the best ways of professional and personal development, where the students learn about the clinical setting but also learn about the healthcare system, culture, and language. This experience can enhance their communication skills to surprisingly great levels.

Research Publications

The students must also look for research opportunities. The research opportunities with no publications will be less valuable; therefore, they should try their best to get some publications. Here again, learning to write is the key to success.

Strong Letters of Recommendation

Many IMGs run after strong letters of recommendation (LoRs), forgetting the fact that LoRs are the effect, while the cause is something else. The cause is their outstanding performance during the clinical or research rotations. Therefore, focusing on the cause is the best approach, the effect will follow. The students then just have to request for the LoRs and the supervisors are usually nice people and do not mind issuing one.

Contacts and Social Connections

Another important aspect of becoming successful in the United States is to ensure that they make strong connections and friendships. When the students get opportunities of research or clinical rotations, they should act like everyone meet is the most important person they have ever met. They should be respectful to everyone and attempt to be good friends with them. The key here is to remain in touch with these contacts even after the rotations are over. These contacts can serve them well for years and may help them in getting some interviews as well. However, the main thing IMGs must remember is that being selfish is never good. The reason of friendships is not just to take, but they should be givers and should also help others getting what they need. Maybe an IMG met another IMG and became friends, and both help each other by using their connections and helping each other get interviews. This is what Stephen Covey called the "Win-Win" strategy. This win-win philosophy will serve them well for the rest of their lives [1].

Professional Help if Necessary

The IMGs must remember that there is no harm in getting professional help to improve their communication and writing skills, and their CV and personal statement writing. The same is true for the USMLE preparation. If they can afford it, then they should consider this option. There are plenty of exam preparation institutes currently working in the United States.

Save Money to Apply

The residency application process is an expensive process for most IMGs. And there is no guarantee that the students will match the first time they apply. They may have to apply the next year as well. Therefore, saving money is the approach that will help them in case they need to apply again. If they have US legal status to work, then working and saving money at the same time will help. However, if they cannot work due to legal restrictions, then they must save money that they already have and spend wisely. They must not be a part of illegal jobs; this can shatter their dreams of becoming a doctor in this country. If money is the issue, the best approach is to go back to their home country and get a job and start saving and then re-apply for the match.

Alternative Career Options

The IMGs must also remember that life is not over if they do not match in the United States. They can always go back to their own country and start practicing medicine or try their luck in the United Kingdom (UK) or other countries. There are other countries – for example, Middle Eastern countries such as Qatar, the United Arab Emirates (UAE), and Israel – that accept IMGs if they have passed USMLEs. A non-Middle Eastern country that accepts USMLE scores is New Zealand. Therefore, the effort of passing USMLEs is not wasted; they have other countries as options to find residency or fellowships. The IMGs must research about these countries and look at the requirements and ask the hospital programs. For example, New Zealand does not accept USMLE Step 2 clinical skills (CS) and you must pass their clinical skill equivalent exam [2].

However, if IMGs do not want to move outside the US after being unable to match and have decided to stay, then there are many other alternate career options they can choose. They can do masters in a field and start an alternate career in that field. Moreover, there are plenty of clinical professions still available that they may choose such as speech pathology or counseling.

Life is more important than anything; therefore, losing hope and getting depressed is not the correct way. The IMGs must remember that there are other options as well. Their life has just begun, and it is not over.

COVID-19 and the Aftermath

The coronavirus pandemic has altered the world like no other problem. The pandemic certainly has reduced the chances of IMGs traveling to the US for clinical and research rotations. However, the IMGs must remember that every problem has a solution, and all of these opportunities are now available online. There are plenty of telemedicine rotations available across the US, and the same is true for research. Many residency programs are expected to switch to online interviews, which will most likely help IMGs mainly by saving the travel expense. Now they can attend interviews sitting home online. Certainly, it is too early to predict how this virtual world will work. Yet, I hope for the best and wish good luck to all the IMGs applying for the US residency.

Conclusion

Adopting the above strategies that include some changes in mindset and taking some actions, IMGs can raise the chances of being successful in one's career. Life does not end with an unsuccessful match. The students can re-apply next year by improving their CVs or can change their plan and find an alternate career option or can move to any other country that accepts USMLEs if becoming a physician is their final decision.

References

1. Covey SR. The 7 habits of highly effective people: powerful lessons in personal change. Free Press; 1989. ISBN 0-7432-6951-9.
2. Registration Exam (NZREX). Medical Council of New Zealand. Available at https://www.mcnz.org.nz/registration/getting-registered/registration-exam-nzrex/

Index